# *Schwartz's* PRINCIPLES OF SURGERY

## SELF-ASSESSMENT AND BOARD REVIEW

**eighth edition**

# Schwartz's
# PRINCIPLES OF
# SURGERY
# SELF-ASSESSMENT AND BOARD REVIEW

**Editor-in-Chief**

## F. Charles Brunicardi, MD, FACS
DeBakey/Bard Professor and Chairman
Michael E. DeBakey Department of Surgery
Baylor College of Medicine
Houston, Texas

**Associate Editors**

## Mary L. Brandt, MD, FACS
Professor of Surgery
Vice Chair and Program Director
Michael E. DeBakey Department of Surgery
Baylor College of Medicine
Texas Children's Hospital
Houston, Texas

## Dana K. Andersen, MD, FACS
Professor and Vice Chairman
Department of Surgery
Johns Hopkins University School of Medicine
Surgeon-in-Chief
Johns Hopkins Bayview Medical Center
Baltimore, Maryland

## Timothy R. Billiar, MD, FACS
George Vance Foster Professor and Chairman
Department of Surgery
University of Pittsburgh School of Medicine
Pittsburgh, Pennsylvania

## David L. Dunn, MD, PhD, FACS
Vice President for Health Sciences
Professor of Surgery, Microbiology, and Immunology
University of Buffalo
Buffalo, New York

## John G. Hunter, MD, FACS
Mackenzie Professor and Chairman of Surgery
Department of Surgery
Oregon Health and Science University
Portland, Oregon

## Raphael E. Pollock, MD, PhD, FACS
Head, Division of Surgery
Professor and Chairman
Department of Surgical Oncology
Senator A.M. Aiken, Jr., Distinguished Chair
The University of Texas M.D. Anderson Cancer Center
Houston, Texas

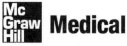

New York  Chicago  San Francisco  Lisbon  London  Madrid  Mexico City
New Delhi  San Juan  Seoul  Singapore  Sydney  Toronto

**Schwartz's Principles of Surgery:**
**Self-Assessment and Board Review, Eighth Edition**

1 2 3 4 5 6 7 8 9 0   QPD/QPD   0 9 8 7 6

ISBN-13: 978-0-07-144687-7
ISBN-10: 0-07-144687-7

This book was set in Times Roman by Silverchair Science + Communications, Inc.
The editors were Martin Wonsiewicz and Christie Naglieri.
The production supervisor was Catherine Saggese.
Project management was provided by Silverchair Science + Communications, Inc.
Quebecor World was printer and binder.

This book is printed on acid-free paper.

**Library of Congress Cataloging-in-Publication Data**

Schwartz's principles of surgery: self-assessment and board review / edited by F. Charles Brunicardi ... [et al.]. – 8th ed.
   p.cm.
  Should be used in conjunction with the 8th ed. of Schwartz's principles of surgery.
  Includes bibliographical references and index.
  ISBN 0-07-144687-7
  1. Surgery–Examinations, questions, etc. I. Schwartz, Seymour I., 1928-II.
Brunicardi, F. Charles. III. Schwartz's principles of surgery. IV. Title: Principles of surgery.
  [DNLM: 1. Surgical Procedures, Operative–Examination Questions. WO 18.2 2006]
RD31.P882 2006
617.0076–dc22
                                                         2006048196

# Contents

# Introduction

This eighth edition of *Schwartz's Principles of Surgery: Self-Assessment and Board Review*, edited by F. Charles Brunicardi and colleagues, has undergone a significant redesign to support the changes that have occurred in surgery and surgical education since this book's last printing. A complete and convenient self-evaluation and review of the surgical discipline, this edition has been chiefly designed for use by residents in preparation for the American Board of Surgery (ABS) Qualifying, In-Training, and Certifying Examinations; however, it is also a useful recertification tool for board-certified surgeons.

This book consists of 861 multiple-choice questions that are representative of the major areas covered in the eighth edition of *Principles of Surgery* by Brunicardi and associates. Viable questions from the seventh edition *PreTest and Self Assessment* have been salvaged and combined with the newly written questions to create a truly comprehensive review of each chapter. Among the additions to this review are seven new chapters: Cell, Genomics, and Molecular Surgery; Soft Tissue Sarcomas; Anesthesia of the Surgical Patient; The Surgical Management of Obesity; Patient Safety, Errors, and Complications in Surgery; Surgical Considerations; and ACGME Core Competencies.

Many factors concerning the practical use and application of this book were considered in its redesign and are reflected in the new columnar layout of questions and answers. The side-by-side placement of questions and answers allows the reader to engage in more efficient study and expedited self-assessment. To maintain the integrity of the practice test, the user is urged to cover the right-hand column of the page to conceal the answer column until review. The style of questioning used mimics that of the ABS board examinations. Additionally, adjacent to each question is the answer, a paragraph-length explanation, and a reference to either *Principles of Surgery*, 8th ed., or *Principles of Surgery*, 7th ed., should the user require a more extensive review of the topic.

# Acknowledgments

Since the last edition, this review has been expanded to include new questions for every chapter while also retaining viable questions from the seventh edition. The editors would like to recognize the enormous effort of Mary L. Brandt, MD, FACS, who created many of the new questions and Liz Lee, MD, for her invaluable assistance in proofreading and fact-checking. We also acknowledge the essential and valuable contribution of Katie Elsbury who worked with Dr. Brandt, the editors, the publisher, and myself during each step of the editorial process.

*F. Charles Brunicardi, MD, FACS*

1. Which of the following would be typical of an enteral hepatic-failure formula?
   A. Lower fluid volume, potassium, phosphorus, and magnesium
   B. Fifty percent reduction of carbohydrates
   C. Fifty percent of proteins are in the form of branched-chain amino acids (leucine, isoleucine, and valine)
   D. Increased arginine, omega-3 fatty acids, and beta-carotene

**Answer: C**
Close to 50% of the proteins in hepatic failure formulae are branched-chain amino acids (e.g., leucine, isoleucine, and valine). The goal of such a formula is to reduce aromatic amino acid levels and increase branched-chain amino acids, which can potentially reverse encephalopathy in patients with hepatic failure. However, the use of this formula is controversial because no clear benefits have been proven by clinical trials. Protein restriction should be avoided in patients with end-stage liver disease because they have significant protein energy malnutrition, predisposing them to additional morbidity and mortality. (See Schwartz 8th ed., p 33.)

2. C-reactive protein
   A. Is secreted in a circadian rhythm with higher levels in the morning
   B. Increases after eating a large meal
   C. Does not increase in response to stress in patients with liver failure
   D. Is less sensitive than erythrocyte sedimentation rate as a marker of inflammation

**Answer: C**
The acute phase proteins are nonspecific biochemical markers produced by hepatocytes in response to tissue injury, infection, or inflammation. Interleukin (IL)-6 is a potent inducer of acute phase proteins that can include proteinase inhibitors, coagulation and complement proteins, and transport proteins. Clinically, only C-reactive protein (CRP) has been consistently used as a marker of injury response due to its dynamic reflection of inflammation. Importantly, CRP levels do not show diurnal variations and are not affected by feeding. Only pre-existing liver failure will impair CRP production. Therefore it has become a useful biomarker of inflammation as well as response to treatment. Its accuracy surpasses that of the erythrocyte sedimentation rate. (See Schwartz 8th ed., p 9.)

3. Which of the following occurs after cortisol administration?
   A. Increase in interleukin-1 (IL-1) and IL-6
   B. Increased capacity for intracellular killing by monocytes
   C. Decreased B-cell function
   D. Decreased T-cell function

**Answer: D**
Immunologic changes associated with glucocorticoid administration include thymic involution, depressed cell-mediated immune responses reflected by decreases in T-killer and natural killer cell functions, T-lymphocyte blastogenesis, mixed lymphocyte responsiveness, graft-versus-host reactions, and delayed hypersensitivity responses. (See Schwartz 8th ed., p 6.)

4. Catecholamine elevation after injury
   A. Is limited to epinephrine only
   B. Is limited to norepinephrine only
   C. Increases by 10- to 20-fold after injury
   D. Is sustained 24 to 48 hours before decreasing

**Answer: D**
Both norepinephrine (NE) and epinephrine (EPI) are increased three- to fourfold in plasma immediately following injury, with elevations lasting 24 to 48 hours before returning toward baseline levels. (See Schwartz 8th ed., p 7.)

5. Healthy patients undergoing uncomplicated surgery can remain n.p.o. (with intravenous fluid support) for how many days before significant protein catabolism occurs?
   A. 2 days
   B. 4 days
   C. 7 days
   D. 10 days

**Answer: D**
Healthy patients without malnutrition undergoing uncomplicated surgery can tolerate 10 days of partial starvation (i.e., maintenance intravenous fluids only) before any significant protein catabolism occurs. (See Schwartz 8th ed., p 32.)

6. Which of the following inflammatory mediators are derived from arachidonic acid?
   A. Leukotrienes
   B. Cytokines
   C. Heat shock proteins
   D. Insulinlike growth factors

**Answer: A**
The eicosanoid class of mediators, which encompasses prostaglandins (PG), thromboxanes (TX), leukotrienes (LT), hydroxy-eicosatetraenoic acids (HETE), and lipoxins (LX), are oxidation derivatives of the membrane phospholipid arachidonic acid (eicosatetraenoic acid). Eicosanoids are secreted by virtually all nucleated cells except lymphocytes. The synthesis of arachidonic acid from phospholipids requires enzymatic activation of phospholipase A2 (Fig. 1-5). Eicosanoids are generated either by the cyclooxygenase or the lipoxygenase pathways. Products of the cyclooxygenase pathway include all of the prostaglandins and thromboxanes. The lipoxygenase pathway generates the leukotrienes and HETE. (See Schwartz 8th ed., p 10.)

7. Enteral nutrition
   A. Results in a reduction of infectious complications in critically ill patients
   B. Is more expensive than parenteral nutrition
   C. Results in faster return of bowel function in healthy patients after gastrointestinal surgery
   D. Has a higher complication rate than parenteral nutrition

**Answer: A**
Most prospectively randomized studies for severe abdominal and thoracic trauma demonstrate significant reductions in infectious complications for patients given early enteral nutrition when compared with those who are unfed or receiving parenteral nutrition. The exception has been in studies for patients with closed-head injury because no significant differences in outcome are demonstrated between early jejunal feeding compared with other nutritional support modalities. Moreover, early gastric feeding following closed-head injury was frequently associated with underfeeding and calorie deficiency due to difficulties overcoming gastroparesis and the high risk of aspiration. (See Schwartz 8th ed., p 31.)

8. Which of the following would be typical of an enteral renal failure formula?
   A. Lower fluid volume, potassium, phosphorus, and magnesium
   B. 50% reduction of carbohydrates
   C. 50% of proteins are in the form of branched-chain amino acids (leucine, isoleucine, and valine)
   D. Increased arginine, omega-3 fatty acids and beta-carotene

**Answer: A**
The primary benefits of the renal formula are the lower fluid volume and concentrations of potassium, phosphorus, and magnesium needed to meet daily calorie requirements. This formulation almost exclusively contains essential amino acids and has a high nonprotein:calorie ratio; however, it does not contain trace elements or vitamins. (See Schwartz 8th ed., p 33.)

9. Adrenocorticotropic hormone
   A. Is synthesized in the hypothalamus
   B. Is superceeded by pain, anxiety, and injury
   C. Continues to be released in a circadian pattern in injured patients
   D. Causes the release of mineralocorticoids from the adrenal in a circadian pattern

**Answer: B**
Adrenocorticotropic hormone (ACTH) is synthesized and released by the anterior pituitary. In healthy humans, ACTH release is regulated by circadian signals such that the greatest elevation of ACTH occurs late at night until the hours immediately before sunrise. This pattern is dramatically altered or obliterated in the injured subject. Most injury is characterized by elevations in corticotropin-releasing hormone and ACTH that are proportional to the severity of injury. Pain, anxiety, vasopressin, angiotensin II, cholecystokinin, vasoac-

tive intestinal polypeptide (VIP), catecholamines, and proinflammatory cytokines are all prominent mediators of ACTH release in the injured patient. (See Schwartz 8th ed., p 6.)

10. Tumor necrosis factor (TNF)
    A. Is primarily produced by hepatocytes
    B. Has a prolonged effect on inflammation due to a half-life of 8 hours
    C. Induces muscle catabolism
    D. Decreased production of prostaglandin $E_2$

**Answer: C**
Following acute injury or during infections, TNF-$\alpha$ is among the earliest and most potent mediators of subsequent host responses. The primary sources of TNF-$\alpha$ synthesis include monocytes/macrophages and T cells, which are abundant in the peritoneum and splanchnic tissues. Furthermore, Kupffer cells represent the single largest concentrated population of macrophages in the human body. Therefore, surgical or traumatic injuries to the abdominal viscera undoubtedly have profound influence on the generation of inflammatory mediators and homeostatic responses such as acute phase protein production. Although the half-life of TNF-$\alpha$ is less than 20 minutes, this brief appearance is sufficient to evoke marked metabolic and hemodynamic changes and activate mediators distally in the cytokine cascade. TNF-$\alpha$ is also a major inducer of muscle catabolism and cachexia during stress by shunting available amino acids to the hepatic circulation as fuel substrates. Other functions of TNF-$\alpha$ include coagulation activation, promoting the expression or release of adhesion molecules, prostaglandin $E_2$, platelet-activating factor (PAF), glucocorticoids, and eicosanoids. (See Schwartz 8th ed., p 12.)

11. Isotonic enteral formulas with fiber
    A. Have approximately 2 kcal/cc
    B. Have a non-protein calorie-to-nitrogen ratio of 90:1
    C. Delay intestinal transit time and may decrease diarrhea associated with enteral formulas
    D. Should not be used in critically ill patients

**Answer: C**
Isotonic formulas with fiber contain soluble and insoluble fiber which are most often soy based. Physiologically, fiber-based solutions delay intestinal transit time and may reduce the incidence of diarrhea compared with nonfiber solutions. Fiber stimulates pancreatic lipase activity and is degraded by gut bacteria into short-chain fatty acids, an important fuel for colonocytes. There are no contraindications for using fiber-containing formulas in critically ill patients. (See Schwartz 8th ed., p 33.)

12. Nitric oxide (NO)
    A. Is primarily made in hepatocytes
    B. Has a half-life of 20–30 minutes
    C. Is formed from oxidation of L-arginine
    D. Can increase thrombosis in small vessels

**Answer: C**
NO is formed from oxidation of L-arginine, a process catalyzed by nitric oxide synthase (NOS). Cofactors of NOS activity include calmodulin, ionized calcium, and reduced nicotinamide adenine dinucleotide phosphate (NADPH). In addition to the endothelium, NO formation also occurs in neutrophils, monocytes, renal cells, Kupffer cells, and cerebellar neurons. (See Schwartz 8th ed., p 21.)

13. Which of the following are the most potent mediators of the inflammatory response?
    A. Corticosteroids
    B. Heat shock proteins
    C. Cytokines
    D. Eicosanoids

**Answer: C**
Cytokines appear to be the most potent mediators of the inflammatory response. When functioning locally at the site of injury or infection, cytokines eradicate invading microorganisms and promote wound healing. However, overwhelming production of proinflammatory cytokines in response to injury can cause hemodynamic instability (i.e., septic shock) or metabolic derangements (i.e., muscle wasting). If uncontrolled, the outcome of these exaggerated responses is end-organ failure and death. The production of anti-inflammatory cytokines as part of the inflammation cascade serves to oppose the excessive

actions of proinflammatory cytokines. However, inappropriate anti-inflammatory mediator release may render the patient immunocompromised and susceptible to overwhelming infections. To view cytokines merely as proinflammatory or anti-inflammatory oversimplifies their functions, and overlapping bioactivity is the rule (Table 1-3). (See Schwartz 8th ed., p 10.)

14. All of the following statements about thyroid hormone function during acute injury are true EXCEPT
   A. Free triiodothyronine ($T_3$) levels are frequently decreased.
   B. Reduced free thyroxine ($T_4$) concentrations are predictors of high mortality.
   C. Thyroid-stimulating hormone (TSH) release undergoes a compensatory rise as $T_3$ levels drop.
   D. Total $T_4$ (protein bound and free) levels may be reduced.

**Answer: C**
TSH release is not increased when $T_3$ levels drop in trauma patients. Free $T_4$ remains relatively constant, although total $T_4$ levels may be reduced. A reduced free $T_4$ level in a severely injured patient is predictive of high mortality. (See Schwartz 7th ed.)

15. The most frequent trace mineral deficiency developing in a patient receiving parenteral alimentation is a deficiency of
   A. Calcium
   B. Chromium
   C. Magnesium
   D. Zinc

**Answer: D**
Zinc deficiency is marked by an eczematoid rash either diffusely or in intertriginous areas. A microcytic anemia can develop from a lack of copper and glucose intolerance and may be associated with a lack of chromium. Daily administration of trace metal supplements obviates these problems. (See Schwartz 7th ed.)

16. A 28-year-old woman who has been on total parenteral nutrition for 4 weeks develops a scaling acrodermatitis and alopecia. This condition is most likely to be a result of
   A. Linoleic acid deficiency
   B. Zinc deficiency
   C. Vitamin C deficiency
   D. Magnesium deficiency

**Answer: A**
Patients who are receiving long-term total parenteral nutrition (TPN) with hypertonic dextrose and amino acids may develop essential fatty acid deficiency. Early signs of the deficiency include scaling of the skin on the digits and shedding of hair with alopecia, and, if left untreated, the condition may be responsible for weakness, lethargy, pruritus, poor wound healing, and thrombocytopenia. The key defect is a decrease in the plasma level of the essential fatty acid linoleic acid. Although arachidonic and linolenic acid levels also are decreased, the former can be synthesized from linoleic acid, and the importance of the latter has not been established, although it is considered to be an essential fatty acid. Zinc deficiency, which is also a possibility with prolonged TPN, produces an eczematoid rash that may be diffuse but is most prominent in intertriginous areas. (See Schwartz 7th ed.)

17. A primary action of aldosterone is to
   A. Convert angiotensinogen to angiotensin
   B. Decrease chloride reabsorption in the renal tubule
   C. Decrease potassium secretion in the renal tubule
   D. Increase sodium reabsorption in the renal tubule
   E. Increase renin release by the juxtaglomerular apparatus

**Answer: D**
Aldosterone, produced by the adrenal zona glomerulosa, acts to preserve hemostasis by maintaining serum sodium and chloride levels and by promoting secretion of excess potassium. (See Schwartz 7th ed.)

18. The appropriate nonprotein calorie to nitrogen ratio in a moderately stressed surgical patient is
   A. 150:1
   B. 120:1
   C. 90:1
   D. 60:1

**Answer: B**
See Table 1-1 on p 5.

**Table 1-1.**
**Caloric Adjustments Above Basal Energy Expenditure (BEE) in Hypermetabolic Conditions**

| Condition | kcal/kg per day | Adjustment Above BEE | Grams of Protein/ kg per day | Nonprotein Calories: Nitrogen |
|---|---|---|---|---|
| Normal/moderate malnutrition | 25–30 | 1.1 | 1.0 | 150:1 |
| Mild stress | 25–30 | 1.2 | 1.2 | 150:1 |
| Moderate stress | 30 | 1.4 | 1.5 | 120:1 |
| Severe stress | 30–35 | 1.6 | 2.0 | 90–120:1 |
| Burns | 35–40 | 2.0 | 2.5 | 90–100:1 |

See Schwartz 8th ed., p 31.

# CHAPTER 2

# Fluid and Electrolyte Management of the Surgical Patient

1. Metabolic acidosis with a normal anion gap (AG) occurs with
   A. Diabetic acidosis
   B. Renal failure
   C. Severe diarrhea
   D. Starvation

**Answer: C**
Metabolic acidosis with a normal anion gap results from either acid administration (HCl or $NH_4^+$) or a loss of bicarbonate from gastrointestinal sources such as diarrhea, fistulas (enteric, pancreatic, or biliary), ureterosigmoidostomy, or from renal loss. The bicarbonate loss is accompanied by a gain of chloride, thus the AG remains unchanged. (See Schwartz 8th ed., p 51.)

2. A serum sodium of 129 seen in the immediate postoperative period
   A. Warrants aggressive treatment with hypertonic saline to prevent seizures
   B. Should be treated with boluses of 0.9% NaCl until corrected
   C. Is a self-limiting problem due to transient increase in antidiuretic hormone secretion
   D. Is due to excessive fluids given intraoperatively

**Answer: C**
A low serum sodium level occurs when there is an excess of extracellular water relative to sodium. Extracellular volume can be high, normal, or low. For most cases of hyponatremia, sodium concentration is decreased as a consequence of either sodium depletion or dilution. Dilutional hyponatremia frequently results from excess extracellular water and, therefore, is associated with a high extracellular volume status. Either intentional (excessive oral water intake) or iatrogenic (intravenous) excess free water administration can cause hyponatremia. Postoperative patients are particularly prone to increased secretion of antidiuretic hormone, which increases reabsorption of free water from the kidneys with subsequent volume expansion and hyponatremia. This is usually self-limiting in that both hyponatremia and volume expansion decrease antidiuretic hormone secretion. Depletional causes of hyponatremia result from either a decreased intake or increased loss of sodium-containing fluids. Etiologies include decreased sodium intake, such as that from a low-sodium diet or enteral feeds that are typically low in sodium, gastrointestinal losses (vomiting, prolonged nasogastric suctioning, or diarrhea), or renal losses (diuretics or primary renal disease). Depletional hyponatremia is often accompanied by extracellular volume deficit. (See Schwartz 8th ed., p 46.)

3. Which of the following is an early sign of hyperkalemia?
   A. Peaked T waves
   B. Peaked P waves
   C. Peaked (shortened) QRS complex
   D. Peaked U waves

**Answer: A**
Symptoms of hyperkalemia are primarily gastrointestinal, neuromuscular, and cardiovascular. Gastrointestinal symptoms include nausea, vomiting, intestinal colic, and diarrhea; neuromuscular symptoms range from weakness to ascending paralysis to respiratory failure; while cardiovascular manifestations range from electrocardiogram (ECG) changes to cardiac arrhythmias and arrest. ECG changes that may be seen with hyperkalemia include:

Peaked T waves (early change)
Flattened P wave
Prolonged PR interval (first-degree block)
Widened QRS complex
Sine wave formation
Ventricular fibrillation

(See Schwartz 8th ed., p 48.)

4. Which of the following drugs causes magnesium depletion?
   A. Amphotericin
   B. Penicillin
   C. Cefuroxime
   D. Ciprofloxacin

**Answer: A**
Additionally, drugs such as amphotericin, aminoglycosides, foscarnet, cisplatin, and ifosfamide that induce magnesium depletion will cause renal potassium wastage. In cases in which potassium deficiency is due to magnesium depletion, potassium repletion is difficult unless hypomagnesemia is first corrected. (See Schwartz 8th ed., p 48.)

5. The next most appropriate test to order in a patient with a pH of 7.1, $Pco_2$ of 40, a sodium of 132, a potassium of 4.2, and a chloride of 105 is
   A. Serum bicarbonate
   B. Serum magnesium
   C. Serum ethanol
   D. Serum salicylate

**Answer: A**
Metabolic acidosis results from an increased intake of acids, an increased generation of acids, or an increased loss of bicarbonate. In evaluating a patient with a low serum bicarbonate level and metabolic acidosis, first measure the anion gap (AG), an index of unmeasured anions.

$$AG = [Na] - [Cl + HCO_3]$$

Metabolic acidosis with an increased AG occurs from either exogenous acid ingestion (ethylene glycol, salicylate, or methanol) or endogenous acid production of β-hydroxybutyrate and acetoacetate in ketoacidosis, lactate in lactic acidosis, or organic acids in renal insufficiency. (See Schwartz 8th ed., p 48.)

6. Lactated Ringer's solution
   A. Is composed of 130 mEq sodium and 130 mEq chloride with a lactate buffer
   B. May induce apoptosis and activate the inflammatory response
   C. Should not be given to patients with acidosis because of the increase in serum lactic acid
   D. Should not be used in patients with liver injury

**Answer: B**
Lactated Ringer's is slightly hypotonic in that it contains 130 mEq of sodium, which is balanced by 109 mEq of chloride and 28 mEq of lactate. Lactate is used rather than bicarbonate because it is more stable in intravenous fluids during storage. It is converted into bicarbonate in the liver following infusion, even in the face of hemorrhagic shock. Recent evidence has suggested that resuscitation using lactated Ringer's may be deleterious because it activates the inflammatory response and induces apoptosis. The component that has been implicated is the D isomer of lactate, which unlike the D isomer is not a normal intermediary in mammalian metabolism. Traditionally, solutions contain a 50:50 mixture of the D and D isomer. In vitro studies show that only the D isomer does not activate neutrophils. (See Schwartz 8th ed., p 52.)

7. Normal saline is
   A. 135 mEq NaCl/L
   B. 145 mEq NaCl/L
   C. 148 mEq NaCl/L
   D. 154 mEq NaCl/L

**Answer: D**
Sodium chloride is mildly hypertonic, containing 154 mEq of sodium that is balanced by 154 mEq of chloride. The high chloride concentration imposes a significant chloride load upon the kidneys and may lead to a hyperchloremic metabolic acidosis. It is an ideal solution, however, for correcting volume deficits associated with hyponatremia, hypochloremia, and metabolic alkalosis. (See Schwartz 8th ed., p 52.)

8. Hydroxyethyl starch solutions (Hetastarch) may cause bleeding from
   A. Decreased platelet counts
   B. Decreased von Willebrand factor
   C. Decreased factor VII
   D. Decreased factor XIII

**Answer: B**
Hydroxyethyl starch solutions are another group of alternative plasma expanders and volume replacement solutions. Hetastarches are produced by the hydrolysis of insoluble amylopectin, followed by a varying number of substitutions of hydroxyl groups for carbon groups on glucose molecules. The molecular weights can range from 1000 to 3,000,000. The high molecular weight hydroxyethyl starch, hetastarch (average molecular weight 480,000), which comes as a 6% solution, is the only hydroxyethyl starch approved for use in the United States. Hemostatic derangements have been related to decreases in von Willebrand factor and factor VIII:c, and its use has been associated with postoperative bleeding in cardiac and neurosurgery patients. (See Schwartz 8th ed., p 53.)

9. Water constitutes what percentage of total body weight?
   A. 30–40%
   B. 40–50%
   C. 50–60%
   D. 60–70%

**Answer: C**
Water constitutes approximately 50% to 60% of total body weight. The relationship between total body weight and total body water (TBW) is relatively constant for an individual and is primarily a reflection of body fat. Lean tissues such as muscle and solid organs have higher water content than fat and bone. As a result, young, lean males have a higher proportion of body weight as water than elderly or obese individuals. An average young adult male will have 60% of his total body weight as TBW, while an average young adult female's will be 50%. The lower percentage of TBW in females correlates with a higher percentage of adipose tissue and lower percentage of muscle mass in most. Estimates of TBW should be adjusted down approximately 10 to 20% in obese individuals and up by 10% in malnourished individuals. The highest percentage of TBW is found in newborns, with approximately 80% of their total body weight comprised of water. This decreases to about 65% by 1 year of age and thereafter remains fairly constant. (See Schwartz 8th ed., p 43.)

10. A patient with a sodium of 132, a glucose of 250, and a blood urea nitrogen of 45 has a serum osmolality of
    A. 226
    B. 256
    C. 294
    D. 304

**Answer: C**
Osmotic pressure is measured in units of osmoles (osm) or milliosmoles (mOsm) that refer to the actual number of osmotically-active particles. For example, one millimole (mmol) of sodium chloride contributes to 2 mOsm (one from sodium and one from chloride). The principal determinants of osmolality are the concentrations of sodium, glucose, and urea (blood urea nitrogen [BUN]):

$$\text{Calculated serum osmolality} = 2\,\text{sodium} + \text{glucose}/18 + \text{BUN}/2.8.$$

(See Schwartz 8th ed., p 44.)

11. What is the actual potassium of a patient with a pH of 7.8 and a serum potassium of 2.2?
    A. 2.2
    B. 2.8
    C. 3.2
    D. 3.4

**Answer: D**
The change in potassium associated with alkalosis can be calculated by the following formula:

Potassium decreases by 0.3 mEq/L for every 0.1 increase in pH above normal.

(See Schwartz 8th ed., p 48.)

12. A hypovolemic patient with a serum sodium of 158 should initially be treated with
    A. 5% dextrose in water
    B. 5 % dextrose in ¼ normal saline
    C. 5% dextrose in ½ normal saline
    D. Normal saline

**Answer: D**
Treatment of hypernatremia usually consists of treatment of the associated water deficit. In hypovolemic patients, volume should be restored with normal saline. Once adequate volume status has been achieved, the water deficit is replaced using a hypotonic fluid such as 5% dextrose, 5% dextrose in ¼ normal saline, or enteral water. This is the formula used to estimate the amount of water required to correct hypernatremia:

$$\text{Water deficit (L)} = \frac{\text{serum sodium} - 140}{140} \times \text{TBW}$$

Estimate TBW (total body weight) as 50% of lean body mass in men and 40% in women. (See Schwartz 8th ed., p 54.)

13. A patient with a serum calcium of 6.8 and an albumin of 1.2 has a corrected calcium of
    A. 7.7
    B. 8.0
    C. 8.6
    D. 9.2

**Answer: D**
When measuring total serum calcium levels, the albumin concentration must be taken into consideration:
Adjust total serum calcium down by 0.8 mg/dL for every 1-g/dL decrease in albumin. (See Schwartz 8th ed., p 49.)

14. The initial treatment in a patient with a serum potassium of 6.4 with electrocardiogram changes is
    A. Kayexalate enema
    B. Kayexalate enema and given orally
    C. Calcium carbonate IV
    D. Calcium gluconate and bicarbonate IV

**Answer: D**

**Table 2-1.**
**Treatment of Symptomatic Hyperkalemia**

| |
|---|
| **Potassium removal** |
|   Kayexalate |
|     Oral administration is 15–30 g in 50–100 mL of 20% sorbitol |
|     Rectal administration is 50 g in 200 mL 20% sorbitol |
|   Dialysis |
| **Shift potassium** |
|   Glucose 1 ampule of $D_{50}$ and regular insulin 5–10 units intravenous |
|   Bicarbonate 1 ampule intravenous |
| **Counteract cardiac effects** |
|   Calcium gluconate 5–10 mL of 10% solution |

See Schwartz 8th ed., p 54.

15. An alcoholic patient with a serum albumin of 3.9, K of 3.1, Mg of 2.4, Ca of 7.8, and PO4 of 3.2 receives three boluses of IV potassium and has a serum potassium of 3.3. You should
    A. Continue to bolus potassium until the serum level is >3.6
    B. Give MgSO4 IV
    C. Check the ionized calcium
    D. Check the blood urea nitrogen and creatinine

**Answer: B**
Magnesium depletion is a common problem in hospitalized patients, particularly in the ICU. The kidney is primarily responsible for magnesium homeostasis through regulation by calcium/magnesium receptors on renal tubular cells that sense serum magnesium levels. Hypomagnesemia results from a variety of etiologies ranging from poor intake (starvation, alcoholism, prolonged use of intravenous fluids, and total parenteral nutrition with inadequate supplementation of magnesium), increased renal excretion (alcohol, most diuretics, and amphotericin B), gastrointestinal losses (diarrhea), malabsorption, acute pancreatitis, diabetic ketoacidosis, and primary aldosteronism. Hypomagnesemia

is important not only for its direct effects on the nervous system but also because it can produce hypocalcemia and lead to persistent hypokalemia. When hypokalemia or hypocalcemia coexist with hypomagnesemia, magnesium should be aggressively replaced to assist in restoring potassium or calcium homeostasis. (See Schwartz 8th ed., p 49.)

16. Insensible water loss from the skin is what percentage of total insensible loss?
    A. 25%
    B. 45%
    C. 60%
    D. 75%

**Answer: D**
The normal person consumes an average of 2,000 mL of water per day, approximately 75% from oral intake and the rest is extracted from solid foods. Daily water losses include about 1 L in urine, 250 mL in stool, and 600 mL as insensible losses. Insensible losses occur through both the skin (75%) and lungs (25%) and, by definition, is pure water. Insensible losses can be increased by such factors as fever, hypermetabolism, and hyperventilation. Sweating, on the other hand, is an active process and involves loss of (hypotonic) electrolytes and water. To clear the products of metabolism, the kidneys must excrete a minimum of 500 to 800 mL of urine per day, regardless of the amount of oral intake. (See Schwartz 8th ed., p 44.)

17. A patient who has spasms in the hand when a blood pressure cuff is blown up most likely has
    A. Hypercalcemia
    B. Hypocalcemia
    C. Hypermagnesemia
    D. Hypomagnesemia

**Answer: B**
Asymptomatic hypocalcemia may occur with hypoproteinemia (normal ionized calcium), but symptoms can develop with alkalosis (decreased ionized calcium). In general, symptoms do not occur until the ionized fraction falls below 2.5 mg/dL, and are neuromuscular and cardiac in origin, including paresthesias of the face and extremities, muscle cramps, carpopedal spasm, stridor, tetany, and seizures. Patients will demonstrate hyperreflexia and positive Chvostek's sign (spasm resulting from tapping over the facial nerve) and Trousseau's sign (spasm resulting from pressure applied to the nerves and vessels of the upper extremity, as when obtaining a blood pressure). Decreased cardiac contractility and heart failure can also accompany hypocalcemia. (See Schwartz 8th ed., p 50.)

18. Metabolic acidosis with a normal anion gap is found in a patient with
    A. Alcohol intoxication
    B. Aspirin ingestion
    C. Diabetic ketoacidosis
    D. Small bowel fistula

**Answer: D**
A normal anion gap occurs in an acidotic patient who is not producing abnormal acid. Increased keto acids are found in alcoholics and diabetics with acidosis. Aspirin ingestion leads to abnormal amounts of sulfuric acid. (See Schwartz 7th ed.)

19. The effective osmotic pressure between the plasma and interstitial fluid compartments is primarily controlled by
    A. Bicarbonate
    B. Chloride ion
    C. Potassium ion
    D. Protein

**Answer: D**
The dissolved protein in plasma does not pass through the semipermeable cell membrane, and this fact is responsible for the effective or colloid osmotic pressure. (See Schwartz 7th ed.)

20. The most common fluid disorder in the surgical patient is
    A. Extracellular fluid deficit
    B. Hyperkalemia
    C. Hyponatremia
    D. Metabolic acidosis
    E. Metabolic alkalosis

**Answer: A**

The most common causes of extracellular fluid deficit in the surgical patient are gastrointestinal fluid losses from vomiting, nasogastric suction, diarrhea, and fistular drainage. These losses consist of water and electrolytes in approximately the same proportion as they are present in extracellular fluid. (See Schwartz 7th ed.)

21. Symptoms and signs of extracellular fluid volume deficit include all of the following EXCEPT
    A. Anorexia
    B. Apathy
    C. Decreased body temperature
    D. High pulse pressure

**Answer: D**

High pulse pressure occurs with extracellular fluid volume excess, but the other symptoms and signs are characteristic of moderate extracellular volume deficit. (See Schwartz 7th ed.)

22. The osmolarity of the extracellular fluid space is determined primarily by the concentration of
    A. Bicarbonate
    B. Chloride ion
    C. Phosphate radicals
    D. Sodium ion

**Answer: D**

Sodium is the prominent extracellular anion, and determination of serum sodium concentrations generally indicates the tonicity of body fluids. (See Schwartz 7th ed.)

23. When lactic acid is produced in response to injury, the body minimizes pH change by
    A. Decreasing production of sodium bicarbonate in tissues
    B. Excreting carbon dioxide through the lungs
    C. Excreting lactic acid through the kidneys
    D. Metabolizing the lactic acid in the liver

**Answer: B**

Lactic acid reacts with base bicarbonate to produce carbonic acid. The carbonic acid is broken down into water and carbon dioxide that is excreted by the lungs. Any diminution in pulmonary function jeopardizes this reaction. (See Schwartz 7th ed.)

24. The simplest effective method of estimating the degree of acidosis in a patient in shock is the measurement of
    A. Arterial pH
    B. End tidal $CO_2$ concentration
    C. pH of mixed venous blood
    D. Serum $CO_2$ level

**Answer: A**

Only the measurement of arterial pH and $P_{CO_2}$ gives an accurate picture of the degree of acid-base imbalances. (See Schwartz 7th ed.)

25. If a patient's arterial $P_{CO_2}$ is found to be 25 mm Hg, the arterial pH will be approximately
    A. 7.52
    B. 7.40
    C. 7.32
    D. 7.28

**Answer: D**

A low $Pa_{CO_2}$ indicates excess elimination of carbon dioxide by the lungs, and the body pH will fall. Within reasonable physiologic ranges a 15 mm Hg fall in $Pa_{CO_2}$ should produce a 0.12 change from the normal body pH of 7.4. (See Schwartz 7th ed.)

26. In a patient with acute renal failure, the LEAST urgent reason for dialysis is
    A. Blood urea nitrogen >100 mL/dL
    B. Hyperkalemia
    C. Severe acidosis
    D. Uremic pericarditis

**Answer: A**

Although all of the listed findings are characteristic of acute renal failure, blood urea nitrogen elevation per se is not a reason for emergency dialysis. Hyperkalemia, severe acidosis, uremic encephalopathy, and uremic pericarditis are all indications of life-threatening problems, and urgent correction is mandatory. (See Schwartz 7th ed.)

27. An elderly diabetic patient who has acute cholecystitis is found to have a serum sodium level of 122 mEq/L and a blood glucose of 600 mg/dL. After correcting the glucose concentration to 100 mg/dL with insulin, the serum sodium concentration would
    A. Decrease significantly unless the patient also received 3% saline
    B. Decrease transiently but return to approximately 122 mEq/L without specific therapy
    C. Remain essentially unchanged
    D. Increase to the normal range without specific therapy

**Answer: D**

A rise in the extracellular fluid concentration of a substance that does not diffuse passively across cell membranes (e.g., glucose or urea) causes an increase in effective osmotic pressure, a transfer of water from cells, and dilutional hyponatremia. For each 100 mg/dL rise in blood glucose above normal, the serum sodium level falls approximately 3 mEq/L. Alternatively, the serum sodium level would increase by about 15 mEq/L if the blood glucose level fell from 600 to 100 mg/dL. (See Schwartz 7th ed.)

28. A decrease in intracellular water can be precipitated by
    A. A decrease in sodium in extracellular fluid
    B. An increase in sodium in extracellular fluid
    C. An increase in sodium in intracellular fluid
    D. An isotonic decrease in extracellular fluid

**Answer: B**

The cell membrane is semipermeable. Potassium concentration is higher within cells than in the extracellular fluid, and sodium concentration is higher in the extracellular space. When sodium rises in the extracellular fluid, water moves out of the cells to maintain osmotic equilibrium. Isotonic gain or loss in extracellular fluid volume does not result in an osmotic gradient. Therefore, intracellular water and electrolyte concentration are not changed significantly. (See Schwartz 7th ed.)

29. The first step in the management of acute hypercalcemia should be
    A. Correction of deficit of extracellular fluid volume
    B. Hemodialysis
    C. Administration of furosemide
    D. Administration of mithramycin

**Answer: A**

Patients with acute hypercalcemia usually have either acute hyperparathyroidism or metastatic breast carcinoma with multiple bony metastases. These patients develop severe headaches, bone pain, thirst, emesis, and polyuria. Unless treatment is instituted promptly the symptoms may be rapidly fatal. Immediate correction of the associated deficit of extracellular fluid volume is the most important step in treatment. When effective, this results in the lowering of the serum calcium level by dilution. Once extracellular fluid volume has been replaced, furosemide is effective treatment. Hemodialysis may also be employed, but its effect is less rapid. Mithramycin is very useful in control of metastatic bone disease, but its effect is slow, and it cannot be depended upon when the patient has acute hypercalcemia. (See Schwartz 7th ed.)

30. Initial administration of fluid during the resuscitation of a patient who has a gunshot wound of the abdomen results in a rise in blood pressure to 110/80 mm Hg. At this point, arterial blood gases are pH, 7.25; $P_{O_2}$, 95 mm Hg; $P_{CO_2}$, 25 mm Hg; $HCO_3^-$, 15 mEq/L. The patient's metabolic acidosis would be treated best with
    A. Tromethamine
    B. Sodium bicarbonate
    C. A balanced salt solution
    D. Hyperventilation

**Answer: C**

In patients suffering from hemorrhagic shock, the presence of a metabolic acidosis early in the postresuscitative period is indicative of tissue hypoxia due to persistent inadequate tissue perfusion. Attempts to correct this problem by administering an alkalizing agent will not solve the basic problem. However, proper volume replacement by means of a balanced salt solution such as Ringer's lactate will restore perfusion and correct the metabolic acidosis by ending anaerobic metabolism. (See Schwartz 7th ed.)

31. Three days after surgery for gastric carcinoma, a 50-year-old alcoholic man exhibits delirium, muscle tremors, and hyperactive tendon reflexes. Magnesium deficiency is suspected. All of the following statements regarding this situation are true EXCEPT
    A. A decision to administer magnesium should be based on the serum magnesium level.
    B. Adequate cellular replacement of magnesium will require 1–3 weeks.
    C. A concomitant calcium deficiency should be suspected.
    D. Calcium is a specific antagonist of the myocardial effects of magnesium.

**Answer: A**
Magnesium deficiency should be suspected in any malnourished patient who exhibits disturbed neuromuscular or cerebral activity in the postoperative period. Laboratory confirmation often is not reliable, and the syndrome may exist in the presence of a normal serum magnesium level. Hypocalcemia often coexists, particularly in patients who have clinical signs of tetany. Intravenous magnesium can be administered safely to a well-hydrated patient for initial treatment of a severe deficit, but concomitant electrocardiographic monitoring is essential. The electrocardiographic changes associated with acute hypermagnesemia resemble those of hyperkalemia, and calcium chloride or gluconate should be readily available to counteract any adverse myocardial effects of excess magnesium ions. Partial or complete relief of symptoms may follow the initial infusion of magnesium, although continued replacement for a period of 1 to 3 weeks is necessary to replenish cellular stores. (See Schwartz 7th ed.)

32. Which of the following best describes the composition of gastric secretions?
    A. Na 60 Cl 60
    B. Na 60 Cl 110
    C. Na 110 Cl 60
    D. Na 110 Cl 110

**Answer: B**
See Table 2-2 on p 15.

**Table 2-2.**
**Composition of Gastrointestinal Secretions**

| Type of Secretion | Volume (mL/24 h) | Na (mEq/L) | K (mEq/L) | Cl (mEq/L) | $HCO_3^-$ (mEq/L) |
|---|---|---|---|---|---|
| Stomach | 1,000–2,000 | 60–90 | 10–30 | 100–130 | 0 |
| Small intestine | 2,000–3,000 | 120–140 | 5–10 | 90–120 | 30–40 |
| Colon | — | 60 | 30 | 40 | 0 |
| Pancreas | 600–800 | 135–145 | 5–10 | 70–90 | 95–115 |
| Bile | 300–800 | 135–145 | 5–10 | 90–110 | 30–40 |

See Schwartz 8th ed., p 46.

# CHAPTER 3

# Hemostasis, Surgical Bleeding, and Transfusion

1. Which of the following is NOT one of the four major physiologic events of hemostasis?
   A. Fibrinolysis
   B. Vasodilatation
   C. Platelet plug formation
   D. Fibrin production

**Answer B:**
Four major physiologic events participate, both in sequence and interdependently, in the hemostatic process. Vascular constriction, platelet plug formation, fibrin formation, and fibrinolysis occur in that general order, but the products of each of these four processes are interrelated in such a way that there is a continuum and multiple reinforcements. (See Schwartz 8th ed., pp 61–62.)

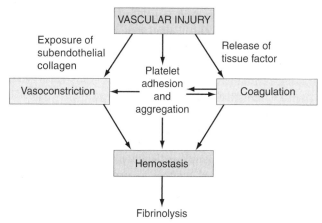

**FIG. 3-1.** *Schematic of processes initiated by vascular injury.*

2. The half-life of platelets is
   A. 2–3 days
   B. 7–10 days
   C. 14–21 days
   D. 30–40 days

**Answer: B**
Platelets are 2 to 4 μm in diameter anucleate fragments of megakaryocytes with normal circulating numbers falling between 150,000 and 400,000/μL. Thrombopoietin is the predominant mediator of platelet production, although other inflammatory mediators, such as interleukin (IL)-6 and IL-11, may play a role. Up to 30% of circulating platelets may be sequestered in the spleen and can be released in response to catecholamines. If not consumed in a clotting reaction, platelets are normally removed by the spleen with an average life span of 7 to 10 days. (See Schwartz 8th ed., p 62.)

3. The primary defect in von Willebrand's disease is
   A. Inadequate production of fibrin
   B. Excessive fibrinolysis
   C. Failure of platelet aggregation
   D. Failure of vessel constriction

**Answer: C**
von Willebrand's disease (vWD) is another disorder with low factor VIII. It is an autosomal dominant disorder, and the primary defect is a low level of the von Willebrand factor (vWF), a large glycoprotein with two functions. One function

is to serve as a carrier for factor VIII; thus when vWF levels are low, factor VIII levels are variably decreased because of loss of the carrier protein. More important, in most patients, vWF is necessary for normal platelet adhesion to exposed subendothelium and for normal aggregation under high shear conditions, so patients with vWD have bleeding that is characteristic of platelet disorders—typically easy bruising and mucosal bleeding. (See Schwartz 8th ed., p 67.)

4. Which congenital factor deficiency is associated with delayed bleeding after initial hemostasis?
   A. Factor VII
   B. Factor IX
   C. Factor XI
   D. Factor XIII

**Answer: D**
Congenital factor XIII deficiency also is rare. It is inherited as an autosomal recessive trait. Bleeding is typically delayed because clots form normally but are susceptible to fibrinolysis. Umbilical stump bleeding is characteristic, and there is a high risk of intracranial bleeding. Spontaneous abortion is usual in women with factor XIII deficiency unless they receive replacement therapy. The half-life of factor XIII is quite long, approximately 9 to 14 days. Replacement can be accomplished with [fresh frozen plasma] FFP, cryoprecipitate, or a factor XIII concentrate. Levels of 1 to 2% are usually adequate for hemostasis. (See Schwartz 8th ed., p 68.)

5. Which of the following is the most common intrinsic platelet defect?
   A. Thrombasthenia
   B. Bernard Soulier syndrome
   C. Cyclooxygenase deficiency
   D. Storage pool disease

**Answer: D**
The most common intrinsic platelet defect is known as storage pool disease. It may involve loss of dense granules (storage sites for adenosine 5′-diphosphate [ADP], adenosine triphosphate [ATP], $Ca^{2+}$, and inorganic phosphate) and $\alpha$-granules (storage sites for a large number of proteins, some of which are specific to platelets [e.g., PF4 and $\beta$-thromboglobulin], while others are present in both platelet $\alpha$-granules and plasma [e.g., fibrinogen, (von Willebrand factor) vWF, and albumin]). Dense granule deficiency is the most prevalent of these. It may be an isolated defect or occur with partial albinism in the Hermansky-Pudlak syndrome. Bleeding is variable, depending on how severe the granule defect is. Bleeding is primarily caused by the decreased release of ADP from these platelets. An isolated defect of the $\alpha$-granules is known as gray platelet syndrome because of the appearance of the platelets on Wright's stain. Bleeding is usually mild with this syndrome. A few patients have been reported who have decreased numbers of both dense and $\alpha$-granules. These patients have a more severe bleeding disorder. Patients with mild bleeding as a consequence of a form of storage pool disease may have decreased bleeding if given DDAVP. It is likely that the high levels of vWF in the plasma after DDAVP somehow compensate for the intrinsic platelet defect. With more severe bleeding, platelet transfusion is required. (See Schwartz 8th ed., p 68.)

6. In a previously unexposed patient, when does the platelet count fall in heparin-induced thrombocytopenia (HIT)?
   A. <24 hours
   B. 24–28 hours
   C. 3–4 days
   D. 5–7 days

**Answer: D**
Heparin-induced thrombocytopenia is a special case of drug-induced immune thrombocytopenia. The platelet count typically begins to fall 5 to 7 days after heparin has been started, but if it is a re-exposure, the decrease in count may occur within 1 to 2 days. Thrombocytopenia is not usually severe. HIT should be suspected if the platelet count falls to less than

100,000 or if it drops by 50 from baseline in a patient receiving heparin. While HIT is more common with full-dose unfractionated heparin (1 to 3%), it can occur with prophylactic doses or with low molecular weight heparins. If it develops with unfractionated heparin, the antibody is likely to cross-react with low molecular weight heparin. (See Schwartz 8th ed., p 69.)

7. A fully heparinized patient develops a condition requiring emergency surgery. After stopping the heparin, what else should be done to prepare the patient?
   A. Nothing, if the surgery can be delayed for 2–3 hours
   B. Immediate administration of protamine 5 mg for every 100 units of heparin most recently administered
   C. Immediate fresh frozen plasma
   D. Transfusion of 10 units of platelets

**Answer: A**

Emergency operations are occasionally necessary in patients who have been heparinized as treatment for deep venous thrombosis. The first step in managing these patients is discontinuation of heparin; this may be sufficient if the operation can be delayed for several hours. For more rapid reversal, 1 mg of protamine sulfate for every 100 units of heparin most recently administered is immediately effective. For each hour that has elapsed since the last heparin dose, the amount of protamine should be halved. The formation of both extrinsic and intrinsic prothrombinase can be retarded, prolonging the [prothrombin time] PT and [activated partial thromboplastin time] aPTT tests. Some patients exhibit the phenomenon of "heparin rebound" after apparently adequate heparin neutralization with protamine; prolongation of the clotting time recurs after adequate postoperative antagonism of the heparin, which can contribute to postoperative bleeding. In one of the author's experience, this is a major cause of "unexplained" postoperative bleeding after cardiac and vascular surgical procedures. Some of the prolongation of the aPTT after heparin neutralization with protamine may also be a result of the anticoagulant effect of protamine. Activation of fibrinolysis and thrombocytopenia may also contribute to the problem of postoperative bleeding. (See Schwartz 8th ed., p 73.)

8. Bank blood is appropriate for replacing each of the following EXCEPT
   A. Factor I (fibrinogen)
   B. Factor II (prothrombin)
   C. Factor VII (proconvertin)
   D. Factor VIII (antihemophilic factor)

**Answer: D**

Factor VIII is labile, and 60–80% of activity is gone 1 week after collection. The other factors listed are stable in banked blood. (See Schwartz 7th ed.)

9. Which of the following clotting factors is consumed during coagulation?
   A. Factor I (fibrinogen)
   B. Factor IX (Christmas factor)
   C. Factor X (Stuart-Prower factor)
   D. Factor XI (plasma thromboplasma antecedent)

**Answer: A**

Factor I, factor II (prothrombin), factor V (proaccelerin), factor VIII (antihemophilic factor), and platelets are consumed during coagulation and must be replaced by the body. The other factors return to their normal levels after coagulation is complete. (See Schwartz 7th ed.)

10. Exsanguinating hemorrhage is most likely to follow which of the following injuries in a previously healthy young adult?
    A. Closed fracture of the femur
    B. Open fracture of the tibia and fibula
    C. Partial transection of the artery from a sharp injury
    D. Severe crush injury of the foot

**Answer: C**

All the injuries would be associated with significant bleeding, but vascular constriction of healthy arteries in a young person would prevent exsanguination. However, if one artery is partially transected, complete constriction of the injured arterial ends is not possible, and spontaneous cessation of bleeding does not occur. (See Schwartz 7th ed.)

11. A prolonged bleeding time may be anticipated in patients with each of the following problems EXCEPT
    A. Aspirin ingestion in the past week
    B. Classic hemophilia
    C. Qualitative platelet dysfunction
    D. von Willebrand's disease

**Answer: B**
Classic hemophilia does not result in an abnormality of platelet plug formation, and bleeding time should be normal. The other conditions listed inhibit the platelet plug necessary for normal homeostasis. (See Schwartz 7th ed.)

12. If a patient is found to have a normal partial thromboplastin time (PTT) and a prolonged one-stage prothrombin time (PT), there may be a deficiency of factor
    A. V (proaccelerin)
    B. VIII (antihemophilic factor)
    C. IX (plasma thromboplastin component)
    D. XI (plasma thromboplastin antecedent)

**Answer: A**
The one-stage prothrombin time, when normal, eliminates the roles of factors VII, IX, XI, XII, and platelets in the coagulation cascade. When PT is prolonged, there may be a deficiency of factors II (prothrombin), V, VII (proconvertin), X (Stuart-Prower), a fibrinogen. Even a small amount of circulating heparin will produce both a long PT and a long PTT. The PTT tells the intrinsic pathway, and a normal value occurs with an intrinsic factor problem because the reagents for the test include the necessary extrinsic factors for clotting. (See Schwartz 7th ed.)

13. Frozen plasma prepared from freshly donated blood is necessary when a patient requires
    A. Fibrinogen
    B. Prothrombin
    C. Antihemophilic factor
    D. Christmas factor
    E. Hageman factor

**Answer: C**
Frozen plasma is required for the transfusion of antihemophilic factor (factor VIII) or proaccelerin (factor V). The other factors are present in banked preparations. (See Schwartz 7th ed.)

14. The most common cause for a transfusion reaction is
    A. Air embolism
    B. Contaminated blood
    C. Human error
    D. Unusual circulating antibodies

**Answer: C**
Although contaminated or outdated blood may cause a reaction, the most common cause is human error—blood drawn for typing from the wrong patient, blood incorrectly crossmatched in the laboratory, blood units mislabeled in the laboratory, blood administered to the wrong patients. Most blood banking programs have instituted elaborate checks and balances to minimize these errors. (See Schwartz 7th ed.)

15. Each of the following is a symptom of a hemolytic transfusion reaction EXCEPT
    A. Constricting chest pain
    B. Flushing of the face
    C. Lumbar pain
    D. Syncope

**Answer: D**
Syncope is not associated with a hemolytic transfusion reaction, whereas the other listed symptoms are common occurrences. (See Schwartz 7th ed.)

16. The most common clinical manifestation of a hemolytic transfusion reaction is
    A. Flank pain
    B. Jaundice
    C. Oliguria
    D. A shaking chill

**Answer: C**
All of the manifestations listed can occur with a hemolytic transfusion reaction. In a large series, oliguria (58%) and hemoglobinuria (56%) were the most common findings. (See Schwartz 7th ed.)

17. The most common fatal infectious complication of a blood transfusion is
    A. Acquired immunodeficiency syndrome
    B. Cytomegalovirus
    C. Malaria
    D. Viral hepatitis

**Answer: D**
Any of the listed diseases can be transmitted by contaminated blood, but posttransfusion viral hepatitis is the most common fatal problem. Hepatitis occurs from infection by hepatitis B virus, hepatitis C, or one of the other non-A, non-B viruses. (See Schwartz 7th ed.)

18. Which of the following factors is labile in acid citrate dextrose (ACD) bank blood?
    A. Antihemophilic globulin
    B. Christmas factor
    C. Fibrinogen
    D. Proconvertin
    E. Prothrombin

**Answer: A**

Antihemophilic globulin (factor VIII) is labile, and only 20–40% remains in ACD bank blood after 1 week. Christmas factor (factor IX), fibrinogen (factor I), proconvertin (factor VII), and prothrombin (factor II) are stable and can be replaced with bank blood. For significant bleeding in a patient with Christmas disease, a bank blood concentrated preparation of factor IX can be used. (See Schwartz 7th ed.)

19. In the awake, nonanesthetized patient suspected of having a hemolytic posttransfusion reaction, the most characteristic signs are
    A. Nausea and vomiting
    B. Fever and chills
    C. Oliguria and hemoglobinuria
    D. Cyanosis and dyspnea

**Answer: C**

Although all the signs listed in the question can be seen in hemolytic transfusion reactions, oliguria and hemoglobinuria are the most common. In one large series, oliguria and hemoglobinuria occurred in 58% and 56% of cases, respectively. Although hypotension occurred in 50% of cases, all the other signs occurred in less than 30%. These data point out the diagnostic value of bladder catheterization as a means of quickly assessing the color and volume of urine. If oliguria and hemoglobinuria are present, prompt measures must be taken to protect the kidney against free hemoglobin, which together with hypotension and acidosis can cause acute tubular necrosis. The most common symptoms in a hemolytic transfusion reaction are the sensation of heat and pain along the vein into which the blood is being transfused, flushing of the face, pain in the lumbar region, and constricting pain in the chest. In patients who are anesthetized, the two signs that may appear are abnormal bleeding and continued hypotension despite adequate replacement. (See Schwartz 7th ed.)

20. A 57-year-old woman who has rheumatic heart disease presents with a 12-h history of increasing right lower quadrant pain associated with nausea and vomiting. A diagnosis of appendicitis is made. History reveals that she suffered a transient ischemic attack 3 years ago and since then has been taking warfarin (Coumadin). Laboratory data are as follows: white blood cell count, 13,000/mm$^3$; hematocrit, 45%; and prothrombin time, 40% of normal. Management of this patient should include
    A. Administration of vitamin K; surgery in 12 h
    B. Administration of vitamin K and fresh frozen plasma; immediate surgery
    C. Administration of vitamin K; immediate surgery with low-dose heparin intraoperatively
    D. Administration of fresh frozen platelets; immediate surgery
    E. None of the above

**Answer: E**

To reverse the effects of warfarin (Coumadin) in the presented patient would be to subject her to an unnecessary risk of recurrent, potentially fatal embolization, and experience has shown that surgery can be performed with relative safety when the prothrombin time is greater than 20% of normal. The performance of a meticulous appendectomy while continuing Coumadin therapy and carefully monitoring the prothrombin time would be the safest course of action to follow in this given case. Certain surgical procedures, however, such as those involving the central nervous system, in which even minor bleeding can cause major morbidity, should not be performed on a patient receiving anticoagulant therapy. (See Schwartz 7th ed.)

21. Each of the following factors requires vitamin K for its production EXCEPT
    A. Factor VIII
    B. Factor X
    C. Factor IX (Christmas factor)
    D. Proconvertin (factor VII)

**Answer: A**

Antihemophilic globulin (factor VIII) is largely synthesized in the liver but does not require vitamin K. Prothrombin, proconvertin (factor VII), plasma thromboplastin component (Christmas factor, factor IX), and factor X all require vitamin K for their production. (See Schwartz 7th ed.)

22. On her third day of hospitalization, a 70-year-old woman who is being treated with antibiotics for acute cholecystitis develops increased pain and tenderness in the right upper quadrant with a palpable mass. Her temperature rises to 40°C (104°F), and her blood pressure falls to 80/60 mm Hg. Hematemesis and melena ensue, and petechiae are noted. Laboratory studies reveal thrombocytopenia, prolonged prothrombin time, and a decreased fibrinogen level. The most important step in the correction of this patient's coagulopathy is
    A. Administration of heparin
    B. Administration of fresh frozen plasma
    C. Administration of whole blood
    D. Exploratory laparotomy

**Answer: D**
The laboratory data given in the question in conjunction with bleeding and sepsis are strongly suggestive of disseminated intravascular coagulation (DIC). Treatment should be directed at eliminating the underlying cause of the consumptive coagulopathy, which in the presented case would involve drainage of the gallbladder and pericolic abscess. Such treatment usually will correct the bleeding diathesis. Heparin has not been found by most studies to be helpful in DIC. The use of fresh frozen plasma or whole blood would not treat the underlying problem, although replacement of clotting factors should proceed judiciously after the cause has been corrected. Aminocaproic acid is contraindicated in DIC as its inhibition of fibrinolysis can aggravate the coagulation defect and result in thrombosis. (See Schwartz 7th ed.)

23. After tissue injury, the first step in coagulation is
    A. Binding of factor XII to subendothelial collagen
    B. Cleavage of factor XI to active factor IX
    C. Complexing of factor IX with factor VIII in the presence of ionized calcium conversion of prothrombin to thrombin
    D. Formation of fibrin from fibrinogen

**Answer: A**
All the listed steps are part of the cascade involved in establishing a firm clot. The process begins with binding of Hageman factor (factor XII) to subendothelial collagen and ends with the conversion of fibrinogen to fibrin. The fibrin forms an insoluble addition that stabilizes the platelet plug. (See Schwartz 7th ed.)

24. Which of the following is NOT in the intrinsic pathway of coagulation?
    A. II
    B. XII
    C. XI
    D. IX

**Answer: A**
The intrinsic pathway begins with factor XII and through a cascade of enzymatic reactions, activates factors XI, IX, and VII in sequence. This pathway is referred to as "intrinsic" because all of the components leading ultimately to fibrin clot formation are intrinsic to the circulating plasma, and no surface is required to initiate the process. In contrast, the extrinsic pathway requires exposure of tissue factor on the surface of the injured vessel wall to initiate the arm of the cascade beginning with factor VII. The two arms of the coagulation cascade merge to a common pathway at factor X, and activation proceeds in sequence of factors II (prothrombin) and I (fibrinogen). Clot formation occurs after proteolytic conversion of fibrinogen to fibrin. (See Schwartz 8th ed., p 63.)
See Figure 3-2 on p 23.

25. The desired initial factor VIII level in a hemophiliac patient undergoing a laparoscopic cholecystectomy is
    A. 25%
    B. 50%
    C. 75%
    D. 100%

**Answer: D**
See Table 3-1 on p 23.

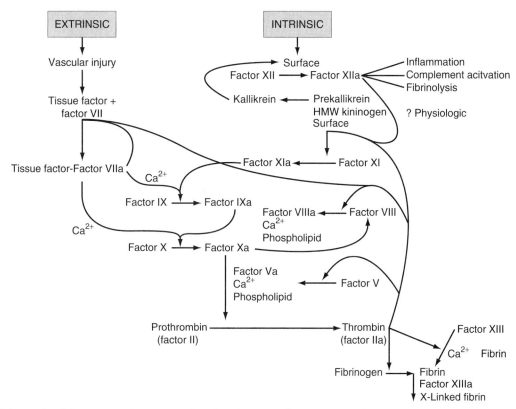

**FIG. 3-2.**   *Schematic of the coagulation system showing the many feedback loops that occur.*

Table 3-1.
**Guidelines for Factors VIII and IX Replacement in Hemophilia**

| Type of Bleeding | Hemostatic Factor Level Desired | Factor VIII Dose (U/kg) | Factor IX Dose (U/kg) |
|---|---|---|---|
| Central nervous system | 100% initially, then 50–100% for 10–14 days | 50 q12h or continuous infusion | 100, then 50 q12h or continuous infusion |
| Trauma or surgery | 100% initially, then 50% until wound healing begins, then 30% until wound healing complete | 50 q12h or continuous infusion | 100, then q24h |
| Retroperitoneal | 100% initially, then 50% until complete resolution | 50 q12h for 6 days | 40 q12h for 6 days |
| Retropharyngeal | 50–70% | 50 q12h for 4 days | 40 qd for 4 days |
| Gastrointestinal | 50–100% | 50 q12h for 3 days or until bleeding subsides | 40 qd for 3 days or until bleeding subsides |
| Hematuria | 40% | 40 qd for 3–5 days | 40 qd for 3 days |
| Tooth extraction | 50% | 40 once, then EACA 100 mg/kg daily for 7–10 days | 30 once, then EACA 100 mg/kg daily for 6 days |
| Mouth | 30–40% | 40 once, then EACA 100 mg/kg daily for 6 days | 20 once, then EACA 100 mg/kg daily for 6 days |
| Intramuscular | 40–50% | 20–30 q12h | 40–60 qod as needed |
| Acute hemarthrosis | 30–50% | 10–20 qd as needed | 15 qod as needed |

EACA = ε-aminocaproic acid.
See Schwartz 8th ed., p 66.

# CHAPTER 4

# Shock

1. In the presence of acute blood loss, adequate preload to the heart is maintained initially by the
   A. Development of tachycardia
   B. Hormonal effects of angiotensin
   C. Hormonal effects of renin
   D. Increase in systemic vascular resistance

**Answer: D**

The effects of angiotensin, antidiuretic hormone, and renin are important in maintaining normal homeostasis, but they are relatively slow in action. Tachycardia drops the effect of preload by decreasing diastolic filling time. Increases in venous time and in systemic vascular resistance augments preload in an effort to maintain cardiac output. (See Schwartz 7th ed.)

2. A patient with acute respiratory distress syndrome (ARDS) exhibits all of the following findings EXCEPT
   A. Decreased pulmonary compliance
   B. Hypercarbia
   C. Hypoxia
   D. Patchy infiltrates in chest X-ray

**Answer: B**

ARDS is characterized by hypoxia despite supplemental oxygen, decreased pulmonary compliance, noncardiac pulmonary edema, and diffuse or patchy infiltrates on chest X-ray. Because of persistent diffusion of $CO_2$ across the pulmonary capillary interface, hypercarbia is not a characteristic finding in this syndrome. (See Schwartz 7th ed.)

3. When a patient with hemorrhagic shock is resuscitated using an intravenous colloid solution rather than lactated Ringer's solution, all of the following statements are true EXCEPT
   A. Circulating levels of immunoglobulins are decreased
   B. Colloid solutions may bind to the ionized fraction of serum calcium
   C. Endogenous production of albumin is decreased
   D. Extracellular fluid volume deficit is restored

**Answer: D**

Because of higher osmotic pressure, colloid solutions draw extracellular fluid into the vascular space, increasing the extracellular fluid deficit. In addition, the ionized fraction of serum calcium is decreased, circulating levels of immunoglobulin drop; and reaction to tetanus toxoid given to the patient suffering from major trauma is decreased. Endogenous production of albumin also decreases. Colloid resuscitation is no more effective than crystalloid resuscitation, and it is more expensive. (See Schwartz 7th ed.)

4. All of the following result from the placement of an intraaortic balloon pump in a patient with acute myocardial failure EXCEPT
   A. Diastolic blood pressure elevation
   B. Increased cardiac output
   C. Increased pulmonary perfusion
   D. Increased probability of survival

**Answer: D**

An intraaortic balloon pump can be inserted at the bedside to provide temporary support for a failing myocardium. It can be anticipated that diastolic blood pressure will increase with associated improvement in pulmonary perfusion. Cardiac output distal to the pump will be increased. There is, however, no convincing evidence that use of the device improves long-term survival in these acutely ill patients. (See Schwartz 7th ed.)

5. Neurogenic shock is characterized by the presence of
   A. Cool, moist skin
   B. Increased cardiac output
   C. Decreased peripheral vascular resistance
   D. Decreased blood volume

**Answer: C**

Neurogenic shock is caused by loss of arteriolar and venular tone in response to paralysis (such as occurs with high spinal anesthesia), acute gastric dilatation, or sudden pain or unpleasant sights; as such, it is characterized by a decrease in peripheral vascular resistance. Affected patients usually present with warm, dry skin, a pulse rate that is slower than normal, and hypotension. A normovolemic state usually exists, and urine output is generally well maintained. Although blood volume measurements indicate a normal intravascular volume, because of the greatly increased reservoir capacity of the arterioles and venules, there is a decrease in cardiac output secondary to decreased venous return to the right side of the heart. (See Schwartz 7th ed.)

6. After drainage of a pelvic abscess, a 45-year-old patient receiving 70% oxygen is found to have the following arterial blood gases: pH, 7.48; $Po_2$, 55 mm Hg; $Pco_2$, 30 mm Hg. These results are most consistent with the diagnosis of
   A. Chronic obstructive pulmonary disease
   B. Postoperative pain and anxiety
   C. Adult respiratory distress syndrome
   D. Postoperative atelectasis

**Answer: C**
The combination of hypoxemia that is resistant to high oxygen concentrations and hyperventilation is characteristic of the adult respiratory distress syndrome (ARDS). There are four general causes of hypoxemia: hypoventilation, a low ventilation-perfusion ratio, diffusion abnormalities, and pulmonary shunting. Although the first three conditions improve in response to an increased inspired oxygen concentration most of the hypoxemia seen in ARDS is secondary to shunting and so is not ameliorated by oxygen. The abnormalities seen in ARDS are thought to result from injury to the alveolar-capillary membrane that causes an increased permeability of the membrane, which in turn leads to interstitial pulmonary edema and decreased pulmonary compliance. (See Schwartz 7th ed.)

7. A patient has a blood pressure of 70/50 mm Hg and a serum lactate level of 30 mg/100 mL (normal: 6 to 16). His cardiac output is 1.9 L/min, and his central venous pressure is 2 cm $H_2O$. The most likely diagnosis is
   A. Congestive heart failure
   B. Cardiac tamponade
   C. Hypovolemic shock
   D. Septic shock

**Answer: C**
The findings given in the question are characteristic of hypovolemic shock, which can be defined as inadequate tissue perfusion secondary to an extracellular fluid loss. The high lactate level is a result of anaerobic metabolism due to decreased blood flow to tissues. The hemodynamic measurements indicate both low blood flow and low venous return. The total combination is most consistent with a diagnosis of hypovolemic shock. Pulmonary embolus, congestive heart failure, and cardiac tamponade are all associated with a high central venous pressure. Septic shock, particularly in its early phases, is usually hyperdynamic, and affected patients have a greater-than-normal cardiac output. Complete hemodynamic monitoring is vital in hypovolemic shock so that prompt diagnosis and rational therapy can be expeditiously carried out. (See Schwartz 7th ed.)

8. A 76-year-old patient who has gram-negative pneumonia becomes hypotensive, and resuscitative measures are started. After 4 L of salt solution are administered, the following measurements are obtained:

    Blood pressure: 60/0 mm Hg
    Pulse: 140 beats per minute
    Central venous pressure: 26 cm $H_2O$
    Pulmonary artery diastolic pressure: 22 mm Hg
    Pulmonary capillary wedge pressure: 22 mm Hg
    Arterial blood gases: pH, 7.33; $P_{O_2}$, 100 mm Hg; $P_{CO_2}$, 35 mm Hg

    A decision is made to commence treatment with an adrenergic agent. An intravenous infusion of which of the following drugs should be started?
    A. Levarterenol
    B. Isoproterenol
    C. Dopamine
    D. Metaraminol

**Answer: C**
The heart is frequently unable to meet the increased circulatory demands of septic shock. Therefore, in a hypotensive patient who has gram-negative pneumonia, when measurements indicate the persistence of hypotension despite an adequate intravascular volume, an inotropic agent such as isoproterenol or dopamine is indicated. Dopamine is a naturally occurring catecholamine biochemical precursor of norepinephrine and is similar to isoproterenol in exerting positive inotropic and chronotropic effects on the heart. Its lower potential for creating tachyarrhythmias and its ability to enhance renal blood flow at low concentrations make dopamine the agent of choice for the patient in the question. (See Schwartz 7th ed.)

9. The $P_{50}$ value (the $P_{O_2}$ at which 50% of hemoglobin is saturated with oxygen) indicates the position of the oxyhemoglobin dissociation curve along the horizontal axis. All of the following conditions can produce a leftward-shifted curve (decreased $P_{50}$) EXCEPT
    A. Carbon monoxide poisoning
    B. Hypothermia
    C. Acidosis
    D. 2,3-diphosphoglycerate deficiency

**Answer: C**
Determinations of $P_{50}$ are used to monitor the affinity of oxygen for hemoglobin, with the normal value being approximately 26 mm Hg. A low $P_{50}$, indicating an increased affinity of oxygen for hemoglobin and a decreased release of oxygen to the tissues, causes a leftward shift in the oxyhemoglobin dissociation curve. Low red blood cell levels of 2,3-diphosphoglycerate (which occur when blood is stored more than 2 weeks), carbon monoxide poisoning, and hypothermia lower the $P_{50}$. Conversely, the natural affinity of hemoglobin for oxygen is decreased by high levels of diphosphoglycerate, by carbon dioxide (Bohr effect), by heat, and by hydrogen ions. In acidosis, shifting of the oxyhemoglobin dissociation curve to the right (increased $P_{50}$) reflects a protective mechanism to improve oxygen supply to the tissues. However, in spite of elevations of the $P_{50}$, severe arterial desaturation (e.g., pulmonary shunting) may offset any potential gains in oxygen availability. (See Schwartz 7th ed.)

10. A patient who is undergoing an elective operation under spinal anesthesia develops a blood pressure of 70/40 mm Hg. There is no evidence of hemorrhage or sepsis. Appropriate initial therapy should consist of administration of
    A. 2 L of saline
    B. Adrenal corticosteroids
    C. A beta-adrenergic stimulator
    D. An alphamimetic drug

**Answer: D**
The hypotension associated with spinal anesthesia is secondary to dilatation of the arterioles and venules resulting in a greatly increased reservoir capacity. Blood volume is known to be normal in this situation, but vascular pooling produces a decrease in venous return to the right side of the heart and a subsequently reduced cardiac output. The preferred initial therapy for an affected patient would be administration of a vasopressor such as ephedrine or phenylephrine (Neo-Synephrine). These agents increase peripheral vascular resistance, which is their most critical therapeutic feature, and restore the blood pressure to normal. Patients who have neurogenic shock that is secondary to central nervous system or spinal cord injury also may incur extracellular fluid losses and therefore require hemodynamic monitoring to establish whether fluid administration is necessary. (See Schwartz 7th ed.)

11. Each of the following indicates adequate pulmonary function in an adult EXCEPT
    A. Effective compliance 40 cm$^3$/cm $H_2O$
    B. Minute volume 11 L/min
    C. $Pa_{CO_2}$ 40 mm Hg
    D. $Pa_{O_2}$ 95 mm Hg
    E. $Pa_{O_2}/Fi_{O_2}$ <200

**Answer: A**
It is important to monitor pulmonary function for critically ill patients, and a number of relatively simple tests are available to monitor oxygenation, ventilation, and pulmonary mechanics. All the listed values are normal except the effective compliance, which should be greater than 50 cm$^3$/cm $H_2O$. The value listed in the item is indicative of "stiff lungs," which provide inefficient gas exchange. (See Schwartz 7th ed.)

12. The effects of the application and inflation of military antishock trousers (MAST) are similar to those after the intravenous administration of
    A. Dopamine
    B. Steroids
    C. Whole blood
    D. Norepinephrine
    E. Digoxin

**Answer: D**
The basic effect of the use of the MAST garment is to increase peripheral resistance, an effect that is achieved pharmacologically by the administration of norepinephrine. Unlike dopamine or digoxin, the device has no direct effect on the myocardium. The use of the MAST garment must not delay fluid therapy. (See Schwartz 7th ed.)

13. In patients with neurogenic shock who are unresponsive to dopamine, the most likely agent to be effective is
    A. Epinephrine
    B. Dobutamine
    C. Phenylephrine
    D. Amrinone

**Answer: C**
After the airway is secured and ventilation is adequate, fluid resuscitation and restoration of intravascular volume will often improve perfusion in neurogenic shock. Most patients with neurogenic shock will respond to restoration of intravascular volume alone, with satisfactory improvement in perfusion and resolution of hypotension. Administration of vasoconstrictors will improve peripheral vascular tone, decrease vascular capacitance, and increase venous return, but should only be considered once hypovolemia is excluded as the cause of the hypotension, and the diagnosis of neurogenic shock established. If the patient's blood pressure has not responded to what is felt to be adequate volume resuscitation, dopamine may be utilized first. A pure α-agonist, such as phenylephrine, may be used primarily or in patients unresponsive to dopamine. Specific treatment for the hypotension is often of brief duration, as the need to administer vasoconstrictors typically lasts 24 to 48 hours. On the other hand, life-threatening cardiac dysrhythmias and hypotension may occur up to 14 days after spinal cord injury. (See Schwartz 8th ed., p 100.)

14. Which of the following is true about anti-diuretic hormone (ADH) production in injured patients?
    A. ADH acts as a potent mesenteric vasoconstrictor.
    B. ADH levels fall to normal within 2–3 days of the initial insult.
    C. ADH decreases hepatic gluconeogenesis.
    D. ADH secretion is mediated by the renin-angiotensin system.

**Answer: A**
The pituitary also releases vasopressin or ADH in response to hypovolemia, changes in circulating blood volume sensed by baroreceptors and left atrial stretch receptors, and increased plasma osmolality detected by hypothalamic osmoreceptors. Epinephrine, angiotensin II, pain, and hyperglycemia increase production of ADH. ADH levels remain elevated for about 1 week after the initial insult, depending on the severity and persistence of the hemodynamic abnormalities. ADH acts on the distal tubule and collecting duct of the nephron to increase water permeability, decrease water and sodium losses, and preserve intravascular volume. Also known as arginine vasopressin, ADH acts as a potent mesenteric vasoconstrictor, shunting circulating blood away from the splanchnic organs during hypovolemia. This may

contribute to intestinal ischemia and predispose to intestinal mucosal barrier dysfunction in shock states. Vasopressin also increases hepatic gluconeogenesis and increases hepatic glycolysis. (See Schwartz 8th ed., p 88.)

15. Cardiogenic shock
    A. Results in a mortality rate of ~25%
    B. Occurs in ~30% of patients with acute myocardial infarctions
    C. Presents ~48 h after the myocardial infarction
    D. Can be caused by mitral stenosis

**Answer: D**

**Table 4-1.**
**Causes of Cardiogenic Shock**

| |
|---|
| *Acute myocardial infarction* |
|    Pump failure |
|    Mechanical complications |
|       Acute mitral regurgitation from papillary muscle rupture |
|       Ventricular septal defect |
|       Free-wall rupture |
|       Pericardial tamponade |
|       Right ventricular infarction |
| *Other causes of cardiogenic shock* |
|    End-stage cardiomyopathy |
|    Myocarditis |
|    Severe myocardial contusion |
|    Prolonged cardiopulmonary bypass |
|    Septic shock with severe myocardial depression |
|    Left ventricular outflow obstruction |
|       Aortic stenosis |
|       Hypertrophic obstructive cardiomyopathy |
|    Obstruction to left ventricular filling |
|       Mitral stenosis |
|       Left atrial myxoma |
|    Acute mitral regurgitation |
|    Acute aortic insufficiency |

See Schwartz 8th ed., p 97.
Source: Adapted with permission from Hollenberg SM, Kavinsky CJ, Parillo JE. Cardiogenic Shock. *Ann Int Med* 131:47, 1999.

16. Which of the following is a cause of vasodilatory shock?
    A. Aspirin poisoning
    B. Carbon monoxide poisoning
    C. Snake bite
    D. Severe muscle injury with rhabdomyolysis

**Answer: B**

In the peripheral circulation, profound vasoconstriction is the typical physiologic response to arterial pressure that is insufficient for tissue perfusion, usually causing cardiogenic or hemorrhagic shock. In vasodilatory shock, hypotension results from failure of the vascular smooth muscle to constrict appropriately. Vasodilatory shock is characterized by both peripheral vasodilatation with resultant hypotension, and resistance to treatment with vasopressors. Despite the hypotension, plasma catecholamine levels are elevated and the renin-angiotensin system is activated in vasodilatory shock. The most frequently encountered form of vasodilatory shock is septic shock. Other causes of vasodilatory shock include hypoxic lactic acidosis, carbon monoxide poisoning, decompensated and irreversible hemorrhagic shock, terminal cardiogenic shock, and postcardiotomy shock (Table 4-3). Thus, vasodilatory shock seems to represent the final common pathway for profound and prolonged shock of any etiology. (See Schwartz 8th ed., p 98.)

17. Which of the following is most likely to be efficacious in a patient with septic shock who is unresponsive to catecholamines?
    A. Amrinone
    B. Nitric oxide
    C. Arginine vasopressin
    D. Intra-aortic balloon pump

**Answer: C**

After first-line therapy of the septic patient with antibiotics, intravenous fluids, and intubation if necessary, vasopressors may be necessary to treat patients with septic shock. Catecholamines are the vasopressors used most often. Occasionally, patients with septic shock will develop arterial resistance to catecholamines. Arginine vasopressin, a potent vasoconstrictor, is often efficacious in this setting. (See Schwartz 8th ed., p 99.)

18. Tight glucose management in critically ill and septic patients
    A. Requires insulin to keep serum glucose <140
    B. Has no effect on mortality
    C. Has no effect on ventilator support
    D. Decreases length of antibiotic therapy

**Answer: D**

Hyperglycemia and insulin resistance are typical in critically-ill and septic patients, including patients without underlying diabetes mellitus. A recent study reported significant positive impact of tight glucose management on outcome in critically-ill patients. The two treatment groups in this randomized, prospective study were assigned to receive intensive insulin therapy (maintenance of blood glucose between 80 and 110 mg/dL) or conventional treatment (infusion of insulin only if the blood glucose level exceeded 215 mg/dL, with a goal between 180 and 200 mg/dL). The mean morning glucose level was significantly higher in the conventional treatment as compared to the intensive insulin therapy group (153 vs. 103 mg/dL). Mortality in the intensive insulin treatment group (4.6%) was significantly lower than in the conventional treatment group (8.0%), representing a 42% reduction in mortality. This reduction in mortality was most notable in the patients requiring longer than 5 days in the ICU. Furthermore, intensive insulin therapy reduced episodes of septicemia by 46%, reduced duration of antibiotic therapy, and decreased the need for prolonged ventilatory support and renal replacement therapy. (See Schwartz 8th ed., p 99.)

19. Which of the following (if present) is a distinguishing feature of neurogenic shock?
    A. Hypotension
    B. Bradycardia
    C. Vasodilation
    D. Vasoconstriction

**Answer: B**

Acute spinal cord injury may result in bradycardia, hypotension, cardiac dysrhythmias, reduced cardiac output, and decreased peripheral vascular resistance. The severity of the spinal cord injury seems to correlate with the magnitude of cardiovascular dysfunction. Patients with complete motor injuries are over five times more likely to require vasopressors for neurogenic shock, as compared to those with incomplete lesions. The classic description of neurogenic shock consists of decreased blood pressure associated with bradycardia (absence of reflexive tachycardia due to disrupted sympathetic discharge), warm extremities (loss of peripheral vasoconstriction), motor and sensory deficits indicative of a spinal cord injury, and radiographic evidence of a vertebral column fracture. Patients with multisystem trauma that includes spinal cord injuries often have head injuries that may make identification of motor and sensory deficits difficult in the initial evaluation. Furthermore, associated injuries may occur that result in hypovolemia, further complicating the clinical presentation. In a subset of patients with spinal cord injuries from penetrating wounds, most of the patients with hypotension had blood loss as the etiology (74%) rather than neurogenic causes, and few (7%) had the classic findings of neurogenic shock. In the multiply injured patient, other causes of hypotension including hemorrhage, tension pneumothorax, and cardiogenic shock must be sought and excluded. (See Schwartz 8th ed., p 100.)

20. Dobutamine
    A. Increases cardiac output and causes peripheral vasodilation
    B. Decreases cardiac output and causes peripheral vasodilation
    C. Increases cardiac output and causes peripheral vasoconstriction
    D. Decreases cardiac output and causes peripheral vasoconstriction

**Answer: A**

When profound cardiac dysfunction exists, inotropic support may be indicated to improve cardiac contractility and cardiac output. Dobutamine primarily stimulates cardiac $\beta_1$ receptors to increase cardiac output, but may also vasodilate peripheral vascular beds, lower total peripheral resistance, and lower systemic blood pressure through effects on $\beta_2$ receptors. Ensuring adequate preload and intravascular volume is therefore essential prior to instituting therapy with dobutamine. Dopamine stimulates $\alpha$ receptors (vasoconstriction), $\beta_1$ receptors (cardiac stimulation), and $\beta_2$ receptors (vasodilation), with its effects on $\beta$ receptors predominating at lower doses. Dopamine may be preferable to dobutamine in treatment of cardiac dysfunction in hypotensive patients. Tachycardia and increased peripheral resistance from dopamine infusion may worsen myocardial ischemia. Titration of both dopamine and dobutamine infusions may be required in some patients. (See Schwartz 8th ed., p 98.)

21. Which of the following is a proinflammatory mediator of shock?
    A. Interleukin-4
    B. Interleukin-6
    C. Interleukin-10
    D. Interleukin-13

**Answer: B**

**Table 4-2.**
**Inflammatory Mediators in Shock**

| Proinflammatory | Anti-Inflammatory |
|---|---|
| IL-1α/β | IL-4 |
| IL-2 | IL-10 |
| IL-6 | IL-13 |
| IL-8 | IL-1ra |
| IFN | PGE$_2$ |
| TNF | TGFβ |
| PAF | |
| TNFR I/TNFR II | |

IL-1α = interleukin 1α; IL-1β = interleukin 1β; IL-1ra = interleukin 1ra; IL-2 = interleukin 2; IL-4 = interleukin 4; IL-6 = interleukin 6; IL-8 = interleukin 8; IL-10 = interleukin 10; IL-13 = interleukin 13; IFN = interferon; PAF = platelet-activating factor; PGE$_2$ = prostaglandin E$_2$; TGF-β = transforming growth factor-β; TNF = tumor necrosis factor; TNFR I = tumor necrosis factor receptor I; TNFR II = tumor necrosis factor receptor II.
See Schwartz 8th ed., p 93.

# CHAPTER 5
## Surgical Infections

1. Transferrin plays a role in host defense by
   A. Sequestering iron, which is necessary for microbial growth
   B. Increasing the ability of fibrinogen to trap microbes
   C. Direct injury to the bacterial cell membrane
   D. Direct injury to the bacterial mitochondria

**Answer: A**
Once microbes enter a sterile body compartment (e.g., pleural or peritoneal cavity) or tissue, additional host defenses act to limit and/or eliminate these pathogens. Initially, several primitive and relatively nonspecific host defenses act to contain the nidus of infection, which may include microbes as well as debris, devitalized tissue, and foreign bodies, depending on the nature of the injury. These defenses include the physical barrier of the tissue itself, as well as the capacity of proteins such as lactoferrin and transferrin to sequester the critical microbial growth factor iron, thereby limiting microbial growth. In addition, fibrinogen within the inflammatory fluid has the ability to trap large numbers of microbes during the process in which it polymerizes into fibrin. Within the peritoneal cavity, unique host defenses exist, including a diaphragmatic pumping mechanism whereby particles including microbes within peritoneal fluid are expunged from the abdominal cavity via specialized structures on the undersurface of the diaphragm. Concurrently, containment by the omentum, the so-called "gatekeeper" of the abdomen and intestinal ileus, serves to wall off infection. However, the latter processes and fibrin trapping have a high likelihood of contributing to the formation of an intra-abdominal abscess. (See Schwartz 8th ed., p 111.)

2. The best method for hair removal from an operative field is
   A. Razor the night before
   B. Depilatory the night before surgery
   C. Razor in the operating room
   D. Hair clippers in the operating room

**Answer: D**
Hair removal should take place using a clipper rather than a razor; the latter promotes overgrowth of skin microbes in small nicks and cuts. Dedicated use of these modalities clearly has been shown to diminish the quantity of skin microflora. (See Schwartz 8th ed., p 114.)

3. Patients with a penicillin allergy are LEAST likely to have a cross-reaction with
   A. Synthetic penicillins
   B. Carbapenems
   C. Cephalosporins
   D. Monobactams

**Answer: D**
Allergy to antimicrobial agents must be considered prior to prescribing them. First, it is important to ascertain whether a patient has had any type of allergic reaction in association with administration of a particular antibiotic. However, one should take care to ensure that the purported reaction consists of true allergic symptoms and signs, such as urticaria, bronchospasm, or other similar manifestations, rather than indigestion or nausea. Penicillin allergy is quite common, the reported incidence ranging from 0.7 to 10%. Although avoiding the use of any beta-lactam drug is appropriate in patients who manifest significant allergic reactions to penicillins, the incidence of cross-

4. The most appropriate prophylactic antibiotic to use in a patient undergoing surgery for a small bowel obstruction is
   A. Cephazolin
   B. Ceftriaxone
   C. Ampicillin-sulbactam
   D. Aminoglycoside

reactivity appears highest for carbapenems, much lower for cephalosporins (~5 to 7%), and extremely small or nonexistent for monobactams. (See Schwartz 8th ed., p 118.)

**Answer: C**

**Table 5-1.**
**Prophylactic Use of Antibiotics**

| Site | Antibiotic | Alternative (e.g., penicillin allergic) |
|---|---|---|
| Cardiovascular surgery | Cefazolin | Vancomycin |
| Gastroduodenal area | Cefazolin, cefotetan, cefoxitin, ampicillin-sulbactam | Fluoroquinolone |
| Biliary tract with active infection (e.g., cholecystitis) | Cefotetan, cefoxitin | Fluoroquinolone plus clindamycin or metronidazole |
| Obstructed small bowel | Ampicillin-sulbactam | |
| Colorectal area | Ticarcillin-clavulanate, piperacillin-tazobactam, carbapenem | |
| Head and neck | Cefazolin | Aminoglycoside plus clindamycin |
| Neurosurgical procedures | Cefazolin | Vancomycin |
| Orthopedic surgery | Cefazolin | Vancomycin |
| Breast | Cefazolin | Vancomycin |

See Schwartz 8th ed., p 118.

5. Closure of an appendectomy wound in a patient with perforated appendicitis who is receiving appropriate antibiotics will result in a wound infection in what percentage of patients?
   A. 3–4%
   B. 8–12%
   C. 15–18%
   D. 22–25%

**Answer: A**
Surgical management of the wound is also a critical determinant of the propensity to develop a surgical site infection (SSI). In healthy individuals, class I and II wounds may be closed primarily, while skin closure of class III and IV wounds is associated with high rates of incisional SSIs (~25 to 50%). The superficial aspects of these latter types of wounds should be packed open and allowed to heal by secondary intention, although selective use of delayed primary closure has been associated with a reduction in incisional SSI rates. It remains to be determined whether [National Nosocomial Infections Surveillance System] NNIS-type stratification schemes can be employed prospectively in order to target specific subgroups of patients who will benefit from the use of prophylactic antibiotic and/or specific wound management techniques. One clear example based on cogent data from clinical trials is that class III wounds in healthy patients undergoing appendectomy for perforated or gangrenous appendicitis can be primarily closed as long as antibiotic therapy directed against aerobes and anaerobes is administered. This practice leads to SSI rates of approximately 3 to 4%. (See Schwartz 8th ed., p 120.)

6. A patient with a localized wound infection after surgery should be treated with
   A. Antibiotics and warm soaks to the wound
   B. Antibiotics alone
   C. Antibiotics and opening the wound
   D. Incision and drainage alone

**Answer: D**
Effective therapy for incisional [surgical site infections] SSIs consists solely of incision and drainage without the addition of antibiotics. Antibiotic therapy is reserved for patients in whom evidence of severe cellulitis is present, or who manifest concurrent sepsis syndrome. The open wound often is allowed to heal by secondary intention, with dressings being changed twice a day. The use of topical antibiotics and antiseptics to further wound healing remains unproven, although anecdotal studies indicate their potential utility in complex wounds that do not heal with routine measures. (See Schwartz 8th ed., p 120.)

7. The most appropriate treatment of a 4-cm hepatic abscess is
   A. Antibiotic therapy alone
   B. Aspiration for culture and antibiotic therapy
   C. Percutaneous drainage and antibiotic therapy
   D. Operative exploration, open drainage of the abscess, and antibiotic therapy

**Answer: C**
Hepatic abscesses are rare, currently accounting for approximately 15 per 100,000 hospital admissions in the United States. Pyogenic abscesses account for approximately 80% of cases, the remaining 20% being equally divided among parasitic and fungal forms. Formerly, pyogenic liver abscesses were caused by pylephlebitis due to neglected appendicitis or diverticulitis. Today, manipulation of the biliary tract to treat a variety of diseases has become a more common cause, although in nearly 50% of patients no cause is identified. The most common aerobic bacteria identified in recent series include *E. coli*, *K. pneumoniae*, and other enteric bacilli, enterococci, and *Pseudomonas* spp., while the most common anaerobic bacteria are *Bacteroides* spp., anaerobic streptococci, and *Fusobacterium* spp. *Candida albicans* and other similar yeasts cause the majority of fungal hepatic abscesses. Small (<1 cm), multiple abscesses should be sampled and treated with a 4- to 6-week course of antibiotics. Larger abscesses invariably are amenable to percutaneous drainage, with parameters for antibiotic therapy and drain removal similar to those mentioned above. Splenic abscesses are extremely rare and are treated in a similar fashion. Recurrent hepatic or splenic abscesses may require operative intervention—unroofing and marsupialization or splenectomy, respectively. (See Schwartz 8th ed., p 121.)

8. Patients with severe, necrotizing pancreatitis should be treated with
   A. No antibiotics unless computed tomography (CT)-guided aspiration of the area yields positive cultures
   B. Empiric cefoxitin or cefotetan
   C. Empiric cefuroxime plus gentamicin
   D. Empiric carbapenems or fluoroquinolones

**Answer: D**
Current care of patients with severe acute pancreatitis includes staging with dynamic, contrast-enhanced helical CT scan with 3-mm tomographs to determine the extent of pancreatic necrosis, coupled with the use of one of several prognostic scoring systems. Patients who exhibit significant pancreatic necrosis (grade >C, Fig. 5-2) should be carefully monitored in the ICU and undergo follow-up CT examination. The weight of current evidence also favors administration of empiric antibiotic therapy to reduce the incidence and severity of secondary pancreatic infection, which typically occurs several weeks after the initial episode of pancreatitis. Several randomized, prospective trials have demonstrated a decrease in the rate of infection and mortality using agents such as carbapenems or fluoroquinolones that achieve high pancreatic tissue levels. (See Schwartz 8th ed., p 121.)

9. A patient with necrotizing pancreatitis undergoes computed tomography (CT)-guided aspiration, which results in growth of *E. coli* on culture. The most appropriate treatment is
   A. Culture appropriate antibiotic therapy
   B. Endoscopic retrograde cholangiopancreatography with sphincterotomy
   C. CT-guided placement of drain(s)
   D. Exploratory laparotomy

**Answer: D**

The presence of secondary pancreatic infection should be suspected in patients whose systemic inflammatory response (fever, elevated [white blood cell] WBC count, or organ dysfunction) fails to resolve, or in those individuals who initially recuperate, only to develop sepsis syndrome 2 to 3 weeks later. CT-guided aspiration of fluid from the pancreatic bed for performance of Gram's stain and culture analysis is of critical importance. A positive Gram's stain or culture from CT-guided aspiration, or identification of gas within the pancreas on CT scan, mandate operative intervention. (See Schwartz 8th ed., p 121.)

10. The first step in the evaluation and treatment of a patient with an infected bug bite on the leg with cellulitis, bullae, thin grayish fluid draining from the wound, and pain out of proportion to the physical findings is
    A. Obtain C-reactive protein
    B. Computed tomographic scan of the leg
    C. Magnetic resonance imaging of the leg
    D. Operative exploration

**Answer: D**

The diagnosis of necrotizing infection is established solely upon a constellation of clinical findings, not all of which are present in every patient. Not surprisingly, patients often develop sepsis syndrome or septic shock without an obvious cause. The extremities, perineum, trunk, and torso are most commonly affected, in that order. Careful examination should be undertaken for an entry site such as a small break or sinus in the skin from which grayish, turbid semipurulent material ("dishwater pus") can be expressed, as well as for the presence of skin changes (bronze hue or brawny induration), blebs, or crepitus. The patient often develops pain at the site of infection that appears to be out of proportion to any of the physical manifestations. Any of these findings mandates immediate surgical intervention, which should consist of exposure and direct visualization of potentially infected tissue (including deep soft tissue, fascia, and underlying muscle) and radical resection of affected areas. Radiologic studies should be undertaken only in patients in whom the diagnosis is not seriously considered, as they delay surgical intervention and frequently provide confusing information. Unfortunately, surgical extirpation of infected tissue frequently entails amputation and/or disfiguring procedures; however, incomplete procedures are associated with higher rates of morbidity and mortality. (See Schwartz 8th ed., p 122.)

11. Which of the following treatments has been shown to be of benefit (reduced mortality) in patients with septic shock?
    A. Antiendotoxin monoclonal antibodies
    B. Drotrecogin alpha (recombinant human-activated protein C)
    C. Anti–tumor necrosis factor (TNF)-α antibodies
    D. High-dose hydrocortisone

**Answer: B**

Over the past several decades, a series of clinical trials have examined the effect of a number of different agents [e.g., antiendotoxin monoclonal antibodies (MABs), interleukin (IL)-1ra, and anti-TNF-α MABs] upon outcome during severe sepsis. Until recently, no agent has shown efficacy. Drotrecogin alpha (activated), also known as Xigris, is a recombinant form of human-activated protein C. The use of this agent in a series of patients with sepsis syndrome has been associated with a 6% overall reduction in mortality (31 to 25%, p = 0.005). This agent has been demonstrated to have antithrombotic, profibrinolytic, and anti-inflammatory properties, although the specific mechanism of action remains to be established. Further analysis of the surgical cohort of patients in this study has demonstrated the benefit of this agent without incurring an increased risk of hemorrhage. The use of this agent should be considered in patients with severe infection who have completed their source control procedure, and who develop severe sepsis with at least one organ failing. Current recommendations are a dose of 24 µg/kg per h given for 96 hours. The infusion should be interrupted for procedures or surgery, or for significant life-threatening bleeding. (See Schwartz 8th ed., p 124.)

12. The most effective post-exposure prophylaxis for a surgeon stuck with a needle while operating on a human immunodeficiency virus (HIV)–positive patient is
    A. None (no effective treatment is known)
    B. Two- or three-drug therapy started within hours of exposure
    C. Single drug therapy started within 24 h of exposure
    D. Triple drug therapy started within 24 h of exposure

**Answer: B**
Postexposure prophylaxis for HIV has significantly decreased the risk of seroconversion for health care workers with occupational exposure to HIV. Steps to initiate postexposure prophylaxis should be initiated within h rather than days for the most effective preventive therapy. Postexposure prophylaxis with a two- or three-drug regimen should be initiated for health care workers with significant exposure to patients with an HIV-positive status. If a patient's HIV status is unknown, it may be advisable to begin postexposure prophylaxis while testing is carried out, particularly if the patient is at high risk for infection due to HIV (e.g., intravenous narcotic use). Generally, postexposure prophylaxis is not warranted for exposure to sources with unknown status, such as deceased persons or needles from a sharps container. (See Schwartz 8th ed., p 124.)

13. The classic chest X-ray finding in anthrax is
    A. Bilateral apical pneumothorax
    B. Basilar pneumonia
    C. Widened mediastinum and effusions
    D. Pulmonary edema

**Answer: C**
Anthrax is a zoonotic disease occurring in domesticated and wild herbivores. The first identification of inhalational anthrax as a disease occurred among woolsorters in England in the late 1800s. The largest recent epidemic of inhalational anthrax occurred in Sverdlovsk, Russia, in 1979 after accidental release of anthrax spores from a military facility. Inhalational anthrax develops after a 1- to 6-day incubation period, with nonspecific symptoms including malaise, myalgia, and fever. Over a short period of time, these symptoms worsen, with development of respiratory distress, chest pain, and diaphoresis. Characteristic chest roentgenographic findings include a widened mediastinum and pleural effusions. A key aspect in establishing the diagnosis is eliciting an exposure history. Rapid antigen tests are currently under development for identification of this gram-positive rod. (See Schwartz 8th ed., p 125.)

14. The rate of seroconversion after an accidental needle stick while operating on a patient with hepatitis C is
    A. <10%
    B. 10–20%
    C. 20–30%
    D. >30%

**Answer: A**
Hepatitis C virus (HCV), previously known as non-A, non-B hepatitis, is an RNA flavivirus first identified specifically in the late 1980s. This virus is confined to humans and chimpanzees. A chronic carrier state develops in 75 to 80% of patients with the infection, with chronic liver disease occurring in three-fourths of patients developing chronic infection. The number of new infections per year has declined since the 1980s due to the incorporation of testing of the blood supply for this virus. Fortunately, HCV virus is not transmitted efficiently through occupational exposures to blood, with the seroconversion rate after accidental needlestick reported to be approximately 2%. (See Schwartz 8th ed., p 124.)

15. Which of the following are *anti*-inflammatory cytokines?
    A. Interleukins 2 and 6
    B. Interleukin 8 and interferon-γ
    C. Interleukins 4 and 10
    D. Interleukin 1β and tumor necrosis factor-α

**Answer: C**

Microbes also immediately encounter a series of host defense mechanisms that reside within the vast majority of tissues of the body. These include resident macrophages and low levels of complement (C) proteins and immunoglobulins (Ig, antibodies). Resident macrophages secrete a wide array of substances in response to the above-mentioned processes, some of which appear to regulate the cellular components of the host defense response. Macrophage cytokine synthesis is upregulated. Secretion of tumor necrosis factor-α (TNF-α), of interleukins (IL)-1β, 6, and 8; and of interferon-γ (INF-γ) occurs within the tissue milieu, and, depending on the magnitude of the host defense response, the systemic circulation. Concurrently, a counterregulatory response is initiated consisting of binding proteins (TNF-BP), cytokine receptor antagonists (IL-1ra), and anti-inflammatory cytokines (IL-4 and IL-10). (See Schwartz 8th ed., p 111.)

16. The best antibiotic for post-exposure prophylaxis to *Bacillus anthracis* (anthrax) is
    A. Rifampin
    B. Clindamycin
    C. Doxycycline
    D. Amoxicillin

**Answer: B**

Anthrax is a zoonotic disease occurring in domesticated and wild herbivores. The first identification of inhalational anthrax as a disease occurred among woolsorters in England in the late 1800s. The largest recent epidemic of inhalational anthrax occurred in Sverdlovsk, Russia, in 1979 after accidental release of anthrax spores from a military facility. Inhalational anthrax develops after a 1- to 6-day incubation period, with nonspecific symptoms including malaise, myalgia, and fever. If an isolate is demonstrated to be penicillin-sensitive, the patient should be switched to amoxicillin. Inhalational exposure followed by the development of symptoms is associated with a high mortality rate. Treatment options include combination therapy with ciprofloxacin, clindamycin, and rifampin, with clindamycin added to block production of toxin, and rifampin for its ability to penetrate the central nervous system and intracellular locations. (See Schwartz 8th ed., p 125.)

17. Infections that require operative treatment include all of the following EXCEPT
    A. Empyema
    B. Infected ascites
    C. Necrotizing fasciitis of the thigh
    D. Vascular graft infection

**Answer: B**

An abscess in any closed space, such as joint space or a lactating breast, requires open drainage. Empyema treatment involves tube thoracostomy or open drainage if this is not effective. Management of necrotizing fasciitis includes radical débridement of infected tissues. An infected vascular graft usually requires removal of the graft or débridement and dressing care if the suture lines are not involved in the infection. Ascites is a diffuse process and is not amenable to surgical drainage. Appropriate antibiotic therapy provides optimal management. However, a localized abscess within the peritoneal cavity should be managed by percutaneous or operative drainage. (See Schwartz 7th ed.)

18. The intense pain associated with a felon occurs because of
    A. Bone involvement
    B. A closed space infection
    C. Digital artery thrombosis
    D. Nail bed involvement

**Answer: B**

A felon is an infection of the distal pulp space of a digit, usually secondary to a puncture wound. This is a closed space at the level of the distal interphalangeal joint. Because the infection cannot spread proximal to this point, pain is throbbing and intense. Late osteomyelitis may develop in the distal phalanx if the felon is not opened appropriately. (See Schwartz 7th ed.)

19. Which of the following is the most commonly acquired infection in hospitalized surgical patients?
    A. Lower gastrointestinal tract
    B. Lower respiratory tract
    C. Nasopharynx
    D. Surgical wound

**Answer: D**

Infection may occur at any site when a patient's immunity is low due to an operation. The surgical wound is the most frequent site of infection for surgical patients, according to a report from the Centers for Disease Control and Prevention. Urinary tract infection represents the second most frequent type of infection. (See Schwartz 7th ed.)

20. Which of the following is the most effective way to prevent post-operative seroma/infection in an obese patient after an open appendectomy?
    A. Leaving the subcutaneous tissue and skin open to heal by secondary intention
    B. Closing the wound over a rubber drain
    C. Closing the wound with a closed suction drain
    D. Closing the wound with multiple sutures in the subcutaneous tissue

**Answer: C**

With a clean-contaminated wound after an appendectomy, it should not be necessary to leave the wound open. In an obese patient, seroma in the wound is a possibility, and primary wound closure might not be appropriate. Rubber drains act as a route for bacteria to enter the wound, and multiple subcutaneous cultures provide foreign bodies as a nidus for possible infection. The best option is to close the wound carefully over a closed-suction drain. Whatever method is used, all devitalized tissue should be removed and careful hemostasis accomplished before the procedure is completed. (See Schwartz 7th ed.)

21. *Staphylococcus aureus* produces each of the following EXCEPT
    A. Cell wall peptidoglycan
    B. Enterotoxin
    C. Epidermolytic toxin
    D. Neuroexotoxin

**Answer: D**

Neuroexotoxin is produced by *Clostridium tetani* and is responsible for the symptoms of tetanus. Staphylococcal cell wall peptidoglycan inhibits edema production and migration of leukocytes in tissue. The coagulase produced by many staphylococcal strains increases the virulence of the organism, but the mechanism involved is food poisoning; and the epidermolytic toxin is present in syndromes involving bulla formation, such as the scalded skin syndrome in children. (See Schwartz 7th ed.)

22. An exotoxin plays an important part in the pathogenicity of infection with each of the following EXCEPT
    A. *Clostridium botulinum*
    B. *Clostridium tetani*
    C. *Escherichia coli*
    D. *Staphylococcus aureus*

**Answer: C**

*Escherichia coli* and other gram-negative bacteria produce endotoxins that are lipopolysaccharide-protein complexes of the cell wall. *Clostridium botulinum* and *Clostridium tetani* elaborate neurotoxins responsible for the clinical syndromes the organisms produce. Some staphylococcal and streptococcal bacteria produce exotoxins important in diseases such as the scalded skin syndrome and toxic shock syndrome. (See Schwartz 7th ed.)

23. A 30-year-old, otherwise healthy woman undergoes an open appendectomy with primary closure of the wound for a perforated appendix. No antibiotics are administered. Should this patient develop an intraabdominal abscess, which of the following organisms would most likely be responsible?
    A. *Escherichia coli*
    B. *Bacteroides*
    C. *Streptococcus faecalis*
    D. *Serratia*

**Answer: B**

A number of organisms can cause abscesses after appendectomy, but *Bacteroides*, either alone or in combination with other organisms, is most commonly responsible. Anaerobes are associated with 90% of cases of intraabdominal abscess and 95% of cases of appendiceal abscess. (See Schwartz 7th ed.)

24. The earliest manifestations of serious gram-negative infection may consist of a triad of signs that includes
    A. Tachypnea, hypotension, and an altered sensorium
    B. Tachypnea, hypotension, and lactic acidosis
    C. Thrombocytopenia, hypotension, and lactic acidosis
    D. Mild hyperventilation, respiratory alkalosis, and an altered sensorium

**Answer: D**

The development of mild hyperventilation, respiratory alkalosis, and an altered sensorium may be the earliest sign of gram-negative infection. This triad may precede the usual signs and symptoms of sepsis by several hours to several days. Although the exact pathophysiology of this manifestation is unknown, the triad of signs is thought to represent a primary response to bacteremia. Early recognition of the findings, followed by a prompt search for the source of infection, may allow diagnosis and treatment prior to the onset of shock. (See Schwartz 7th ed.)

25. The drug of choice for clostridial myonecrosis is
    A. Penicillin G
    B. Ampicillin
    C. Amikacin
    D. Cephalosporin

**Answer: A**

*Clostridium perfringens* is the most important of the pathogenic clostridial organisms. Five types, A through E, can be differentiated on the basis of production of toxins. All five types produce alpha toxin, a lethal, necrotizing hemolytic exotoxin, which is also a lecithinase, but type A produces the greatest amount. In addition, some strains produce variable amounts of hemolysin, collagenase, and hyaluronidase. Clostridia may cause cellulitis, which presents as a gassy, crepitant infection, or a much more serious infection called clostridial myonecrosis (or gas gangrene), which may be crepitant or noncrepitant. Early treatment of the latter condition is the most effective means of managing it as even a 24-h delay in treatment may be fatal. Antibiotic therapy with penicillin G or tetracycline is effective as an adjunct to multiple longitudinal incisions for decompression and drainage and aggressive débridement. Antitoxin is of no value therapeutically. (See Schwartz 7th ed.)

26. An infection with *Staphylococcus aureus* acquired in an intensive care unit should be treated initially with
    A. Aztreonam
    B. Erythromycin
    C. Methicillin
    D. Vancomycin

**Answer: D**

Most nosocomial staphylococcal infections are resistant to erythromycin, methicillin, and penicillin G. Aztreonam is useful against gram-negative, not gram-positive, organisms. Once organisms' sensitivities are known, therapy may be changed. In the unlikely event that the staphylococcus is sensitive to penicillin G or methicillin, these agents are substantially less costly than vancomycin and should be substituted. (See Schwartz 7th ed.)

27. Cefuroxime is a
    A. 1st generation cephalosporin
    B. 2nd generation cephalosporin
    C. 3rd generation cephalosporin
    D. 4th generation cephalosporin

**Answer: B**

See Table 5-2 on p 41.

**Table 5-2.**
**Antimicrobial Agents**

| Antibiotic Class, Generic Name | Trade Name | Mechanism of Action | Organism | | | | | | | | |
|---|---|---|---|---|---|---|---|---|---|---|---|
| | | | S. pyogenes | MSSA | MRSA | S. epidermidis | Enterococcus | VRE | E. coli | P. aeruginosa | Anaerobes |
| Penicillins | | Cell wall synthesis inhibitors (bind penicillin-binding protein) | | | | | | | | | |
| Penicillin G | | | 1 | 0 | 0 | 0 | +/- | 0 | 0 | 0 | 1 |
| Nafcillin | Nallpen, Unipen | | 1 | 1 | 0 | +/- | 0 | 0 | 0 | 0 | 0 |
| Piperacillin | Pipracil | | 1 | 0 | 0 | 0 | +/- | 0 | 1 | 1 | +/- |
| Penicillin/beta lactamase inhibitor combinations | | Cell wall synthesis inhibitors/beta lactamase inhibitors | | | | | | | | | |
| Ampicillin-sulbactam | Unasyn | | 1 | 1 | 0 | +/- | 1 | +/- | 1 | 0 | 1 |
| Ticarcillin-clavulanate | Timentin | | 1 | 1 | 0 | +/- | +/- | 0 | 1 | 1 | 1 |
| Piperacillin-tazobactam | Zosyn | | 1 | 1 | 0 | 1 | +/- | 0 | 1 | 1 | 1 |
| First-generation cephalosporins | | Cell wall synthesis inhibitors (bind penicillin-binding protein) | | | | | | | | | |
| Cephazolin, cephalexin | Ancef, Keflex | | 1 | 1 | 0 | +/- | 0 | 0 | 1 | 0 | 0 |
| Second-generation cephalosporins | | Cell wall synthesis inhibitors (bind penicillin-binding protein) | | | | | | | | | |
| Cefoxitin | Mefoxin | | 1 | 1 | 0 | +/- | 0 | 0 | 1 | 0 | 1 |
| Cefotetan | Cefotan | | 1 | 1 | 0 | +/- | 0 | 0 | 1 | 0 | 1 |
| Cefuroxime | Ceftin | | 1 | 1 | 0 | +/- | 0 | 0 | 1 | 0 | 0 |
| Third- and fourth-generation cephalosporins | | Cell wall synthesis inhibitors (bind penicillin-binding protein) | | | | | | | | | |
| Ceftriaxone | Rocephin | | 1 | 1 | 0 | +/- | 0 | 0 | 1 | 0 | 0 |
| Ceftazidime | Fortaz | | 1 | +/- | 0 | +/- | 0 | 0 | 1 | 1 | 0 |
| Cefepime | Maxipime | | 1 | 1 | 0 | +/- | 0 | 0 | 1 | 1 | 0 |
| Cefotaxime | Cefotaxime | | 0 | 1 | 0 | +/- | 0 | 0 | 1 | +/- | 0 |
| Carbapenems | | Cell wall synthesis inhibitors (bind penicillin-binding protein) | | | | | | | | | |
| Imipenem-cilastatin | Primaxin | | 1 | 1 | 0 | 1 | +/- | 0 | 1 | 1 | 1 |
| Meropenem | Merrem | | 1 | 1 | 0 | 1 | 0 | 0 | 1 | 1 | 1 |
| Ertapenem | Invanz | | 1 | 1 | 0 | 1 | 0 | 0 | 1 | +/- | 1 |
| Aztreonam | Azactam | Cell wall synthesis inhibitor (bind penicillin-binding protein) | 0 | 0 | 0 | 0 | 0 | 0 | 1 | 1 | 0 |
| Aminoglycosides | | Alteration of cell membrane, binding and inhibition of 30S ribosomal unit | | | | | | | | | |
| Gentamicin | | | 0 | 1 | 0 | +/- | 1 | 0 | 1 | 1 | 0 |
| Tobramycin, amikacin | | | 0 | 1 | 0 | +/- | 0 | 0 | 1 | 1 | 0 |
| Fluoroquinolones | | Inhibit topoisomerase II and IV (DNA synthesis inhibition) | | | | | | | | | |
| Ciprofloxacin | Cipro | | +/- | 1 | 0 | 1 | 0 | 0 | 1 | 1 | 0 |
| Gatifloxacin | Tequin | | 1 | 1 | +/- | 1 | +/- | 0 | 1 | +/- | +/- |
| Levofloxacin | Levaquin | | 1 | 1 | 0 | 1 | 0 | 0 | 1 | +/- | 0 |
| Glycopeptides | | Cell wall synthesis inhibition (peptidoglycan synthesis inhibition) | | | | | | | | | |
| Vancomycin | Vancocin | | 1 | 1 | 1 | 1 | 1 | 0 | 0 | 0 | 0 |

*(continued)*

**Table 5-2.**
**Antimicrobial Agents (Continued)**

| Antibiotic Class, Generic Name | Trade Name | Mechanism of Action | Organism | | | | | | | | |
|---|---|---|---|---|---|---|---|---|---|---|---|
| | | | S. pyogenes | MSSA | MRSA | S. epidermidis | Entero-coccus | VRE | E. coli | P. aeruginosa | Anaerobes |
| Quinupristin-Dalfopristin | Synercid | Inhibits 2 sites on 50S ribosome (protein synthesis inhibition) | 1 | 1 | 1 | 1 | 1 | 1 | 0 | 0 | +/- |
| Linezolid | Zyvox | Inhibits 50S ribosomal activity (protein synthesis inhibition) | 1 | 1 | 1 | 1 | 1 | 1 | 0 | 0 | +/- |
| Daptomycin | Cubicin | Binds bacterial membrane, results in depolarization, lysis | 1 | 1 | 1 | 1 | 1 | 1 | 0 | 0 | 0 |
| Rifampin | | Inhibits DNA-dependent RNA polymerase | 1 | 1 | 1 | 1 | +/- | 0 | 0 | 0 | 0 |
| Clindamycin | Cleocin | Inhibits 50S ribosomal activity (protein synthesis inhibition) | 1 | 1 | 0 | 0 | 0 | 0 | 0 | 0 | 1 |
| Metronidazole | Flagyl | Production of toxic intermediates (free radical production) | 0 | 0 | 0 | 0 | 0 | 0 | 0 | 0 | 1 |
| Macrolides | | | | | | | | | | | |
| Erythromycin | | Inhibit 50S ribosomal activity (protein synthesis inhibition) | 1 | +/- | 0 | +/- | 0 | 0 | 0 | 0 | 0 |
| Azithromycin | Zithromax | | 1 | 1 | 0 | 0 | 0 | 0 | 0 | 0 | 0 |
| Clarithromycin | Biaxin | | 1 | 1 | 0 | 0 | 0 | 0 | 0 | 0 | 0 |
| Trimethoprim-sulfamethoxazole | Bactrim, Septra | Inhibits sequential steps of folate metabolism | +/- | 1 | 0 | +/- | 0 | 0 | 1 | 0 | 0 |
| Tetracyclines | | | | | | | | | | | |
| Minocycline | Minocin | Bind 30S ribosomal unit (protein synthesis inhibition) | 1 | 1 | 0 | 0 | 0 | 0 | 0 | 0 | +/- |
| Doxycycline | Vibramycin | | 1 | +/- | 0 | 0 | 0 | 0 | 1 | 0 | +/- |

*E. coli* = *Escherichia coli*; MRSA = methicillin-resistant *Staphylococcus aureus*; MSSA = methicillin-sensitive *Staphylococcus aureus*; *P. aeruginosa* = *Pseudomonas aeruginosa*; *S. epidermidis* = *Staphylococcus epidermidis*; *S. pyogenes* = *Streptococcus pyogenes*; VRE = vancomycin-resistant enterococcus.

1 = Reliable activity; +/– = variable activity; 0 = no activity.

The sensitivities presented are generalizations. The clinician should confirm sensitivity patterns at the locale where the patient is being treated since these patterns may vary widely depending on location. See Schwartz 8th ed., pp 116–117.

# CHAPTER 6

# Trauma

1. Which of the following would lead you to an arteriogram and/or exploration of a possible femoral artery injury from a gunshot wound?
   A. Proximity of the probable bullet path to the neurovascular bundle
   B. A small hematoma at the entrance site
   C. Systolic blood pressure 5% different in the two legs
   D. A bruit over the injury

**Answer: A**

Physical diagnosis will serve to identify and localize arterial injuries in many instances. Physical findings are classified as either hard signs or soft signs (Table 6-4). In general, hard signs constitute indications for operative exploration, whereas soft signs are indications for observation or further testing. Arteriography may be helpful to localize the injury in some patients with penetrating injuries and hard signs. For example, a bullet which enters the lateral hip and exits below the knee medially and is associated with a femoral shaft fracture and absent popliteal pulse could have injured either the femoral or popliteal artery almost anywhere. Arteriography would be useful to localize the injury and limit the dissection.

In vascular trauma, controversy exists regarding the management of patients with soft signs of injury, particularly in those with injuries in proximity to major vessels. It is known that some of these patients will have arterial injuries that require repair. One approach has been to measure systolic blood pressure (SBP) using Doppler ultrasound (US) and compare the injured side with the uninjured side. If the pressures are within 10% of each other, a significant injury is excluded and no further evaluation is performed. If the difference is greater than 10%, an arteriogram is indicated. Others argue that there are occult injuries, such as pseudoaneurysms or injuries of the profunda femoris or peroneal arteries, which may not be detected with this technique. If hemorrhage occurs from these injuries, compartment syndrome and limb loss may occur. While busy trauma centers continue to debate this issue, the surgeon who is obliged to treat the occasional injured patient may be better served by performing angiography in selected patients with soft signs. (See Schwartz 8th ed., p 144.)

2. Cricothyroidotomy
   A. Should not be performed in children younger than 12 years of age
   B. Should only be performed in patients who are not good candidates for a tracheostomy
   C. Requires the use of an endotracheal tube smaller than 4 mm in diameter
   D. Is preferable to the use of percutaneous transtracheal ventilation

**Answer: A**

Patients in whom attempts at intubation have failed or are precluded from intubation due to extensive facial injuries require a surgical airway. Cricothyroidotomy (Fig. 6-1) and percutaneous transtracheal ventilation are preferred over tracheostomy in most emergency situations because of their simplicity and safety. One disadvantage of cricothyroidotomy is the inability to place a tube greater than 6 mm in diameter due to the limited aperture of the cricothyroid space. Cricothyroidotomy is also relatively contraindicated in patients under the age of 12 because of the risk of damage to the cricoid cartilage and the subsequent risk of subglottic stenosis. (See Schwartz 8th ed., p 130.)

3. A patient with a palpable carotid pulse but no femoral pulses has an approximate systolic blood pressure of
   A. 60 mm Hg
   B. 70 mm Hg
   C. 80 mm Hg
   D. 90 mm Hg

**Answer: B**
With a secure airway and adequate ventilation established, circulatory status is addressed next. A rough first approximation of the patient's cardiovascular status is obtained by palpating peripheral pulses. In general, a systolic blood pressure (SBP) of 60 mm Hg is required for the carotid pulse to be palpable, 70 mm Hg for the femoral pulse, and 80 mm Hg for the radial pulse. At this point in the patient's treatment, hypotension is assumed to be caused by hemorrhage. Blood pressure and pulse should be measured at least every 15 min. (See Schwartz 8th ed., p 131.)

4. Which of the following is a cause of cardiogenic shock in a trauma patient?
   A. Hemothorax
   B. Penetrating injury to the aorta
   C. Air embolism
   D. Iatrogenic increased afterload due to pressors

**Answer: C**
In trauma patients the differential diagnosis of cardiogenic shock is a short list:

   (1) tension pneumothorax,
   (2) pericardial tamponade,
   (3) myocardial contusion or infarction, and
   (4) air embolism.

Tension pneumothorax is the most frequent cause of cardiac failure. Traumatic pericardial tamponade is most often associated with penetrating injury to the heart. As blood leaks out of the injured heart, it accumulates in the pericardial sac. Because the pericardium is not acutely distensible, the pressure in the pericardial sac will rise to match that of the injured chamber. Since this pressure is usually greater than that of the right atrium, right atrial filling is impaired and right ventricular preload is reduced. This leads to decreased right ventricular output and increased central venous pressure (CVP). Increased intrapericardial pressure also impedes myocardial blood flow, which leads to subendocardial ischemia and a further reduction in cardiac output. This vicious cycle may progress insidiously with injury of the vena cava or atria, or precipitously with injury of either ventricle. With acute tamponade, as little as 100 mL of blood within the pericardial sac can produce life-threatening hemodynamic compromise. Patients usually present with a penetrating injury in proximity to the heart, and they are hypotensive and have distended neck veins or an elevated CVP. The classic findings of Beck's triad (hypotension, distended neck, and muffled heart sounds) and pulsus paradoxus are not reliable indicators of acute tamponade. Ultrasonography (US) in the ED using a subxiphoid or parasternal view is extremely helpful if the findings are clearly positive (Fig. 6-5); however, equivocal findings are common. Early in the course of tamponade, blood pressure and cardiac output will transiently improve with fluid administration. This may lead the surgeon to question the diagnosis or be lulled into a false sense of security. (See Schwartz 8th ed., p 133.)

5. What percentage of blood volume must be lost in healthy patients before hypotension occurs?
   A. 10–20%
   B. 20–30%
   C. 30–40%
   D. 40–50%

**Answer: C**
There are several caveats that must be considered when making this presumption. Although tachycardia may be the earliest sign of ongoing blood loss, individuals in good physical condition, particularly trained athletes with a low resting pulse rate, may manifest only a relative tachycardia. Patients on

beta-blocking medications may not be able to increase their heart rate in response to stress. In children, bradycardia or relative bradycardia can occur with severe blood loss, and is an ominous sign often heralding cardiovascular collapse. On the other hand, hypoxia, pain, apprehension, and stimulant drugs (cocaine, amphetamines) will produce a tachycardia unrelated to physiologic demands. Hypotension is not a reliable early sign of hypovolemia. In healthy patients blood volume must decrease by 30 to 40% before hypotension occurs (Table 6-1). Younger patients with good sympathetic tone can maintain systemic blood pressure with severe intravascular deficits until they are on the verge of cardiac arrest. In contrast, pregnancy increases circulating blood volume and a relatively larger volume of blood loss must occur before signs and symptoms become apparent. (See Schwartz 8th ed., p 132.)

6. A patient with spontaneous eye opening, who is confused and localizes pain has a Glasgow Coma Score of
   A. 9
   B. 11
   C. 13
   D. 15

**Answer: C**
The Glasgow Coma Score (GCS) should be determined for all injured patients (Table 6-2). It is calculated by adding the scores of the best motor response, best verbal response, and eye opening. Scores range from 3 (the lowest) to 15 (normal). Scores of 13 to 15 indicate mild head injury, 9 to 12 moderate injury, and less than 9 severe injury. The GCS is useful for both triage and prognosis. (See Schwartz 8th ed., p 137.)

7. Appropriate treatment for a bite from a wild animal that was not captured includes giving either human diploid cell rabies vaccine or rabies vaccine adsorbed
   A. By intramuscular injection in the gluteal muscle immediately and again at 3, 7, 14, and 28 days
   B. By intramuscular injection in the deltoid muscle immediately and again at 3, 7, 14, and 28 days
   C. By subcutaneous injection daily for 21 days
   D. By subcutaneous injection every 5 days for 8 doses

**Answer: B**
Postexposure prophylaxis in addition to local wound treatment consists of both human rabies immune globulin (HRIG) (Imogam Rabies) and vaccine. There are two rabies vaccines currently available in the United States: human diploid cell rabies vaccine (HDCV) and rabies vaccine adsorbed (RVA) (Imovax). Either is administered in conjunction with HRIG at the beginning of postexposure therapy. A regimen of five 1-mL doses of HDCV or RVA is given intramuscularly. The first dose of the five-dose course is given as soon as possible after exposure. Additional doses are given on days 3, 7, 14, and 28 after the first vaccination. For adults, the vaccine is always administered intramuscularly in the deltoid area. For children, the anterolateral aspect of the thigh is also acceptable. The gluteal area should never be used for HDCV or RVA injections since administration in this area results in lower neutralizing antibody titers. (See Schwartz 8th ed., p 180.)

8. Fusion of a cervical spine injury is performed in patients with
   A. An unstable fracture at any level
   B. C-1 or C-2 fractures
   C. Neurologic deficits
   D. Distraction of greater than 5° on flexion/extension films

**Answer: C**
Blunt trauma may involve the cervical spine, spinal cord, larynx, carotid and vertebral arteries, and the jugular veins. Treatment of injuries to the cervical spine is based on the level of injury, the stability of the spine, the presence of subluxation, the extent of angulation, and the extent of neurologic deficit. In general, cautious axial traction in line with the mastoid process is used to reduce subluxations. A halo-vest combination can accomplish this and also provide rigid external fixation for definitive treatment when left in place for 3 to 6 months. Today this device is the treatment of choice for many cervical spine injuries. Surgical fusion is usually reserved for those with neurologic deficit, those who

9. Which of the following statements about blunt carotid injuries is true?
    A. Magnetic resonance imaging is the diagnostic modality of choice in patients at risk.
    B. Approximately 50% of patients have a delayed diagnosis.
    C. The mechanism of injury is usually cervical flexion and rotation.
    D. Such injuries are always treated operatively when identified.

10. A patient with penetrating injury to the chest should undergo thoracotomy if
    A. There is more than 1000 mL of blood which drains from the chest tube when placed
    B. There is more than 200 mL/hour of blood for 3 h from the chest tube
    C. There is an air leak that persists >48 h
    D. There is documented lung injury on computed tomography scan

11. Appropriate surgical management of a through-and-through gunshot wound to the lung with minimal bleeding and some air leak is
    A. Chest tube only
    B. Oversewing entrance and exit wounds to decrease the air leak
    C. Pulmonary tractotomy with a stapler and oversewing of vessels or bronchi
    D. Wedge resection of the injured lung

demonstrate angulation greater than 11° on flexion and extension X-rays, or those who remain unstable after external fixation. (See Schwartz 8th ed., p 154.)

**Answer: B**

Blunt injury to the carotid or vertebral arteries may cause dissection, thrombosis, or pseudoaneurysm. More than one half of patients have a delayed diagnosis. Facial contact resulting in hypertension and rotation appears to be the mechanism. To reduce delayed recognition, the authors employ computed tomography (CT) angiography in patients at risk, to identify these injuries before neurologic symptoms develop. The injuries frequently occur at or extend into the base of the skull and are usually not surgically accessible. Currently accepted treatment for thrombosis and dissection is anticoagulation with heparin followed by warfarin for 3 months. Pseudoaneurysms also occur near the base of the skull. If they are small, they can be followed with repeat angiography. If enlargement occurs, consideration should be given to the placement by an interventional radiologist of a stent across the aneurysm. Another possibility is to approach the intracranial portion of the carotid by removing the overlying bone and performing a direct repair. This method has only recently been described and has been performed in a limited number of patients. (See Schwartz 8th ed., p 154.)

**Answer: B**

**Table 6-1.**
**Indications for Operative Treatment of Penetrating Thoracic Injuries**

| |
| --- |
| Caked hemothorax |
| Large air leak with inadequate ventilation or persistent collapse of the lung |
| Drainage of more than 1500 mL of blood when chest tube is first inserted |
| Continuous hemorrhage of more than 200 mL/h for ≥3 consecutive hours |
| Esophageal perforation |
| Pericardial tamponade |

See Schwartz 8th ed., p 158.

**Answer: C**

Pulmonary injuries requiring operative intervention usually result from penetrating injury. Formerly the entrance and exit wounds were oversewn to control hemorrhage. This set the stage for air embolism which occasionally caused sudden death in the operating room or in the immediate postoperative period. A recent development, pulmonary tractotomy, has been employed to reduce this problem as well as the need for pulmonary resection (Fig. 6-38). Linear stapling devices are inserted directly into the injury tract and positioned to cause the least degree of devascularization. Two staple lines are created and the lung is divided between. This allows direct access to the bleeding vessels and leaking bronchi. No effort is made to close the defect. Lobectomy or pneumonectomy is rarely necessary. Lobectomy is only indicated for a completely devascularized or destroyed lobe. Parenchymal injuries severe enough to require pneumonectomy are rarely survivable, and major pulmonary hilar injuries necessitating pneumonectomy are usually lethal in the field. (See Schwartz 8th ed., p 158.)

12. The most appropriate treatment for a duodenal hematoma that occurs from blunt trauma is
    A. Exploratory laparotomy and bypass of the duodenum
    B. Exploratory laparotomy and evacuation of the hematoma
    C. Exploratory laparotomy to rule out associated injuries
    D. Observation

**Answer: D**
Duodenal hematomas are caused by a direct blow to the abdomen and occur more often in children than adults. Blood accumulates between the seromuscular and submucosal layers, eventually causing obstruction. The diagnosis is suspected by the onset of vomiting following blunt abdominal trauma; barium examination of the duodenum reveals either the coiled spring sign or obstruction. Most duodenal hematomas in children can be managed nonoperatively with nasogastric suction and parenteral nutrition. Resolution of the obstruction occurs in the majority of patients if this therapy is continued for 7 to 14 days. If surgical intervention becomes necessary, evacuation of the hematoma is associated with equal success but fewer complications than bypass procedures. Despite few existing data on adults, there is no reason to believe that their hematomas should be treated differently from those of children. A new approach is laparoscopic evacuation if the obstruction persists more than 7 days. (See Schwartz 8th ed., p 167.)

13. The most appropriate treatment for a gunshot wound to the hepatic flexure of the colon that cannot be repaired primarily is
    A. End colostomy and mucous fistula
    B. Loop colostomy
    C. Exteriorized repair
    D. Resection of the right colon with ileocolostomy

**Answer: D**
Numerous large retrospective and several prospective studies have now clearly demonstrated that primary repair is safe and effective in the majority of patients with penetrating injuries. Colostomy is still appropriate in a few patients, but the current dilemma is how to select them. Exteriorized repair is probably no longer indicated since most patients who were once candidates for this treatment are now successfully managed by primary repair. Two methods have been advocated that result in 75 to 90% of penetrating colonic injuries being safely treated by primary repair. The first is to repair all perforations not requiring resection. If resection is required due to the local extent of the injury, and it is proximal to the middle colic artery, the proximal portion of the right colon up to and including the injury is resected and an ileocolostomy performed. If resection is required distal to the middle colic artery, an end colostomy is created and the distal colon oversewn and left within the abdomen. The theory behind this approach is that an ileocolostomy heals more reliably than colocolostomy, because in the trauma patient who has suffered shock and may be hypovolemic, assessing the adequacy of the blood supply of the colon is much less reliable than in elective procedures. The blood supply of the terminal ileum is never a problem. The other approach is to repair all injuries regardless of the extent and location (including colocolostomy), and reserve co-

lostomy for patients with protracted shock and extensive contamination. The theory used to support this approach is that systemic factors are more important than local factors in determining whether a suture line will heal. Both of these approaches are reasonable and result in the majority of patients being treated by primary repairs. When a colostomy is required, regardless of the theory used to reach that conclusion, performing a loop colostomy proximal to a distal repair should be avoided because a proximal colostomy does not protect a distal suture line. All suture lines and anastomoses are performed with the running single-layer technique described in Fig. 6-57. (See Schwartz 8th ed., p 171.)

14. Appropriate initial treatment of a patient with a severe closed head (Glasgow Coma Score <8) injury includes
    A. Hyperventilation to a $P_{CO_2}$ <30 mm Hg
    B. Lasix to decrease cerebral swelling
    C. Placement of a ventriculostomy
    D. Barbiturate coma

**Answer: C**
General principles of the management of cerebral injuries have changed in recent years. Attention is now focused on maintaining or enhancing cerebral perfusion rather than merely lowering intracranial pressure (ICP). For example, it has been found that hyperventilation to a $P_{CO_2}$ less than 30 mm Hg to induce cerebral vasoconstriction actually exacerbates cerebral ischemia in spite of decreasing ICP. These secondary iatrogenic cerebral injuries cause more harm than previously appreciated. Other treatments or conditions that must be avoided include decreased cardiac output due to the excessive use of osmotic diuretics, sedatives, or barbiturates, and hypoxia. Nevertheless, the measurement of ICP is still important and is efficiently accomplished with a ventriculostomy tube. The tube also permits the withdrawal of cerebrospinal fluid, which is the safest method for lowering ICP. Although an ICP of 10 mm Hg is believed to be the upper limit of normal, therapy is not usually initiated until the ICP reaches 20 mm Hg. Cerebral perfusion pressure (CPP) is an important measurement which is used to monitor therapy. CPP is equal to the mean arterial pressure (MAP) minus the ICP, and 60 mm Hg is the lowest acceptable pressure. This figure can be adjusted by either lowering ICP or raising MAP. In practice, both are manipulated. Paralysis, sedation, osmotic diuresis, and barbiturate coma are all still used, with coma being the last resort. The goal of fluid therapy is to achieve a euvolemic state, and arbitrary fluid restriction is avoided. Whether boosting MAP with pressors or inotropes in patients with an elevated ICP resistant to treatment improves outcome is unclear, although recent data suggest it does. Moderate hypothermia may also be helpful by decreasing metabolic requirements. (See Schwartz 8th ed., p 153.)

15. The lowest acceptable cerebral perfusion pressure in a patient with a closed head injury is
    A. 40 mm Hg
    B. 60 mm Hg
    C. 80 mm Hg
    D. 100 mm Hg

**Answer: B**
See Answer text for Question 14.

16. Therapy for increased intracranial pressure (ICP) in a patient with a closed head injury is instituted when the ICP is greater than
    A. 10
    B. 20
    C. 30
    D. 40

**Answer: B**

See Answer text for Question 14.

17. Patients with acute spinal cord injuries
    A. May recover function in up to 10% of cases (concussive injury)
    B. May have improved outcome if methylprednisolone is given within 24 h of injury
    C. Have an increased risk of deep venous thrombosis
    D. Should not have a Foley placed due to increased risk of urinary tract infection

**Answer: C**

Injuries of the spinal cord, particularly complete injuries, remain essentially untreatable. Approximately 3% of patients who present with flaccid quadriplegia actually have concussive injuries, and these patients represent the very few who seem to have miraculous recoveries. A recent prospective randomized study comparing methylprednisolone with placebo demonstrated a significant improvement in outcome (usually one or two spinal levels) for those who received the corticosteroid within 8 h of injury. The standard dosage is 30 mg/kg given as an IV bolus, followed by a 5.4-mg/kg infusion administered over the next 23 hours. Patients with spinal cord injuries are also at high risk for deep venous thrombosis and pulmonary embolus. Prophylactic anticoagulation is essential. (See Schwartz 8th ed., p 154.)

18. Laryngeal fractures
    A. Should be suspected in any patient with a hoarse voice
    B. Are treated conservatively with steroids and antibiotics
    C. Rarely result in airway compromise
    D. May be associated with flexion injuries of the cervical spine

**Answer: A**

The larynx may be fractured by a direct blow, which can result in airway compromise. A hoarse voice is highly suggestive. A cricothyroidotomy, or tracheostomy if time permits, should be done to protect the airway in cases of severe fracture. The larynx is anatomically repaired with fine wires and sutures. If direct repair of internal laryngeal structures is necessary, the thyroid cartilage is split longitudinally in the midline and opened like a book. This is referred to as a laryngeal fissure. (See Schwartz 8th ed., p 154.)

19. Primary repair of the trachea should be carried out with
    A. Wire suture
    B. Absorbable monofilament suture
    C. Nonabsorbable monofilament suture
    D. Absorbable braided suture

**Answer: B**

Injuries of the trachea are repaired with a running 3-0 absorbable monofilament suture. Tracheostomy is not required in most patients. Esophageal injuries are repaired in a similar fashion. If an esophageal wound is large or if tissue is missing, a sternocleidomastoid muscle pedicle flap is warranted, and a closed suction drain is a reasonable precaution. The drain should be near but not in contact with the esophageal or any other suture line. It can be removed in 7 to 10 days if the suture line remains secure. Care must be taken when exploring the trachea and esophagus to avoid iatrogenic injury to the recurrent laryngeal nerve. (See Schwartz 8th ed., p 156.)

20. At what pressure is operative decompression of a compartment mandatory?
    A. 15 mm Hg
    B. 25 mm Hg
    C. 35 mm Hg
    D. 45 mm Hg

**Answer: D**

In comatose or obtunded patients, the diagnosis is more difficult to secure. A compatible history, firmness of the compartment to palpation, and diminished mobility of the joint are suggestive. The presence or absence of a pulse distal to the affected compartment is notoriously unreliable in the diagnosis of a compartment syndrome. A frozen joint and myoglobinuria are late signs and suggest a poor prognosis. As in the abdomen, compartment pressure can be measured. The small, hand-held Stryker device is a convenient tool for this purpose. Pressures greater than 45 mm Hg usually require operative intervention. Patients with pressures between 30 and 45 mm Hg should be carefully evaluated and closely watched. (See Schwartz 8th ed., p 178.)

21. Exposure for injury to the proximal left subclavian artery is best achieved through
    A. A left posterolateral thoracotomy
    B. A left 3rd intercostal space anterior thoracotomy
    C. A median sternotomy
    D. Two horizontal incisions (supraclavicular and 3rd intercostal space) connected by a median sternotomy

**Answer: D**
If angiography has identified an arterial injury, a more direct approach can be employed. Fig. 6-35 shows the various incisions that are used depending on the location of the arterial injury. A median sternotomy is used for exposure of the innominate, proximal right carotid and subclavian, and the proximal left carotid arteries. The proximal left subclavian artery presents a unique challenge. Because it arises from the aortic arch far posteriorly, it is not readily approached via median sternotomy. A posterolateral thoracotomy provides excellent exposure but severely limits access to other structures and is not recommended. The best option is to create a full-thickness flap of the upper chest wall. This is accomplished with a third or fourth interspace anterolateral thoracotomy for proximal control, a supraclavicular incision with a resection of the medial third of the clavicle, and a median sternotomy, which links the two horizontal incisions. The ribs can be cut laterally for additional exposure, which allows the flap to be folded laterally with little effort. This incision has been referred to as a book or trap-door thoracotomy for obvious reasons (Fig. 6-36). The mid-portion of the subclavian artery is accessible by removing the proximal third of either clavicle, with the skin incision made directly over the clavicle. Muscular attachments are stripped away, and the clavicle is divided with a Gigli saw. The medial remnant of the clavicle is forcefully elevated. The periosteum is dissected from the posterior aspect of the bone until the sternoclavicular joint is reached. The capsular attachments are cut with a heavy scissors or knife and the bone is discarded. The periosteum and underlying fascia are very tough and must be sharply incised along the direction of the vessel. The subclavian vein is mobilized and the artery is directly underneath. The anterior scalene is divided for injuries just proximal to the thyrocervical trunk; the relatively small phrenic nerve should be identified on its anterior aspect and spared. Iatrogenic injury to cords of the brachial plexus can occur. (See Schwartz 8th ed., p 156.)

22. A 24-year-old man is brought into the emergency department after a fall from a ladder. His breathing is labored, and he is cyanotic. No breath sounds can be heard, even in the right lung field, which is resonant to percussion. The first step in his management should be
    A. Cricothyroidotomy
    B. Obtaining a stat chest X-ray
    C. Passing an oral endotracheal tube
    D. Tube thoracostomy

**Answer: D**
This patient has a tension pneumothorax and immediate management by right tube thoracostomy is imperative. This diagnosis is a clinical one, and treatment should not await X-ray confirmation. (See Schwartz 7th ed.)

23. After an automobile accident, a 19-year-old man is admitted to the emergency department with an extensive central facial injury. His breathing is labored, and he is coughing up blood and mucus with each breath. He is thrashing about and is combative despite efforts to restrain him. The first step in his management should be to maintain in-line cervical traction and
    A. Pass an endotracheal tube by the nasal route
    B. Pass an endotracheal tube by the oral route
    C. Perform a cricothyroidotomy
    D. Perform a tracheostomy

**Answer: C**

Immediate airway control is vital in this patient. Time should not be spent trying to pass a nasal endotracheal tube blindly or an oral endotracheal tube through a pharynx filled with blood. A cricothyroidotomy is a faster way to obtain surgical airway than a tracheostomy. Cricothyroidotomy buys time, and another airway can be established later. (See Schwartz 7th ed.)

24. A 19-year-old man is admitted to the emergency department with a stab wound just below the right inguinal ligament. There is profuse bleeding from the wound, and he is in shock. The first step in local wound control should be to
    A. Apply compression of the bleeding vessel with a gloved finger
    B. Place a tourniquet on the right thigh above the wound
    C. Use clamps and ligatures to control the bleeding
    D. Wrap the wound and upper thigh in a bulky pressure dressing

**Answer: A**

In all likelihood, this patient has a lateral partial transection of a major artery or vein. Immediate control of this type of bleeding is mandatory if life and limb are to be saved. Clamping and ligating bleeding vessels in the wound should only be done under controlled circumstances in the operating room. A proximal tourniquet, even if one can be applied, is damaging to tissue and is a poor choice. A pressure dressing might control bleeding, but this is not likely with a major bleeding vessel. Application of medical antishock trousers in these circumstances takes too long, although the maneuver might provide temporary control. The most effective technique is for the surgeon to place a gloved finger directly through the wound to apply gentle pressure to the bleeding vessel. The patient can then be appropriately resuscitated and moved to the operating room for definitive repair, with the surgeon maintaining finger control of the bleeding. (See Schwartz 7th ed.)

25. After an automobile accident, a 20-year-old woman is found by a retrograde urethrogram to have an extraperitoneal bladder rupture. Initial management of this injury should be
    A. Celiotomy and open repair of the injury
    B. Insertion of a Foley catheter through the urethra
    C. Observation for evidence of a continuing urinary leak
    D. Suprapubic cystostomy

**Answer: B**

With Foley catheter drainage, an extraperitoneal bladder injury should close spontaneously. Celiotomy and bladder repair is appropriate for intraperitoneal bladder injury. Suprapubic cystostomy may be required if a Foley catheter cannot be passed safely through an injury in the posterior urethra. (See Schwartz 7th ed.)

26. A 20-year-old man has an injury to the posterior urethra. After appropriate initial management and follow-up care of this injury, the most likely late complication is
    A. Ascending urinary tract infection
    B. Retrograde ejaculation
    C. Sterility
    D. Urethral stricture

**Answer: D**

Initial management involves passage of catheters through the urethral meatus and through an incision in the bladder. After this has been accomplished, a Foley catheter is threaded through the urethra into the bladder and left in situ. Urethral healing occurs as the hematoma resolves, but a posterior urethral stricture is not uncommon. If the stricture is not managed appropriately, ascending urinary tract infection may result. (See Schwartz 7th ed.)

27. After an automobile accident, a 30-year-old woman is discovered to have a posterior pelvic fracture. Hypotension and tachycardia respond marginally to volume replacement. Once it is evident that her major problem is free intraperitoneal bleeding and a pelvic hematoma in association with the fracture, appropriate management would be
    A. Application of medical antishock trousers with inflation of the extremity and abdominal sections
    B. Arterial embolization of the pelvic vessels
    C. Celiotomy and ligation of the internal iliac arteries bilaterally
    D. Celiotomy and pelvic packing
    E. External fixation application to stabilize the pelvis

**Answer: D**
Severe pelvic bleeding is a major problem in the trauma patient. Neither external fixation nor the use of medical antishock trousers control free intraabdominal hemorrhage regardless of its source. In the unstable patient, celiotomy is mandatory. If there is a ruptured retroperitoneal hematoma bleeding into the peritoneal cavity, control is a major problem. Internal iliac artery ligation has been abandoned as it is rarely effective. Angiography and arterial embolization may be effective with an arterial bleeding problem, but most severe pelvic hemorrhage is venous in origin. If the hematoma is stable, it is best to leave it undisturbed. However, if the hematoma has ruptured into the peritoneal cavity, pelvic packing offers the best hope of control. (See Schwartz 7th ed.)

28. Bites of the following wild animals have caused rabies in the United States EXCEPT
    A. Bats
    B. Foxes
    C. Rats
    D. Raccoons
    E. Skunks

**Answer: C**
Although dog bites account for rabies exposure in much of the world, this is not true in the United States. Bats, foxes, raccoons, and skunks account for more than 85% of animal rabies in the United States. There are no known cases of human rabies after rodent bites in this country. (See Schwartz 7th ed.)

29. A 25-year-old man has multiple intra-abdominal injuries after a gunshot wound. Celiotomy reveals multiple injuries to small and large bowel and major bleeding from the liver. After repair of the bowel injuries, the abdomen is closed with towel clips, leaving a large pack in the injured liver. Within 12 h, there is massive abdominal swelling with edema fluid, and intra-abdominal pressure exceeds 35 mm Hg. The immediate step in managing this problem is to
    A. Administer albumin intercavernously
    B. Give an intravenous diuretic
    C. Limit intravenous fluid administration
    D. Open the incision to decompress the abdomen

**Answer: D**
Cardiac, pulmonary, and renal problems develop when invasive ascites compresses the diaphragm and the inferior vena cava. Dialysis, diuresis, and increasing serum oncotic pressure will not correct this problem rapidly enough to save the patient's life. Opening the incision relieves the intra-abdominal pressure. There are few reports of sudden hypotension after this maneuver, but volume loading has largely eliminated this problem. (See Schwartz 7th ed.)

30. An early sign of anterior compartment syndrome in the calf is
    A. Absence of pulses in the foot
    B. Firm calf muscles
    C. Foot drop
    D. Paresthesia between the great and second toes

**Answer: D**
Anterior compartment syndrome can produce all of these signs, but the presence of paresthesia between the great toe and the second toe is an early sign, which mandates surgical intervention. The paresthesia is caused by pressure on the deep peroneal nerve, and it is relieved by decompressing the compartment. (See Schwartz 7th ed.)

31. Significant vascular injury is likely to occur with all of the following fractures or dislocations EXCEPT
    A. Fracture of the midshaft of the humerus
    B. Supracondylar fracture of the humerus
    C. Fracture of the femoral shaft
    D. Supracondylar fracture of the femur

**Answer: A**
Arterial injuries should always be considered whenever a fracture or dislocation of an extremity is encountered. Fractures of the femoral shaft, supracondylar fractures of the humerus and femur, and posterior dislocations of the knee are particularly prone to produce vascular injury. In any of these circumstances, arteriography should be done unless the distal circulation is entirely normal. Although fractures of the humeral shaft are frequently associated with radial nerve injury, damage to the accompanying deep brachial artery is not usually a problem because of the rich collateral circulation around the elbow. (See Schwartz 7th ed.)

32. A 55-year-old woman sustains closed fractures of the right tibia and fibula in a skiing accident, and she is noted to have a loss of sensation over the lateral aspect of the affected calf and foot. The fractures are non-displaced. The patient's leg is casted, and the fractures heal without complication. Six months after the injury, the patient develops intense burning, hyperesthesia, and cyanosis of the right foot. The treatment of choice for her would be
    A. Local exploration of the peroneal nerve
    B. Narcotics
    C. Ganglionic blockade
    D. Paravertebral sympathetic block

**Answer: D**
The treatment of causalgia should use a paravertebral sympathetic block with local anesthesia as soon as the diagnosis is made. Repetitive blocks may provide permanent relief, or sympathectomy can be performed to relieve recurrent pain. Local exploration of the nerve, narcotics, muscle relaxants, and ganglionic blockade are not effective in the treatment of reflex sympathetic dystrophy. (See Schwartz 7th ed.)

33. An 18-year-old man is admitted to the emergency department shortly after being involved in an automobile accident. He is in a coma (Glasgow Coma Score = 7). His pulse is barely palpable at a rate of 140 beats per minute, and blood pressure is 60/0. Breathing is rapid and shallow, aerating both lung fields. His abdomen is moderately distended with no audible peristalsis. There are closed fractures of the right forearm and the left lower leg. After rapid intravenous administration of 2 L of lactated Ringer's solution in the upper extremities, his pulse is 130 and blood pressure 70/0. The next immediate step should be to
    A. Obtain cross-table lateral X-rays of the cervical spine
    B. Obtain head and abdominal computed tomography (CT) scans
    C. Obtain supine and lateral decubitus X-rays of the abdomen
    D. Obtain an arch aortogram
    E. Explore the abdomen

**Answer: E**
Ideally, a patient seriously injured in an automobile accident should undergo X-rays of the cervical spine, the chest, and the abdomen. When he has a Glasgow Coma Score of 7, CT scans of the head are certainly desirable. If the chest X-ray shows a widened mediastinum, arch aortograms are indicated. However, this patient has had no response to a rapid fluid challenge, and if he is to survive, bleeding must be controlled immediately. The head injury, although severe, is not responsible for his hypotension and tachycardia. The most likely problem is uncontrolled abdominal hemorrhage. Immediate abdominal exploration offers the best chance for survival. (See Schwartz 7th ed.)

34. A 28-year-old man undergoes an uncomplicated splenectomy after blunt abdominal trauma. During anesthesia, he is given oxygen, nitrous oxide, a narcotic, and a muscle relaxant. No other significant injuries are found during surgery, and transfusion of blood products is not required. In the recovery room after extubation, the patient is noted to have a blood pressure of 170/100 mm Hg, a pulse of 140 beats per minute, and a respiratory rate of 8 breaths per minute. Shortly thereafter, his blood pressure is found to have dropped to 100/60 mm Hg and his pulse to 60 beats per minute; he is not arousable. The diagnostic maneuver most likely to define this patient's problem is
    A. Measurement of central venous pressure
    B. Measurement of pulmonary capillary wedge pressure
    C. Spirometry
    D. Analysis of arterial blood gas
    E. Chest X-ray

**Answer: D**
Delayed emergence from anesthesia after surgery for trauma is frequently characterized by hypoventilation, clinical signs of which include diminution of respiration, hypertension progressing to hypotension, tachycardia progressing to bradycardia, restlessness or stupor, and pallor or cyanosis. The diagnosis is best established by analysis of arterial blood gas, which will reveal acidosis, hypercapnia, and arterial desaturation. Additionally, spirometry can help to confirm the diagnosis by showing diminished tidal ventilation. Pneumothorax, hemothorax, or volume overload may all cause or contribute to postanesthetic hypoventilation but are less frequently associated with the condition than anesthetic, relaxant, or narcotic overdosage. The postoperative recovery room should be equipped to permit analysis of blood gas, measurement of central venous pressure, X-ray examination, and spirometry without undue delay. (See Schwartz 7th ed.)

1. Which of the following patients should be transferred to a burn center?
   A. A 9-year-old with a 12% partial thickness burn
   B. A 25-year-old with an 18% deep partial thickness burn
   C. A 62-year-old with 8% deep partial thickness burn
   D. A 36-year-old with hypertension and a 16% deep partial thickness burn

**Answer: A**

The American Burn Association (ABA) has identified the following injuries as those requiring referral to a burn center after initial assessment and stabilization at an emergency department:

1. Partial-thickness and full-thickness burns totaling greater than 10% total body surface area (TBSA) in patients under 10 or over 50 years of age.
2. Partial-thickness and full-thickness burns totaling greater than 20% TBSA in other age groups.
3. Partial-thickness and full-thickness burns involving the face, hands, feet, genitalia, perineum, or major joints.
4. Full-thickness burns greater than 5% TBSA in any age group.
5. Electrical burns, including lightning injury.
6. Chemical burns.
7. Inhalation injury.
8. Burn injury in patients with preexisting medical disorders that could complicate management, prolong the recovery period, or affect mortality.
9. Any burn with concomitant trauma (e.g., fractures) in which the burn injury poses the greatest risk of morbidity or mortality. If the trauma poses the greater immediate risk, the patient may be treated initially in a trauma center until stable, before being transferred to a burn center. The physician's decisions should be made with the regional medical control plan and triage protocols in mind.
10. Burn injury in children admitted to a hospital without qualified personnel or equipment for pediatric care.
11. Burn injury in patients requiring special social, emotional, and/or long-term rehabilitative support, including cases involving suspected child abuse.

(See Schwartz 8th ed., p 191.)

2. Which of the following is a clear indication for intubation in a burn patient?
   A. History of being in a closed room
   B. Coughing up carbonaceous sputum
   C. Carbon monoxide level of >2%
   D. P:F ratio of <250

**Answer: D**

A decreased P:F ratio, the ratio of arterial oxygen pressure ($Pa_{O_2}$) to the percentage of inspired oxygen ($Fi_{O_2}$), is one of the earliest indicators of smoke inhalation. A ratio of 400 to 500 is normal; patients with impending pulmonary problems have a ratio of less than 300. A ratio of less than 250 is

3. A patient with a 90% burn encompassing the entire torso develops an increasing $P_{CO_2}$ and peak inspiratory pressure. Which of the following is most likely to resolve this problem?
   A. Increase the delivered tidal volume
   B. Increase the respiratory rate
   C. Increase the $F_{IO_2}$
   D. Perform a thoracic escharotomy

4. What percentage burn does a patient have who has suffered burns to one leg (circumferential), one arm (circumferential), and the anterior trunk?
   A. 18%
   B. 27%
   C. 36%
   D. 45%

5. The appropriate management of a deep partial-thickness burn is
   A. Early excision and grafting
   B. Surgical débridement and dressings
   C. Dressings only
   D. Observation

an indication for endotracheal intubation rather than for increasing the inspired oxygen concentration. (See Schwartz 8th ed., p 192.)

**Answer: D**
The adequacy of respiration must be monitored continuously throughout the resuscitation period. Early respiratory distress may be due to the compromise of ventilation caused by chest wall inelasticity related to a deep circumferential burn wound of the thorax. Pressures required for ventilation increase and arterial $P_{CO_2}$ rises. Inhalation injury, pneumothorax, or other causes can also result in respiratory distress and should be appropriately treated.

Thoracic escharotomy is seldom required, even with a circumferential chest wall burn. When required, escharotomies are performed bilaterally in the anterior axillary lines. If there is significant extension of the burn onto the adjacent abdominal wall, the escharotomy incisions should be extended to this area by a transverse incision along the costal margins. (See Schwartz 8th ed., p 193.)

**Answer: D**
A general idea of the burn size can be made by using the rule of nines. Each upper extremity accounts for 9% of the total body surface area (TBSA), each lower extremity accounts for 18%, the anterior and posterior trunk each account for 18%, the head and neck account for 9%, and the perineum accounts for 1%. Although the rule of nines is reasonably accurate for adults, a number of more precise charts have been developed that are particularly helpful in assessing pediatric burns. Most emergency rooms have such a chart. A diagram of the burn can be drawn on the chart, and more precise calculations of the burn size made from the accompanying TBSA estimates given.

Children under 4 years of age have much larger heads and smaller thighs in proportion to total body size than do adults. In infants the head accounts for nearly 20% of the TBSA; a child's body proportions do not fully reach adult percentages until adolescence. Even when using precise diagrams, interobserver variation may vary by as much as ±20%. An observer's experience with burned patients, rather than educational level, appears to be the best predictor of the accuracy of burn size estimation. For smaller burns, an accurate assessment of size can be made by using the patient's palmar hand surface, including the digits, which amounts to approximately 1% of TBSA. (See Schwartz 8th ed., p 194.)

**Answer: A**
For deeper burns (i.e., deep partial-thickness and full-thickness burns), rather than waiting for spontaneous separation, the eschar is surgically removed and the wound closed via grafting techniques and/or immediate flap procedures tailored to the individual patient. This aggressive surgical approach to burn wound management has become known as early excision and grafting (E&G). Several technical ad-

vances have made this possible, including a safer autologous blood supply, better monitoring equipment and methods, and a better understanding of the deranged physiology of patients with major burns. The ability to stabilize the patient within a few days of the injury has enabled the surgeon to remove deep burn wounds before invasive infection occurs. The optimal timing of early E&G has yet to be definitively determined; however, E&G within 3 to 7 days, and certainly by 10 days, following injury appears prudent. (See Schwartz 8th ed., p 204.)

6. Pulse oximetry readings in a patient with carbon monoxide poisoning will be
   A. Unchanged
   B. Falsely high
   C. Falsely low
   D. Unobtainable

**Answer: B**

Patients burned in an enclosed space or having any signs or symptoms of neurologic impairment should be placed on 100% oxygen via a nonrebreather face mask while waiting for measurement of COHb levels. The use of pulse oximetry ($SpO_2$) to assess arterial oxygenation in the CO-poisoned patient is contraindicated, as the COHb results in erroneously elevated $SpO_2$ measurements. (See Schwartz 8th ed., p 201.)

7. The half-life of carboxyhemoglobin in a patient breathing 100% oxygen is
   A. 10 min
   B. 1 h
   C. 3 h
   D. 10 h

**Answer: B**

CO is reversibly bound to the heme molecules of Hb, and despite intense affinity, readily dissociates according to the laws of mass action. The half-life ($t_{1/2}$) of COHb when breathing room air is approximately 4 h. On 100% oxygen, the $t_{1/2}$ is reduced to 45 to 60 min. In a hyperbaric oxygen chamber at 2 atm, it is approximately 30 min, and at 3 atm it is about 15 to 20 min. (See Schwartz 8th ed., p 201.)

8. Which of the following is a common sequelae of electrical injury?
   A. Cardiac arrhythmias
   B. Paralysis
   C. Brain damage
   D. Cataracts

**Answer: D**

Myoglobinuria frequently accompanies electrical burns, but the clinical significance appears to be trivial. Disruption of muscle cells releases cellular debris and myoglobin into the circulation to be filtered by the kidney. If this condition is untreated, the consequence can be irreversible renal failure. However, modern burn resuscitation protocols alone appear to be sufficient treatment for myoglobinuria.

Cardiac damage, such as myocardial contusion or infarction, may be present. More likely, the conduction system may be deranged. Household current at 110 V either does no damage or induces ventricular fibrillation. If there are no electrocardiographic rhythm abnormalities present upon initial emergency department evaluation, the likelihood that they will appear later is minuscule. Even with high-voltage injuries, a normal cardiac rhythm on admission generally means that subsequent dysrhythmia is unlikely. Studies confirm that commonly measured cardiac enzymes bear little correlation to cardiac dysfunction, and elevated enzymes may be from skeletal muscle damage. Mandatory electrocardiogram (ECG) monitoring and cardiac enzyme analysis in an ICU setting for 24 h following injury is unnecessary in patients with electrical burns, even those resulting from high-voltage current, in patients who have stable cardiac rhythms on admission.

The nervous system is exquisitely sensitive to electricity. The most devastating injury with frequent brain damage occurs when current passes through the head, but spinal cord damage is possible whenever current has passed from one side of the body to the other. Schwann cells are quite susceptible, and delayed transverse myelitis can occur days or weeks after injury. Conduction initially remains normal through existing myelin, but as myelin wears out, it is not replaced and conduction ceases. Anterior spinal artery syndrome from vascular dysregulation can also precipitate spinal cord dysfunction. Damage to peripheral nerves is common and may cause permanent functional impairment. Every patient with an electrical injury must have a thorough neurologic exam as part of the initial assessment. Persistent neurologic symptoms may lead to chronic pain syndromes, and posttraumatic stress disorders are apparently more common after electrical burns than thermal burns.

Cataracts are a well-recognized sequela of high-voltage electrical burns. They occur in 5 to 7% of patients, frequently are bilateral, occur even in the absence of contact points on the head, and typically manifest within 1 to 2 years of injury. Electrically injured patients should undergo a thorough ophthalmologic examination early during their acute care. (See Schwartz 8th ed., p 214.)

9. How long does it take 140°F water to create a scald burn?
   A. 3 sec
   B. 15 sec
   C. 1 min
   D. 3 min

**Answer: A**
Scalds, usually from hot water, are the most common cause of burns in civilian practice. Water at 140°F (60°C) creates a deep partial-thickness or full-thickness burn in 3 sec. At 156°F (69°C), the same burn occurs in 1 sec. As a reference point, freshly brewed coffee generally is about 180°F (82°C). Boiling water always causes deep burns; likewise, thick soups and sauces, which remain in contact with the skin longer, invariably cause deep burns. Exposed areas of skin tend to be burned less deeply than clothed areas, as the clothing retains the heat and keeps the hot liquid in contact with the skin for a longer period of time. Immersion scalds are always deep, severe burns. The liquid causing an immersion scald may not be as hot as with a spill scald; however, the duration of contact with the skin is longer during immersion, and these burns frequently occur in small children or elderly patients who have thinner skin. (See Schwartz 7th ed.)

10. A 25-year-old man is admitted shortly after being rescued from a house fire. He is hoarse and dyspneic with expiratory wheezes. His P:F ratio is 200 on 40% inspired oxygen by non-rebreather mask. The first step in management of his airway should be
    A. Administration of oxygen by mask
    B. Administration of oxygen and racemic epinephrine by mask
    C. Fiberoptic bronchoscopy and bronchial lavage
    D. Intubation and administration of oxygen

**Answer: D**
The P:F ratio is the ratio of arterial $P_{O_2}$ to inspired oxygen ($F_{IO_2}$) and a ratio of 200 would indicate a $Pa_{O_2}$ of 80 mm Hg at an $F_{IO_2}$ of 0.4. This $Pa_{O_2}$ is dangerous, and immediate intubation is in order. If secretions remain a problem after oxygenation has been improved, fiberoptic bronchoscopy and bronchial lavage may be in order. (See Schwartz 7th ed.)

11. A 30-year-old man is admitted with full thickness burns covering both upper extremities and the anterior chest. Fluid resuscitation should be begun through
    A. An antecubital vein
    B. A femoral vein
    C. An internal jugular vein
    D. A subclavian vein

**Answer: A**

Venous access should not be established through the lower extremities because of the danger of septic thrombophlebitis. In an adult the antecubital route should be used even with burns of the overlying skin. (See Schwartz 7th ed.)

12. The best way to relieve pain for an individual with a large area burn is by
    A. Intramuscular meperidine
    B. Intravenous morphine
    C. Oral ibuprofen
    D. Subcutaneous Dilaudid

**Answer: B**

Absorption and perfusion from subcutaneous or intramuscular sites are unreliable in a burned individual. Oral medication will not be rapidly absorbed and inhalation agents are evanescent in their effects. The intravenous route is preferred, and 2 to 5 mg of morphine given slowly is usually adequate for a burned adult. (See Schwartz 7th ed.)

13. Successful antibiotic penetration of a burn eschar can be achieved with
    A. Mafenide acetate
    B. Neomycin
    C. Silver nitrate
    D. Silver sulfadiazine

**Answer: A**

Mafenide acetate is the antibiotic agent that penetrates burn eschar to reach the interface with the patient's viable tissue. This agent has the disadvantages that it is quite painful on any partial thickness areas, and it is a carbonic anhydrase inhibitor that interferes with renal buffering mechanisms. Chloride is retained, and metabolic acidosis results. For these reasons, silver sulfadiazine is more commonly used in burn centers unless a major problem with burn wound sepsis is present. (See Schwartz 7th ed.)

14. After a burn, the agent responsible for early increased capillary permeability is
    A. Bradykinin
    B. Histamine
    C. Prostacyclin prostaglandin $I_2$ ($PGI_2$)
    D. Serotonin

**Answer: B**

Burn injury releases a cascade of vasoactive products. Bradykinin increases vascular permeability, especially in the venule. Histamine is primarily responsible for increased capillary permeability. Prostaglandins such as $PGI_2$ result in arterial dilatation and increased wound edema. Serotonin, released on postburn platelet aggregation, increases pulmonary vascular resistance. Thromboxane $A_2$ is a vasoconstrictor found in burn blister fluid and lymph. (See Schwartz 7th ed.)

15. All of the following statements concerning early tangential excision of a burn wound are true EXCEPT
    A. The procedure entails significant blood loss.
    B. In a patient with severe smoke inhalation the procedure should be done under local anesthesia.
    C. By expediting healing in burns around joints the procedure preserves joint function.
    D. The procedure is carried out sequentially until good capillary bleeding indicates viable tissue.

**Answer: B**

Tangential excision is technically easy to perform, but the procedure entails significant blood loss. It cannot be performed under local anesthesia, and significant smoke inhalation frequently delays the process. It is particularly applicable with burns around joints as early healing provides better joint function. Excision is carried out sequentially unless good bleeding is encountered. When a burn extends into subcutaneous fat, the relative avascularization of the tissue makes it hard to judge proper excision depth. (See Schwartz 7th ed.)

16. Whether the nutritional needs of a patient 10 days after a major burn are being met is best assessed by
    A. Calorie counts
    B. Measurement of daily body weight
    C. Measurement of serum albumin levels
    D. Nitrogen balance studies

**Answer: B**

Once the initial wound edema is resolved, measurement of body weight on a daily basis is in order. The patient who is recovering should gain slowly and steadily. Other measurements are inaccurate or hard to perform in the severely burned patient. (See Schwartz 7th ed.)

17. A 45-year-old firefighter who weighs 74 kg (163 lb) sustains a third-degree burn to 64% of his total body surface area. The patient arrives in the emergency department approximately 30 min after the time of the accident.

    When the patient's intravenous fluid requirements are calculated using the Parkland formula, the initial orders for choice of fluid and rate of infusion should be
    A. Ringer's lactate, 200 mL/h for $7\frac{1}{2}$ h
    B. Ringer's lactate, 1250 mL/h for $7\frac{1}{2}$ h
    C. Ringer's lactate, 600 mL/h, and colloid solution, 200 mL/h, for $7\frac{1}{2}$ h
    D. Ringer's lactate, 800 mL/h, and colloid solution, 200 mL/h, for $7\frac{1}{2}$ h

**Answer: B**

The Parkland formula for calculating the amount of fluid needed for resuscitation of burned patients calls for 4 mL of Ringer's lactate per kilogram of body weight per percentage of total body surface area of second- and third-degree burns. Ringer's lactate solution alone is administered for the first 24 h after injury, and one-half of the 24-h requirement should be administered in the first 8 h from the time of injury. In the case described in the question, in which the patient weighed 74 kg, suffered a third-degree burn to 64% of his total body surface area, and arrived for treatment a half hour after injury, fluid requirements would be calculated as follows:

$$4 \text{ mL} \times 74 \text{ kg} \times 64 = 18,944 \text{ mL}$$
$$18,944/2 = 9,472 \text{ mL over the next } 7\frac{1}{2} \text{ h}$$
$$9,472/7.5 = 1,262 \text{ mL/h}$$

(See Schwartz 7th ed.)

18. The most frequent nonbacterial, opportunistic organism recovered from burn wounds is
    A. *Aspergillus*
    B. *Candida*
    C. *Fusarium*
    D. *Phycomycetes*

**Answer: B**

The most common nonbacterial, opportunistic organism recovered from burn wounds is *Candida*. Although this imperfect fungus has the potential to invade viable tissue and colonize deep layers of the eschar, it rarely does so. Systemic spread of candidal infection also appears to be rare. Other fungi colonize burn wounds less commonly than *Candida* but, when they do so, often produce extensive invasion. After *Candida*, the most common types of fungi that invade burn wounds are *Aspergillus* and *Fusarium*. (See Schwartz 7th ed.)

19. A 14-year-old girl sustains a steam burn measuring 6 by 7 inches over the ulnar aspect of her right forearm. Blisters develop over the entire area of the burn wound, and by the time the patient is seen 6 h after the injury, some of the blisters have ruptured spontaneously. All of the following therapeutic regimens might be considered appropriate for this patient EXCEPT
    A. Application of silver sulfadiazine cream (Silvadene) and daily washes, but no dressing
    B. Application of mafenide acetate cream (Sulfamylon), but no daily washes or dressing
    C. Homograft application without sutures to secure it in place, but no daily washes or dressing
    D. Heterograft (pigskin) application with sutures to secure it in place and daily washes, but no dressing

**Answer: D**

A number of different acceptable regimens exist for treating small, superficial second-degree burn injuries. In all cases, the necrotic epithelium is first débrided. Topical antibacterial agents then may be applied and the wounds treated open or closed with dressings changed daily or every other day. Biologic dressings (homografts or heterografts) may be applied to superficial second-degree burns at the time of initial débridement. Typically, these dressings quickly adhere to the wounds, relieve pain, and promote rapid epithelialization. These dressings should not be sutured in place, however, because suturing creates the potential for a closed-space infection and for conversion of a second-degree to a full-thickness injury. If a biologic dressing does not adhere, it should be removed immediately, and the wound should then be treated with topical antibacterial agents. (See Schwartz 7th ed.)

20. A man who weighs 70 kg (154 lb) is transferred to a burn center 4 weeks after sustaining a second- and third-degree burn injury to 45% of his total body surface area. Prior to the accident, the patient's weight was 90 kg (198 lb). The patient has not been given anything by mouth since the injury, except for antacids because of a previous ulcer history. On physical examination, the patient's burn wounds are clean, but only minimal healing is evident, and thick adherent eschar is present. The patient's abdomen is soft and nondistended, and active bowel sounds are heard. His stools are trace-positive for blood. He has poor range of motion of all involved joints and has developed early axillary and popliteal fossae flexion contractures. In managing this patient at this stage of his injury, top priority must be given to correcting
    A. The contractures and poor range of motion in joints—by aggressive physical therapy
    B. The open, poorly healing burn wounds—by surgical excision and grafting
    C. The presence of blood in the stools—by increasing the dose of antacids and adding cimetidine
    D. The nutritional status—by enteral supplementation or parenteral hyperalimentation

**Answer: D**
Healthy persons usually can tolerate an acute loss of no more than one-third of their lean body weight before death ensues. Thus, extensively burned patients who are in a hypermetabolic state may rapidly develop a life-threatening nutritional problem in the absence of adequate oral or parenteral caloric intake. (The patient presented in the question would have an energy requirement of approximately 4000 kcal/day: 40 kcal × 45% body surface area burned + 25 kcal × 90 kg preburn body weight = 4050 kcal.) Because most of the early energy requirements of bedridden burn patients are devoted to maintenance of normal respiratory function, the most common cause of death in these patients is pulmonary sepsis, secondary to insufficient respiratory effort resulting in atelectasis. In a severely burned patient who has acutely lost a large amount of weight owing to inadequate caloric intake, the top priority in management must be to supply adequate nutrition. Any surgical procedure at this stage carries an inordinately high mortality and must be avoided until the weight loss is stopped or reversed. (See Schwartz 7th ed.)

21. A 45-year-old woman is admitted to a hospital because of a third-degree burn injury to 40% of her total body surface area, and her wounds are treated with topical silver sulfadiazine cream (Silvadene). Three days after admission, a burn wound biopsy semiquantitative culture shows $10^4$ *Pseudomonas* organisms per gram of tissue. The patient's condition is stable at this time. The most appropriate management for this patient would be to
    A. Repeat the biopsy and culture in 24 h
    B. Start subeschar clysis with antibiotics
    C. Administer systemic antibiotics
    D. Surgically excise the burn wounds

**Answer: B**
Bacterial proliferation in a burn wound may occur despite topical antibacterial agents. When bacterial proliferation has escaped control, as proved by quantitative burn wound biopsy, administration of antibiotics by needle clysis beneath the eschar is indicated. This therapy is most effective if initiated early, before invasive burn wound sepsis has developed or wound colonization has reached greater than $10^4$ organisms per gram of tissue. Systemic antibiotics usually are ineffective at this point because by the third day after a burn, blood flow to a burn wound is markedly decreased. Thus, adequate levels of antibiotic are not achieved at the eschar-viable tissue interface where the bacterial proliferation is occurring. Before the use of subeschar antibiotics, *Pseudomonas* sepsis of burn wounds accompanied by ecthyma gangrenosum was uniformly fatal in children. Once colonization of a burn wound has occurred, surgical excision is extremely dangerous, as systemic seeding will occur. (See Schwartz 7th ed.)

22. Twelve days after admission to the hospital for a 30% partial thickness burn, a patient develops a spiking temperature curve, and blood cultures are found to be positive for gram-positive organisms (*Staphylococcus*) sensitive to methicillin, vancomycin, and clindamycin. On physical examination, the only positive finding is a small amount of pus that can be expressed above the ankle from the right greater saphenous vein, at the site where a venous infusion catheter was removed 1 week ago. The best treatment for this complication is to
    A. Apply warm compresses to and elevate the affected leg while maintaining the patient on bed rest
    B. Elevate the affected leg and start a 10-day course of intravenous vancomycin
    C. Locally excise the offending vein by removing at least 4 cm above and below the point of entry and leave the wound open
    D. Completely excise the offending vein, leave the entire wound open

**Answer: D**

Suppurative thrombophlebitis, as a complication of prolonged venous cannulation, occurs more frequently in patients who have massive thermal injuries than in other trauma patients. Commonly, affected patients have neither calf tenderness nor edema and present only with evidence of bacteremia of unknown origin. When the diagnosis is suspected, all peripheral veins that have been cannulated during hospitalization must be surgically explored. The affected veins must be opened and milked in a retrograde manner, and if pus is expressed, the diagnosis is confirmed. The offending vein must be excised in its entirety because "skip areas" of involvement commonly occur. Failure to perform prompt, complete excision usually results in fatal bacteremia. (See Schwartz 7th ed.)

23. Seven days after injury, a 45-year-old man who has sustained a second- and third-degree burn injury to 34% of his total body surface develops acute gastric stress bleeding, which is confirmed by gastroscopy. Local control by the endoscopist is unsuccessful × 2. Assuming that the patient is stable and has no previous existing diseases, the next stage of management should consist of
    A. Ligation of the left gastric artery
    B. Gastrotomy and open ligation of bleeding points
    C. Ligation of bleeding points, vagotomy, and hemigastrectomy
    D. Total gastrectomy

**Answer: C**

The incidence of Curling's ulcers as a complication of serious burn injuries has been greatly reduced in recent years. The decreased incidence is attributable to the reduced frequency of major septic complications in burns, the prophylactic introduction of antacids into the stomach after burns, and the improved provision of nutritional supplements to burn patients. When hemorrhage from acute stress gastritis does occur and cannot be controlled by conservative measures, prompt surgical intervention is indicated. The bleeding sources are first oversewn to achieve hemostasis. Then, blood volume replacement is continued until the patient's condition is stable, and a vagotomy and hemigastrectomy are performed. Lesser procedures are associated with an unacceptably high incidence of rebleeding, and later reoperation has an extremely high mortality. (See Schwartz 7th ed.)

24. Three hours after a burn injury that consisted of circumferential, third-degree burns at the wrist and elbow of the right arm, a patient loses sensation to light touch in his fingers. Motor function of his digits, however, remains intact. The most appropriate treatment for this patient now would consist of
    A. Elevation of the extremity, Doppler ultrasonography every 4 h, and if distal pulses are absent 8 h later, immediate escharotomy
    B. Palpation for distal pulses and immediate escharotomy if pulses are absent
    C. Doppler ultrasonography for assessment of peripheral flow and immediate escharotomy if flow is decreased
    D. Immediate escharotomy under general anesthesia from above the elbow to below the wrist on both medial and lateral aspects of the arm

**Answer: C**

Third-degree burn injuries are characterized by almost complete loss of elasticity of the skin. Thus, as soft tissue swelling progresses, neurovascular compromise may occur. Failure to recognize this problem may result in the loss of distal extremities. The most reliable signs of decreased peripheral blood flow in burned patients are slow capillary refill as observed in the nail beds, the onset of neurologic deficits, and decreased or absent Doppler ultrasonic pulse detection. When vascular impairment is diagnosed, immediate escharotomies are indicated. Anesthesia is not required for escharotomy—the burn area is insensate because skin nerve endings are destroyed by third-degree burns. (See Schwartz 7th ed.)

1. The proliferative phase of wound healing occurs how long after the injury?
   A. 1 day
   B. 2 days
   C. 7 days
   D. 14 days

**Answer: C**

Normal wound healing follows a predictable pattern that can be divided into overlapping phases defined by the cellular populations and biochemical activities: (a) hemostasis and inflammation, (b) proliferation, and (c) maturation and remodeling.

The proliferative phase is the second phase of wound healing and roughly spans days 4 through 12. It is during this phase that tissue continuity is re-established. Fibroblasts and endothelial cells are the last cell populations to infiltrate the healing wound, and the strongest chemotactic factor for fibroblasts is platelet-derived growth factor (PDGF). Upon entering the wound environment, recruited fibroblasts first need to proliferate, and then become activated, to carry out their primary function of matrix synthesis remodeling. This activation is mediated mainly by the cytokines and growth factors released from wound macrophages. (See Schwartz 8th ed., p 224.)

2. Which type of collagen is most important in wound healing?
   A. Type III
   B. Type V
   C. Type VII
   D. Type XI

**Answer: A**

Although there are at least 18 types of collagen described, the main ones of interest to wound repair are types I and III. Type I collagen is the major component of extracellular matrix in skin. Type III, which is also normally present in skin, becomes more prominent and important during the repair process. (See Schwartz 8th ed., p 227.)

3. The tensile strength of a wound reaches normal (pre-injury) levels
   A. 10 days after injury
   B. 3 months after injury
   C. 1 year after injury
   D. Never

**Answer: D**

Wound strength and mechanical integrity in the fresh wound are determined by both the quantity and quality of the newly deposited collagen. The deposition of matrix at the wound site follows a characteristic pattern: fibronectin and collagen type III constitute the early matrix scaffolding; glycosaminoglycans and proteoglycans represent the next significant matrix components; and collagen type I is the final matrix. By several weeks postinjury the amount of collagen in the wound reaches a plateau, but the tensile strength continues to increase for several more months. Fibril formation and fibril cross-linking result in decreased collagen solubility, increased strength, and increased resistance to enzymatic degradation of the collagen matrix. Scar remodeling continues for many (6 to 12) months postinjury, gradually resulting in a mature, avascular, and acellular scar. The mechanical strength of the scar never achieves that of the uninjured tissue. (See Schwartz 8th ed., p 228.)

4. Which of the following is commonly seen in Ehlers-Danlos syndrome?
   A. Small bowel obstructions
   B. Spontaneous thrombosis
   C. Direct hernia in children
   D. Abnormal scarring of the hands with contractures

**Answer: C**
Ehlers-Danlos syndrome (EDS) is a group of 10 disorders that present as a defect in collagen formation. Characteristics include thin, friable skin with prominent veins, easy bruising, poor wound healing, abnormal scar formation, recurrent hernias, and hyperextensible joints. Gastrointestinal problems include bleeding, hiatal hernia, intestinal diverticula, and rectal prolapse. Small blood vessels are fragile, making suturing difficult during surgery. Large vessels may develop aneurysms, varicosities, arteriovenous fistulas, or may spontaneously rupture. EDS must be considered in every child with recurrent hernias and coagulopathy, especially when accompanied by platelet abnormalities and low coagulation factor levels. Inguinal hernias in these children resemble those seen in adults. Great care should be taken to avoid tearing the skin and fascia. The transversalis fascia is thin and the internal ring is greatly dilated. An adult-type repair with the use of mesh or felt may result in a lower incidence of recurrence. Table 8-3 presents a description of EDS subtypes. (See Schwartz 8th ed., p 230.)

5. Steroids impair wound healing by
   A. Decreasing angiogenesis and macrophage migration
   B. Decreasing platelet plug integrity
   C. Increasing release of lysosomal enzymes
   D. Increasing fibrinolysis

**Answer: A**
Large doses or chronic usage of glucocorticoids reduce collagen synthesis and wound strength. The major effect of steroids is to inhibit the inflammatory phase of wound healing (angiogenesis, neutrophil and macrophage migration, and fibroblast proliferation) and the release of lysosomal enzymes. The stronger the anti-inflammatory effect of the steroid compound used, the greater the inhibitory effect on wound healing. Steroids used after the first 3 to 4 days postinjury do not affect wound healing as severely as when they are used in the immediate postoperative period. Therefore if possible, their use should be delayed or, alternatively, forms with lesser anti-inflammatory effects should be administered. (See Schwartz 8th ed., p 235.)

6. Supplementation of which of the following micronutrients improves wound healing in patients without micronutrient deficiency?
   A. Vitamin C
   B. Vitamin A
   C. Selenium
   D. Zinc

**Answer: B**
The vitamins most closely involved with wound healing are vitamin C and vitamin A. Scurvy or vitamin C deficiency leads to a defect in wound healing, particularly via a failure in collagen synthesis and cross-linking. Biochemically, vitamin C is required for the conversion of proline and lysine to hydroxyproline and hydroxylysine, respectively. The recommended dietary allowance is 60 mg daily. This provides a considerable safety margin for most healthy nonsmokers. In severely injured or extensively burned patients this requirement may increase to as high as 2 g daily. There is no evidence that excess vitamin C is toxic; however, there is no evidence that supertherapeutic doses of vitamin C are of any benefit.

Vitamin A deficiency impairs wound healing, while supplemental vitamin A benefits wound healing in nondeficient humans and animals. Vitamin A increases the inflammatory response in wound healing, probably by increasing the lability of lysosomal membranes. There is an increased influx of macrophages, with an increase in their activation and increased collagen synthesis. Vitamin A directly increases collagen production and epidermal growth factor receptors when it is added in vitro to cultured fibroblasts. As mentioned before, supplemental vitamin A can reverse the inhibitory effects of corticosteroids on wound healing. Vitamin A also can restore wound healing that has been impaired by diabetes, tumor formation, cyclophosphamide, and radiation. Serious injury or stress leads to increased vitamin A requirements. In the severely injured patient, supplemental doses of vitamin A have been recommended. Doses ranging from 25,000 to 100,000 IU per day have been advocated.

Zinc is the most well-known element in wound healing and has been used empirically in dermatologic conditions for centuries. It is essential for wound healing in animals and humans. There are over 150 known enzymes for which zinc is either an integral part or an essential cofactor, and many of these enzymes are critical to wound healing. With zinc deficiency there is decreased fibroblast proliferation, decreased collagen synthesis, impaired overall wound strength, and delayed epithelialization. These defects are reversed by zinc supplementation. To date, no study has shown improved wound healing with zinc supplementation in patients who are not zinc deficient. (See Schwartz 8th ed., p 237.)

7. Signs of malignant transformation in a chronic wound include
   A. Persistent granulation tissue with bleeding
   B. Overturned wound edges
   C. Non-healing after 2 weeks of therapy
   D. Distal edema

**Answer: B**
Malignant transformation of chronic ulcers can occur in any long-standing wound (Marjolin's ulcer). Any wound that does not heal for a prolonged period of time is prone to malignant transformation. Malignant wounds are differentiated clinically from nonmalignant wounds by the presence of overturned wound edges. In patients with suspected malignant transformations, biopsy of the wound edges must be performed to rule out malignancy. Cancers arising de novo in chronic wounds include both squamous and basal cell carcinomas. (See Schwartz 8th ed., p 239.)

8. The treatment of choice for keloids is
   A. Excision alone
   B. Excision with adjuvant therapy (e.g., radiation)
   C. Pressure treatment
   D. Intralesional injection of steroids

**Answer: B**
Excision alone of keloids is subject to a high recurrence rate, ranging from 45 to 100%. There are fewer recurrences when surgical excision is combined with other modalities such as intralesional corticosteroid injection, topical application of silicone sheets, or the use of radiation or pressure. Surgery is recommended for debulking large lesions or as second-line therapy when other modalities have failed. Silicone application is relatively painless and should be maintained for 24 h a day for about 3 months to prevent rebound hypertrophy. It may be secured with tape or worn beneath a pressure garment. The mechanism of action is not understood, but increased hydration of the skin, which decreases capillary activity, inflammation, hyperemia, and collagen deposition, may be involved. Silicone is more effective than other occlusive dressings and is an especially good treatment for children and others who cannot tolerate the pain involved in other modalities. (See Schwartz 8th ed., p 241.)

9. The major cause of impaired wound healing is
   A. Anemia
   B. Diabetes mellitus
   C. Local tissue infection
   D. Malnutrition

**Answer: C**
All the factors listed impair wound healing, but local infection is the major problem. The surgeon should make every effort to remove all devitalized tissue and leave a clean wound for closure. (See Schwartz 7th ed.)

10. Bradykinin, serotonin, and histamine in wounds are released from
    A. Lymphocytes
    B. Mast cells
    C. Polymorphonuclear leukocytes
    D. Platelets

**Answer: B**
Bradykinin, serotonin, and histamine are released from tissue mast cells. They facilitate diapedesis of intravascular cells through vessel walls into the extravascular space of the wound. (See Schwartz 7th ed.)

11. Platelets in the wound form a hemostatic clot and release clotting factors to produce
    A. Fibrin
    B. Fibrinogen
    C. Thrombin
    D. Thromboplastin

**Answer: A**
Platelet clotting factors initiate a healing cascade by producing hemostatic fibrin. A mesh is produced, and inflammatory cells and fibroblasts migrate into the mesh. Fibrin is formed from fibrinogen, which is formed by the action of thrombin in the presence of thromboplastin. (See Schwartz 7th ed.)

12. In a healing wound, metalloproteinases are responsible for
    A. Establishing collagen cross-links
    B. Glycosylation of collagen molecules
    C. Incorporation of hydroxyproline into the collagen chain
    D. Initiating collagen degradation

**Answer: D**
In a healing wound, collagen is both synthesized and degraded. Specific enzymes called metalloproteinases initiate degradation. The other processes listed are involved in collagen synthesis. (See Schwartz 7th ed.)

13. Severe cases of hidradenitis suppurativa in the groin area are best managed by excision of the involved area and
    A. Closure by secondary intention
    B. Delayed primary closure
    C. Primary closure
    D. Split thickness skin grafting

**Answer: A**
Healing of these wounds is difficult because of the indolent infection in the area. Closure by secondary intention is the preferred method, allowing the wound margins to come together spontaneously after the infection is controlled. (See Schwartz 7th ed.)

14. All of the following statements about keloids are true EXCEPT
    A. A keloid does not regress spontaneously.
    B. A keloid extends beyond the boundaries of the original wound.
    C. Keloids or hypertrophic scars are best managed by excision and careful reapproximation of the wound.
    D. Keloid tissue contains an abnormally large amount of collagen.

**Answer: C**
Keloids and hypertrophic scars both occur after injuries or operations. Hypertrophic scars remain confined to the original injury site and usually regress spontaneously. By contrast, keloids extend beyond the original wound and rarely regress. Keloids contain abnormally large amounts of soluble collagen and water. Keloids tend to recur after excision, and any surgical therapy should be undertaken cautiously, with the patient aware that the result may not be ideal. (See Schwartz 7th ed.)

15. When a long bone fracture is repaired by internal fixation with plates and screws,
    A. Callus at the fracture site forms more rapidly
    B. Delayed union is prevented
    C. Direct bone-to-bone healing occurs without soft callus formation
    D. Endochondral ossification is more complete

**Answer: C**
Precise fracture reduction and fixation allows the fracture to heal bone-to-bone without the soft callus formation and endochondral ossification, which are characteristic of closed fracture management. However, internal reduction does not prevent delayed union, especially when infection or poor blood supply are present. (See Schwartz 7th ed.)

1. The highest incidence of breast cancer in the world is in
   A. Africa
   B. North America
   C. South America
   D. Asia

**Answer: B**
The incidence of breast cancer is high in all of the most highly developed regions except Japan, including the United States and Canada, Australia, and Northern and Western Europe, ranging from 67.3 to 86.3 per 100,000 women per year. In comparison, the rates are relatively low (less than 30 per 100,000 women) in sub-Saharan Africa (except South Africa) and Asia. The highest breast cancer incidence is in the United States and the lowest is in China. Although breast cancer has been linked to cancer susceptibility genes, mutations in these genes account for only 5 to 10% of breast tumors, suggesting that the wide geographic variations in breast cancer incidence are not due to geographic variations in the prevalence of these genes. Most of the differences, therefore, are attributed to differences in reproductive factors, diet, and other environmental differences. Indeed, breast cancer risk increases significantly in females who have migrated from Asia to America. Overall, the incidence of breast cancer is rising in most countries. (See Schwartz 8th ed., p 252.)

2. Which of the following is a tyrosine kinase oncogene?
   A. HER2/*neu*
   B. c-*myc*
   C. k-ras
   D. *p*53

**Answer: A**
Protein tyrosine kinases account for a large portion of known oncogenes. HER2/*neu*, also known as c-*erb*B-2, is a member of the epidermal growth factor (EGF) receptor (EGFR) family and is one of the best characterized tyrosine kinases. Unlike other receptor tyrosine kinases, HER2/*neu* does not have a direct soluble ligand. It plays a key role in signaling, however, as it is the preferred partner in heterodimer formation with all the other EGFR family members (EGFR/c-*erb*B-1, HER2/c-*erb*B-3, and HER3/c-*erb*B-4), which bind at least 30 ligands including EGF, transforming growth factor alpha (TGF-α), heparin-binding EGF-like growth factor, amphiregulin, and heregulin. Heterodimerization with HER2/*neu* potentiates recycling of receptors rather than degradation, enhances signal potency and duration, increases affinity for ligands, and increases catalytic activity. (See Schwartz 8th ed., p 257.)

3. Li-Fraumeni syndrome is associated with a mutation of which of the following genes?
   A. BRCA-1
   B. APC
   C. *p*53
   D. PTEN

**Answer: C**
Li-Fraumeni syndrome (LFS) was first defined on the basis of observations of clustering of malignancies, including early-onset breast cancer, soft-tissue sarcomas, brain tumors, adrenocortical tumors, and leukemia. Criteria for classic LFS in an individual (the proband) include: (1) a bone or soft-

tissue sarcoma when younger than 45 years, (2) a first-degree relative with cancer before age 45 years, and (3) another first- or second-degree relative with either a sarcoma diagnosed at any age or any cancer diagnosed before age 45 years. Approximately 70% of LFS families have been shown to have germline mutations in the tumor suppressor *p*53 gene. Breast carcinoma, soft-tissue sarcoma, osteosarcoma, brain tumors, adrenocortical carcinoma, Wilms' tumor, and phyllodes tumor of the breast are strongly associated; pancreatic cancer is moderately associated; and leukemia and neuroblastoma are weakly associated with germline *p*53 mutations. Mutations of *p*53 have not been detected in approximately 30% of LFS families, and it is hypothesized that genetic alterations in other proteins interacting with *p*53 function may play a role in these families. (See Schwartz 8th ed., p 262.)

**Answer: D**

4. Aflatoxin exposure is associated with which of the following cancers?
   A. Lung cancer
   B. Vaginal clear cell carcinoma
   C. Endometrial cancer
   D. Liver cancer

**Table 9-1.**
**Selected IARC Group 1 Chemical Carcinogens**

| Chemical | Predominant Tumor Type |
|---|---|
| Aflatoxins | Liver cancer |
| Arsenic | Skin cancer |
| Benzene | Leukemia |
| Benzidine | Bladder cancer |
| Beryllium | Lung cancer |
| Cadmium | Lung cancer |
| Chinese-style salted fish | Nasopharyngeal carcinoma |
| Chlorambucil | Leukemia |
| Chromium [VI] compounds | Lung cancer |
| Coal tar | Skin cancer, scrotal cancer |
| Cyclophosphamide | Bladder cancer, leukemia |
| Diethylstilbestrol (DES) | Vaginal and cervical clear cell adenocarcinomas |
| Ethylene oxide | Leukemia, lymphoma |
| Estrogen replacement therapy | Endometrial cancer, breast cancer |
| Nickel | Lung cancer, nasal cancer |
| Tamoxifen | Endometrial cancer |
| Vinyl chloride | Angiosarcoma of the liver, hepatocellular carcinoma, brain tumors, lung cancer, malignancies of lymphatic and hematopoietic system |
| TCDD (2,3,7,8-tetrachlorodibenzo-para-dioxin) | Soft-tissue sarcoma |
| Tobacco products, smokeless | Oral cancer |
| Tobacco smoke | Lung cancer, oral cancer, pharyngeal cancer, laryngeal cancer, esophageal cancer (squamous cell, pancreatic cancer, bladder cancer, liver cancer, renal cell carcinoma, cervical cancer, leukemia) |

5. The origin of carcinoembryonic antigen is embryonic
   A. Endoderm
   B. Mesoderm
   C. Ectoderm
   D. Mesenchyme

**Answer: A**

Carcinoembryonic antigen (CEA) is a glycoprotein found in the embryonic endodermal epithelium. Elevated CEA levels have been detected in patients with primary colorectal cancer, as well as patients with breast, lung, ovarian, prostate, liver, or pancreatic cancer. Levels of CEA also may be elevated in benign conditions such as diverticulitis, peptic ulcer disease, bronchitis, liver abscess, and alcoholic cirrhosis, especially in smokers and in elderly persons. (See Schwartz 8th ed., p 273.)

6. Elevation of cancer antigen 15-3 is useful in detecting metastatic
   A. Liver cancer
   B. Pancreatic cancer
   C. Thyroid cancer
   D. Breast cancer

**Answer: D**

Cancer antigen 15-3 (CA 15-3) is an epitope of a large membrane glycoprotein, encoded by the *MUC1* gene, which tumor cells shed into the bloodstream. The CA 15-3 epitope is recognized by two monoclonal antibodies in a sandwich radioimmunoassay. CA 15-3 levels are most useful in following the course of treatment in women diagnosed with advanced breast cancer. The CA 15-3 levels are infrequently elevated in early breast cancer. Only 9% of patients with stage I breast cancer and 19% of women with stage II cancer have elevated CA 15-3 levels. The predictive value of a positive test result is calculated to be 0.7% for stage I disease and 1.5% for stage II disease emphasizing that CA 15-3 is not an appropriate screening tool. CA 15-3 levels can be elevated in benign conditions such as chronic hepatitis, tuberculosis, sarcoidosis, pelvic inflammatory disease, endometriosis, systemic lupus erythematosus, pregnancy and lactation, and in other types of cancer such as lung, ovarian, endometrial, and gastrointestinal cancers. (See Schwartz 8th ed., p 273.)

7. Which of the following tumor markers is the best to monitor recurrence of colon cancer?
   A. α-fetoprotein
   B. Carcinoembryonic antigen
   C. Cancer antigen 15-3
   D. 5-hydroxyindoleacetic acid

**Answer: B**

Efforts to develop serum tumor markers useful in screening for various cancers have been of limited value. However, these markers may be helpful in following patients during and after therapy. Carcinoembryonic antigen is not specific for colon cancer, but rising values after treatment are suggestive of recurrence. α-Fetoprotein is associated with hepatocellular adenocarcinoma. Calcitonin is a marker for medullary thyroid cancer. Cancer antigen 15-3 is being studied in patients with breast cancer. Carcinoid tumors are associated with elevations in 5-hydroxyindoleacetic acid. (See Schwartz 7th ed.)

8. Postoperative wound infections after operations for head and neck cancer are most frequently caused by
   A. *Bacillus fragilis*
   B. *Escherichia coli*
   C. Gram-negative anaerobes
   D. *Staphylococcus aureus*

**Answer: D**

Because the nasal and oral pharyngeal cavities are open during operation on many head and neck cancers, postoperative wound infections are frequent complications of these operations, with incidence figures between 15% and 40%. *Staphylococcus aureus* is the most frequent pathogen, and gram-negative anaerobes are also common problems. (See Schwartz 7th ed.)

9. The multidrug resistance gene
   A. Blocks drug activation
   B. Blocks intracellular DNA synthesis
   C. Causes efflux of drugs from intracellular space of target host cells
   D. Interferes with DNA repair in target host cells

**Answer: C**

A multidrug resistance gene has been identified. Its protein product is a P-glycoprotein, which causes an efflux of several drugs from the intracellular space of host cells. This protein is found in high levels in normal cells leaving the luminal spaces of the gastrointestinal tract, liver, and kidney where it is preserved to induce an active efflux of environmental toxins from the body. (See Schwartz 7th ed.)

10. When a woman develops pulmonary metastases from a breast carcinoma, she will most frequently complain of
    A. Chronic cough
    B. Hemoptysis
    C. Shortness of breath
    D. No specific symptoms

**Answer: D**

Most pulmonary metastases are asymptomatic. If a metastatic lesion involves a main bronchus, any of the listed symptoms may develop. However, the metastatic lesions are most frequently discovered on a follow-up radiograph of the chest. (See Schwartz 7th ed.)

11. Emergency radiation therapy is used for each of the following EXCEPT
    A. Sigmoid colon obstruction from carcinoma
    B. Spinal cord compression from metastatic prostatic carcinoma
    C. Superior vena caval obstruction from carcinoma of the lung
    D. Vertebral bone pain from metastatic breast cancer

**Answer: A**

Colonic obstruction from a sigmoid carcinoma is a surgical emergency. When malignant disease is responsible for upper airway obstruction, superior vena caval obstruction or spinal cord compression tumor response to radiation therapy provides effective palliation. The relief of bone pain after radiation therapy for metastatic vertebral disease is dramatic. (See Schwartz 7th ed.)

12. A chemotherapeutic agent to be used in a patient with diffuse peritoneal metastases should produce all of the following effects EXCEPT
    A. Lipid solubility
    B. Little or no toxicity
    C. Low rate of peritoneal absorption
    D. Rapid plasma clearance

**Answer: B**

Chemotherapeutic agents affect normal cells as well as cancer cells, and toxicity must be anticipated from an effective agent. If an agent has high lipid solubility, tumoricidal activity, and a low rate of peritoneal absorption, it should be an effective agent. If it is cleared rapidly from plasma, systemic toxicity should be limited. Cisplatin fulfills these characteristics. (See Schwartz 7th ed.)

13. Survivors of the nuclear bombs dropped on Japan in 1945 have an increased incidence of each of the following EXCEPT
    A. Carcinoma of the breast
    B. Carcinoma of the colon
    C. Carcinoma of the lung
    D. Carcinoma of the thyroid

**Answer: B**

Long-term side effects of radiation represent important health problems. Survivors of the nuclear explosions in Hiroshima and Nagasaki show increased incidence of breast, lung, and thyroid cancer and of chronic myeloid leukemia after a latent period of over 10 years. No increase in colon cancer has been observed. (See Schwartz 7th ed.)

14. Characteristic findings in a malignant lesion include all of the following EXCEPT
    A. Cellular polymorphism
    B. Loss of cell polarity
    C. Nuclear polymorphism
    D. Polyclonal origin

**Answer: D**

Although the cells in a malignant lesion show loss of cell polarity and marked polymorphism both in the cells themselves and in their nuclei, it is believed that most malignant tumors originate in multiplication of a single abnormal cell with deranged growth regulation. (See Schwartz 7th ed.)

15. Epstein-Barr virus has been associated with the development of each of the following malignancies EXCEPT
    A. B-cell lymphoma
    B. Burkitt's lymphoma
    C. Cancer of the pancreas
    D. Nasopharyngeal carcinoma

**Answer: C**

There are a number of tumor-associated viruses recognized in human malignancies. Epstein-Barr virus (EBV) is a DNA virus that is associated with several diseases of the lymphatic system, among them are B-cell lymphoma, Burkitt's lymphoma, and Hodgkin's disease. Nasopharyngeal carcinoma is also associated with EBV. Carcinoma of the pancreas has been increasing in incidence, but no etiologic agent has been implicated in this process. (See Schwartz 7th ed.)

16. A tumor with much higher incidence in the United States than in Africa is cancer of the
    A. Bladder
    B. Colon
    C. Liver
    D. Stomach

**Answer: B**

Colon cancer in the United States is significantly more common than it is in Africa. It is believed that the high roughage diet among African natives produces a more rapid transit time in the colon, thus reducing the time of mucosal exposure to luminal carcinogens secondary to high fat content of the U.S. diet. Bladder cancer is more frequent in the United States than in Japan, whereas the incidence of gastric cancer is much higher among Japanese. Buccal cavity cancer is prevalent in all areas where tobacco chewing is a common practice. Primary cancer of the liver is most frequent in southeast Asia and Africa, where it is associated with hepatitis B virus infection. (See Schwartz 7th ed.)

17. The effectiveness of radiation therapy of carcinoma is decreased by
    A. Administration of actinomycin D
    B. Decrease in local tissue temperature
    C. Increased radiation dose during each treatment
    D. Low-tissue oxygen tension

**Answer: D**

Low-tissue oxygen tension secondary to such effects as fibrosis around the tumor, or necrosis within the tumor, decreases the effectiveness of radiation. This is true because molecular oxygen must be present for maximal cell killing by ionizing radiation. Increasing the radiation dose during each treatment kills more tumor cells, but the normal surrounding tissues receive greater injury, and the overall effect does not favor the host. Actinomycin D and doxorubicin therapy, as well as increased local heat to 42°C or 45°C, increase cell killing by inhibiting repair processes. Target DNA is more radiosensitive when thymidine is replaced by a halogenated pyrimidine analogue such as 5-bromodeoxyuridine (BUdR) or 5-fluorodeoxyuridine (FUdR). (See Schwartz 7th ed.)

18. The high prevalence of gastric cancer in Japan is
    A. Equally a hereditary and an environmental issue
    B. Primarily an environmental issue
    C. Primarily a hereditary issue
    D. Unrelated to hereditary or environmental issues

**Answer: B**

When Japanese move to Hawaii, the prevalence of gastric cancer falls to the level of Hawaiians of American or European descent within two generations. This suggests that an environmental factor, probably dietary, is responsible for the high gastric cancer prevalence in Japan. At the same time, Japanese who move to Hawaii experience an increase in colon cancer, and, again, this is probably due to dietary change. (See Schwartz 7th ed.)

19. After resection of a high-risk (stage II-B) melanoma from the right thigh, the most promising management is currently
    A. Administration of bovine tuberculosis bacillus vaccine
    B. Administration of a recombinant cytokine (interferon-α-2b)
    C. Limb perfusion chemotherapy
    D. Radiation therapy to the thigh and groin
    E. Wider local resection and regional lymph node resection

**Answer: B**

All the modalities listed have been used in managing high-risk melanoma. A randomized controlled trial use of interferon-α-2b, a recombinant cytokine, has shown a significant increase in both median disease-free and median overall survival. (See Schwartz 7th ed.)

20. All of the following conditions are known to have a familial pattern associated with a predisposition to cancer EXCEPT
    A. Colonic polyposis
    B. Breast cancer
    C. Peutz-Jeghers syndrome
    D. Gardner's syndrome

**Answer: C**
Patients who have either familial polyposis or Gardner's syndrome are predisposed to develop carcinoma of the colon or rectum. Although the gene for Gardner's syndrome is thought to be distinct from that determining familial polyposis, the possibility exists that there is only one gene with variable expressivity and that patients with familial polyposis do not have the extracolonic abnormalities of Gardner's syndrome expressed. Breast cancer is also associated with a familial predisposition and occurs three times more commonly in the daughters of affected women than in the general population. Retinoblastoma has a distinct familial predisposition. In Peutz-Jeghers syndrome, the intestinal polyps now are believed to be hamartomas rather than adenomas, and whether the malignant gastrointestinal tract tumors that have been reported represent coincidence or a malignant potential is not yet clear. (See Schwartz 7th ed.)

21. In a 20-year-old woman with an asymptomatic 2-cm mass in the lower pole of the right thyroid lobe, the most appropriate initial maneuver is
    A. Excisional biopsy
    B. Incisional biopsy
    C. Needle aspiration cytology
    D. Radioiodine uptake study

**Answer: C**
Needle aspiration cytology of the thyroid has become the method of choice for diagnosis of thyroid nodules. Radio-immunoassay uptake and thyroid ultrasonography have been largely replaced. Needle aspiration cytology is quite accurate for identifying a papillary neoplasm. Follicular lesions are more difficult to evaluate because it is hard to define the capsule of the nodule without a larger specimen. (See Schwartz 7th ed.)

22. The first step in carcinogenesis produced by an RNA virus is
    A. Alteration in the cell wall
    B. Destruction of the cell nuclear membrane
    C. Integration into host chromosomal DNA
    D. Transcription into cellular DNA

**Answer: D**
Viral RNA is transcribed into cellular DNA by reverse transcriptase. It then becomes part of the host chromosomal DNA. It is for this reason that management of RNA-induced tumor is difficult; an agent that destroys the viral RNA destroys the DNA of the host cell. (See Schwartz 7th ed.)

23. Which of the following is recommended for cancer screening?
    A. Annual mammography for women older than age 35
    B. Annual prostate-specific antigen for men starting at age 50
    C. Annual flexible sigmoidoscopy starting at age 50
    D. Annual PAP smear for women starting at age 30

**Answer: B**
See Table 9-2 on p 73.

**Table 9-2.**
**American Cancer Society Recommendations for Early Detection of Cancer in Average-Risk, Asymptomatic People**

| Cancer Site | Population | Test or Procedure | Frequency |
|---|---|---|---|
| Breast | Women, age 20+ | Breast self-examination | Monthly, starting at age 20 |
| | | Clinical breast examination | Every 3 years, ages 20–39 |
| | | | Annual, starting at age 40 |
| | | Mammography | Annual, starting at age 40 |
| Colorectal | Men and women, age 50+ | Fecal occult blood test (FOBT) *or* | Annual, starting at age 20 |
| | | Flexible sigmoidoscopy *or* | Every 5 years, starting at age 50 |
| | | Fecal occult blood test and flexible sigmoidoscopy *or* | Annual FOBT and flexible sigmoidoscopy every 5 years, starting at age 50 |
| | | Double-contrast barium enema (DCBE) *or* | DCBE every 5 years, starting at age 50 |
| | | Colonoscopy | Colonoscopy every 10 years, starting at age 50 |
| Prostate | Men, age 50+ | Digital rectal examination (DRE) and prostate-specific antigen test (PSA) | Offer PSA and DRE annually, starting at age 50, for men who have life expectancy of at least 10 years |
| Cervix | Women | Pap test | Cervical cancer screening beginning 3 years after first vaginal intercourse, but no later than 21 years of age; screening every year with conventional Pap tests or every 2 years using liquid-based Pap tests; at or after age 30, women who have had three or more normal Pap tests and no abnormal Pap tests in the last 10 years, and women who have had a total hysterectomy, may choose to stop cervical cancer screening |
| Cancer-related check-up | Men and women, age 20+ | On the occasion of a periodic health examination, the cancer-related check-up should include examination of the thyroid, testicles, ovaries, lymph nodes, oral cavity, and skin, as well as health counseling about tobacco, sun exposure, diet and nutrition, risk factors, sexual practices, and environmental and occupational exposures. | |

Source: Modified with permission from Smith RA, Cokkinides V, Eyre HJ: American Cancer Society guidelines for the early detection of cancer, 2003. *CA Cancer J Clin* 53:27, 2003.
See Schwartz 8th ed., p 269.

1. Hyperacute rejection is caused by
   A. Preformed antibodies
   B. B-cell–generated antidonor antibodies
   C. T-cell–mediated allorejection
   D. Nonimmune mechanism

**Answer: A**

Hyperacute rejection, which usually occurs within minutes after the transplanted organ is reperfused, is due to the presence of preformed antibodies in the recipient, antibodies that are specific to the donor. These antibodies may be directed against the donor's HLA antigens or they may be anti-ABO blood group antibodies. Either way, they bind to the vascular endothelium in the graft and activate the complement cascade, leading to platelet activation and to diffuse intravascular coagulation. The result is a swollen, darkened graft, which undergoes ischemic necrosis. This type of rejection is generally not reversible, so prevention is key.

Prevention is best done by making sure the graft is ABO-compatible and by performing a pretransplant cross-match. The cross-match is an in vitro test that involves mixing the donor's cells with the recipient's serum to look for evidence of donor cell destruction by recipient antibodies. A positive cross-match indicates the presence of preformed antibodies in the recipient that are specific to the donor, thus a high risk of hyperacute rejection if the transplant is performed. (See Schwartz 8th ed., p 298.)

2. The mechanism of action of azathioprine is
   A. Inhibition of calcineurin
   B. Interference with DNA synthesis
   C. Binding of FK-506 binding proteins
   D. Inhibition of P7056 kinase

**Answer: B**

Azathioprine (AZA) acts late in the immune process, affecting the cell cycle by interfering with DNA synthesis, thus suppressing proliferation of activated B and T lymphocytes. AZA is valuable in preventing the onset of acute rejection, but is not effective in the treatment of rejection episodes themselves.

Cyclosporine binds with its cytoplasmic receptor protein, cyclophilin, which subsequently inhibits the activity of calcineurin. Doing so impairs expression of several critical T-cell activation genes, the most important being for interleukin-2 (IL-2). As a result, T-cell activation is suppressed. The metabolism of cyclosporine is via the cytochrome P450 system, therefore several drug interactions are possible. Inducers of P450 such as phenytoin decrease blood levels; drugs such as erythromycin, cimetidine, ketoconazole, and fluconazole increase them.

Tacrolimus, like cyclosporine, is a calcineurin inhibitor and has a very similar mechanism of action. Cyclosporine acts by binding cyclophilins, while tacrolimus acts by binding FK506-binding proteins (FKBPs). The tacrolimus-FKBP complex inhibits the enzyme calcineurin, which is essential for activating transcription factors in response to the rise in intracellular calcium seen with stimulation of the T-cell receptor (TCR). The net effect of tacrolimus is to inhibit T-cell function by preventing synthesis of IL-2 and other important cytokines.

Sirolimus (previously known as rapamycin) is structurally similar to tacrolimus and binds to the same immunophilin (FKBP). Unlike tacrolimus, it does not affect calcineurin activity, and therefore does not block the calcium-dependent activation of cytokine genes. Rather, the active complex binds so-called target of rapamycin (TOR) proteins (Fig. 10-2), resulting in inhibition of P7056 kinase (an enzyme linked to cell division). The net result is to prevent progression from the $G_1$ to the S phase of the cell cycle, halting cell division.

Mycophenolate mofetil works by inhibiting inosine monophosphate dehydrogenase, which is a crucial, rate-limiting enzyme in de novo synthesis of purines. Specifically, this enzyme catalyzes the formation of guanosine nucleotides from inosine. Many cells have a salvage pathway and therefore can bypass this need for guanosine nucleotide synthesis by the de novo pathway. Activated lymphocytes, however, do not possess this salvage pathway and require de novo synthesis for clonal expansion. The net result is a selective, reversible antiproliferative effect on T and B lymphocytes. (See Schwartz 8th ed., p 300.)

3. Which of the following is NOT a side effect of cyclosporine?
   A. Interstitial fibrosis of the renal parenchyma
   B. Gingival hyperplasia
   C. Headache
   D. Pancreatitis

**Answer: D**

Adverse effects of cyclosporine can be classified as renal or nonrenal. Nephrotoxicity is the most important and troubling adverse effect of cyclosporine. Cyclosporine has a vasoconstrictor effect on the renal vasculature. This vasoconstriction (likely a transient, reversible, and dose-dependent phenomenon) may cause early posttransplant graft dysfunction or may exaggerate existing poor graft function. Also, long-term cyclosporine use may result in interstitial fibrosis of the renal parenchyma, coupled with arteriolar lesions. The exact mechanism is unknown, but renal failure may eventually result.

A number of nonrenal side effects may also be seen with the use of cyclosporine. Cosmetic complications, most commonly hirsutism and gingival hyperplasia, may result in considerable distress, possibly leading to noncompliant behavior, especially in adolescents and women. Several neurologic complications, including headaches, tremor, and seizures, also have been reported. Other nonrenal side effects include hyperlipidemia, hepatotoxicity, and hyperuricemia. (See Schwartz 8th ed., p 300.)

4. Lymphoceles occur how long after a renal transplant?
   A. Within 48 h
   B. ~1 week after surgery
   C. 2–4 weeks after surgery
   D. 3 months after surgery

**Answer: C**

The reported incidence of lymphoceles (fluid collections of lymph that generally result from cut lymphatic vessels in the recipient) is 0.6 to 18%. Lymphoceles usually do not occur until at least two weeks posttransplant. Symptoms are generally related to the mass effect and compression of nearby structures (e.g., ureter, iliac vein, allograft renal artery), and patients develop hypertension, unilateral leg swelling on the side of the transplant, and elevated serum creatinine. Ultrasound is used to confirm a fluid collection, although percutaneous aspiration may be necessary to exclude presence of other collections such as urinomas, hematomas, or abscesses. The standard surgical treatment is creation of a peritoneal window to allow for drainage of the lymphatic fluid into the peritoneal cavity where it can be absorbed. Either a laparoscopic or an open approach may be used. Another option is percutaneous insertion of a drainage catheter, with or without sclerotherapy; however, it is associated with some risk of recurrence or infection. (See Schwartz 8th ed., pp 309–310.)

5. The 5-year graft survival rate after renal transplantation is
   A. 35–40%
   B. 50–55%
   C. 75–80%
   D. 90–95%

**Answer: C**
The incidence of acute rejection has declined steadily since the early 1990s. Most centers now report acute rejection rates of 10 to 20% at 1 year posttransplant. This decline has been a major factor in the improvement in graft survival rates, which are now about 75 to 80% at 5 years and 60 to 65% at 10 years posttransplant for all kidney recipients. Currently, the most common cause of graft loss is recipient death (usually from cardiovascular causes) with a functioning graft. The second most common cause is chronic allograft nephropathy. Characterized by a slow, unrelenting deterioration of graft function, it likely has multiple causes (both immunologic and nonimmunologic). The graft failure rate due to surgical technique has remained at about 2%. (See Schwartz 8th ed., pp 310–311.)

6. After completion of the vascular anastomoses, drainage of a transplanted pancreas is accomplished by anastomosis to
   A. Right colon
   B. Left colon
   C. Duodenum
   D. Bladder or small bowel

**Answer: D**
Once the pancreas is revascularized, a drainage procedure must be performed to handle the pancreatic exocrine secretions. Options include anastomosing the donor duodenum to the recipient bladder or to the small bowel, with the small bowel either in continuity or connected to a Roux-en-Y limb. Some centers always use enteric drainage, others always use bladder drainage, and others tailor the approach according to the recipient category. Both enteric drainage and bladder drainage now have a relatively low surgical risk. The main advantage of bladder drainage is the ability to directly measure enzyme activity in the pancreatic graft exocrine secretions by measuring the amount of amylase in the urine. A decrease in urine amylase is a sensitive marker for rejection, even though it is not entirely specific. Urine amylase always decreases before hyperglycemia ensues. A rise in serum amylase may precede a decrease in urine amylase, but serum amylase by itself is less sensitive (it does not always rise, but urine amylase always decreases), and is no more specific for the diagnosis of rejection. The leak rate is the same whether the pancreas is drained to the bladder or to the bowel, but the consequences of a bladder leak are much less severe than those associated with a bowel leak. The disadvantages of bladder drainage include complications such as dehydration and acidosis (from loss of alkalotic pancreatic secretions in the urine), and local problems with the bladder such as infection, hematuria, stones, and urethritis. Because of these chronic complications, between 10 and 20% of bladder-drained graft recipients are ultimately converted to enteric drainage.

Enteric drainage is more physiologic and has fewer long-term complications. However, the ability to monitor for rejection is decreased, given the absence of urinary amylase. Rejection in simultaneous pancreas and kidney (SPK) transplant recipients almost always affects both the kidney and the pancreas; therefore, the serum creatinine level can be used as a marker for rejection of the pancreas. Hence, most centers now use enteric drainage for SPK transplants. If the kidney and the pancreas are from different donors, or if a pancreas transplant alone (PTA) is performed, then bladder drainage is preferred, so rejection of the pancreas can be detected earlier. (See Schwartz 8th ed., p 313.)

7. All of the following are absolute contraindications in considering a candidate for orthotopic cardiac transplantation EXCEPT
   A. Active infection
   B. Age over 65 years
   C. History of medical noncompliance
   D. Severe renal insufficiency

**Answer: A**
Active infection is considered a potentially reversible contraindication to cardiac transplantation. The other conditions listed are absolute contraindications to orthotopic cardiac transplantation. Heterotopic cardiac transplantation, in which the patient's right heart continues to work against the pulmonary hypertension while the donor heart supplies systemic circulation, is used for a certain number of patients with pulmonary hypertension. (See Schwartz 7th ed.)

8. Absolute contraindications for donation of a heart include all of the following EXCEPT
   A. Carbon monoxide-hemoglobin level >20%
   B. Prolonged cardiac arrest
   C. Prolonged high-dopamine requirement
   D. Significant smoking history

**Answer: C**
The use of high doses of dopamine for more than 24 h before death is a relative contraindication to transplantation of the heart. The other listed items are all absolute contraindications to cardiac donation. Severe structural heart disease and human immunodeficiency virus seropositivity are other absolute contraindications. (See Schwartz 7th ed.)

9. Required laboratory tests in evaluation of a patient under consideration for heart transplantation include all of the following EXCEPT
   A. Blood type
   B. Cardiac catheterization
   C. Complete blood count
   D. Prothrombin time and activated partial thromboplastin time

**Answer: B**
Cardiac catheterization may be indicated in some patients to evaluate cardiac function. The other tests are required in any patient under consideration for cardiac transplantation. (See Schwartz 7th ed.)

10. Immunologic rejection is mediated by the recipient's
    A. Eosinophils
    B. Lymphocytes
    C. Neutrophils
    D. Plasma cells

**Answer: B**
Early work in the transplantation field showed that graft rejection was mediated by the recipient's white blood cells. Refinement of the techniques involved demonstrated that the lymphocytes played the major role in this phenomenon. The development of antilymphocyte serum was an early step in controlling the rejection process. (See Schwartz 7th ed.)

11. In the prevention of graft rejection, cyclosporine
    A. Blocks transcription of interleukin-1 (IL-1) and tumor necrosis factor-α (TNF-α)
    B. Inhibits lymphocyte nucleic acid metabolism
    C. Results in rapid decrease in the number of circulatory T lymphocytes
    D. Selectively inhibits T-cell activation

**Answer: D**
There are a number of different agents used to control graft rejection, and they function in different ways. Cyclosporine, the mainstay of immunosuppression, selectively inhibits T-cell activation. Corticosteroids block the transcription of IL-1 and TNF-α. Azathioprine inhibits lymphocyte nucleic acid metabolism. Mycophenolate mofetil inhibits RNA and DNA synthesis. OKT3 results in a rapid decrease in circulatory T lymphocytes. (See Schwartz 7th ed.)

12. The most common cause of renal failure in the United States is
    A. Chronic glomerulonephritis
    B. Chronic pyelonephritis
    C. Diabetes mellitus
    D. Obstructive uropathy

**Answer: C**
Because the life expectancy of patients with diabetes mellitus has dramatically lengthened by appropriate use of insulin, diabetes is now the leading cause of renal failure and contributes to blindness, neuropathies, and early atherosclerosis. These problems have led to the continued interest in the possibility of pancreatic transplantation as a form of disease control. (See Schwartz 7th ed.)

13. The best method of monitoring the development of acute rejection in a patient after cardiac transplantation is
    A. Dipyridamole thallium study
    B. Electrocardiogram
    C. Endomyocardial biopsy
    D. Ultrasound examination of the heart

**Answer: C**
It would be desirable to follow possible rejection by some noninvasive procedure, but none has given timely results. Endomyocardial biopsies allow rejection to be diagnosed before significant organ damage and dysfunction occur. (See Schwartz 7th ed.)

14. Absolute contraindications to renal transplantation for a patient with chronic renal failure include all of the following EXCEPT
    A. Chronic active hepatitis
    B. Human immunodeficiency virus infection
    C. Recent operation of cancer of the colon
    D. Sickle cell disease

**Answer: D**
Sickle cell disease is a relative contraindication to renal transplantation because of the associated high incidence of recurrence. The other listed conditions are considered absolute contraindications because of the patient's generally poor health prognosis. (See Schwartz 7th ed.)

15. All of the following conditions in a potential donor are absolute contraindications to the use of a kidney for transplantation EXCEPT
    A. Age older than 70 years
    B. Chronic renal insufficiency
    C. Long-standing hypertension
    D. Presence of hepatitis C

**Answer: D**
Cadaveric kidneys make up 75% of all donor kidneys, and the demand far exceeds the supply. For this reason, donor criteria have been liberalized in recent years. Advanced age, chronic renal insufficiency, intravenous drug abuse, and long-standing hypertension remain absolute contraindications. Human immunodeficiency virus seropositivity and the presence of surface antigens against hepatitis B are also absolute contraindications. Although there is risk associated with using a kidney from a donor with evidence of hepatitis C, this condition is not considered an absolute contraindication to kidney use. (See Schwartz 7th ed.)

16. The single most important factor in determining whether to perform a transplant between a specific donor and recipient is
    A. Mixed lymphocyte culture assays of the donor and recipient
    B. HLA types of the donor and recipient
    C. ABO blood types of the donor and recipient
    D. Peripheral T-cell count of the recipient

**Answer: C**
Although mixed lymphocyte culture assays and HLA typing of the donor and recipient to determine compatibility have been shown to enhance long-term graft survival, immediate graft function has been correlated to the absence of the presensitized state. This presensitization can be with respect to lymphocytotoxic antibodies or preformed isoagglutinins. ABO compatibility is essential in renal and cardiac transplantation because incompatibility leads to prompt destruction of the transplanted organ. In liver transplantation, the presensitized state is of less importance, but diminished graft survival has been demonstrated in ABO-incompatible combinations. (See Schwartz 7th ed.)

17. A 24-year-old woman is admitted to the intensive care unit for sudden collapse with progressive neurologic deficits. A computed tomography scan reveals an intracranial tumor with evidence of acute hemorrhage. Emergent craniotomy is done for decompression, and tissue obtained reveals high-grade malignant astrocytoma. On postoperative day 1, the patient is placed on large doses of phenobarbital for seizure activity but continues to deteriorate. On day 3, she requires dopamine support at 10 mg/kg/min to maintain a systolic blood pressure of 90 mm Hg. She develops diabetes insipidus, and her urine output is adequate, although her creatinine rises to 1.5 mg/dL and the blood urea nitrogen (BUN) is 40 mg/dL. A urine culture from a Foley specimen yields *Escherichia coli* at 100,000/mL. On day 4, she becomes unresponsive, without evidence of cortical or brainstem function. An electroencephalogram (EEG) is isoelectric. Which of the following is an absolute contraindication for consideration of this woman as a potential organ donor?
    A. Presence of high-grade intracranial malignancy
    B. Requirement of pressor support
    C. Elevated BUN and creatinine
    D. Presence of supratherapeutic phenobarbital levels

**Answer: D**
The presence of phenobarbital, narcotics or alcohol, or of hypothermia is a contraindication to organ donation, even with an isoelectric EEG. This is because these factors may suppress spontaneous electric activity of the brain. Intracranial tumors are not considered a contraindication, mainly because of their lack of systemic metastasis. Other malignancies do contraindicate donation. The need for pressor is not necessarily a contraindication, especially if these drugs are used in the terminal period to maintain blood pressure and urine output. Elevations of BUN and creatinine are not uncommon, especially in the face of diabetes insipidus with prerenal azotemia. Adequate urine output is the most important factor in consideration of renal organ donation. Lower urinary tract infection caused by instrumentation is not a contraindication to donation of kidneys, whereas systemic or peritoneal sepsis is. (See Schwartz 7th ed.)

18. An absolute contraindication to cardiac transplantation is
    A. Active peptic ulcer disease
    B. Age older than 60 years
    C. Fixed pulmonary vascular resistance
    D. Heavy cigarette smoking

**Answer: C**
Although the other three items are relative contraindications to cardiac transplantation, fixed pulmonary vascular resistance is the only absolute contraindication among those listed. A heart accustomed to low pulmonary artery pressure and resistance will fail immediately if placed in a recipient with fixed pulmonary vascular resistance. (See Schwartz 7th ed.)

19. All of the following are side effects of cyclosporine A administration for prevention of organ rejection EXCEPT
    A. Hepatotoxicity
    B. Hirsutism
    C. Tremor
    D. Bone marrow depression

**Answer: D**
Bone marrow depression has often been seen with azathioprine but is not seen in patients on cyclosporine. Hepatotoxicity, hirsutism, tremor, and nephrotoxicity are complications of prolonged use of cyclosporine A. Nephrotoxicity is the most clinically important and most frequently seen side effect and may limit the drug's use in some patients. (See Schwartz 7th ed.)

20. Postoperative indicators of primary nonfunction of a liver allograft include all of the following EXCEPT
    A. Hypokalemia
    B. Hypoglycemia
    C. Elevated prothrombin time
    D. Alkalosis

**Answer: A**
Primary graft failure is a very serious complication. The patient decompensates quickly, and urgent transplantation is indicated. Severe central nervous system changes, with acid-base changes (early alkalosis due to inability to metabolize citrate and acidosis as a terminal event), hyperkalemia, coagulopathy, hypoglycemia, and oliguria are often terminal events of this acute hepatic decompensation. (See Schwartz 7th ed.)

21. Currently, which of the following infectious illnesses is most likely to compromise patients after renal transplantation?
    A. Coli sepsis
    B. Pneumococcal sepsis
    C. Candidiasis
    D. Cytomegalovirus sepsis

**Answer: D**

Immunosuppression for transplantation increases the risk for all types of infection. Use of cyclosporine, along with broad-spectrum antibiotics, has reduced the incidence of bacterial infections. Most serious posttransplant infections arise when rejection is being treated, and in the past, these led to high mortality. Both *Candida* and *Aspergillus* infections can occur but are relatively rare compared with viral infection. Cytomegalovirus (CMV) can produce a spectrum of illness characterized by fever, neutropenia, arthralgias, malaise, gastrointestinal ulcerations, and decreased renal function. CMV itself produces a state of immunosuppression, and many serious infections are superinfections in patients already experiencing CMV infections. Treatment of CMV sepsis includes decreasing immunosuppression and administering ganciclovir, a new antiviral drug. (See Schwartz 7th ed.)

# CHAPTER 11

# Patient Safety, Errors, and Complications in Surgery

1. Which of the following is the most appropriate diagnostic study to order for a patient who develops laryngospasm after a thyroidectomy?
   A. Lateral neck radiograph
   B. Lateral chest radiograph
   C. Bronchoscopy
   D. Serum calcium

**Answer: D**
Surgery of the thyroid and parathyroid glands can lend itself to various complications. Bleeding should be obvious, but specific electrolyte abnormalities will also contribute to postoperative morbidity, and possibly mortality, if not followed closely. Electrolyte abnormalities largely involve calcium and to a lesser extent phosphate. During thyroidectomy—whether subtotal or total—close follow-up of serum calcium levels (preferably ionized calcium) is warranted. Acutely, patients can have frank manifestations of hypocalcemia in the immediate postoperative period. These include electrocardiogram changes (shortened P-R interval), muscle spasm (tetany, Chvostek's sign, and Trousseau's sign), paresthesias, and laryngospasm. Treatment includes calcium gluconate infusion, and if tetany ensues, chemical paralysis with intubation. Maintenance treatment is thyroid hormone replacement in addition to calcium carbonate and vitamin D. (See Schwartz 8th ed., p 343.)

2. Which of the following is the most appropriate treatment for a seroma after a soft-tissue biopsy?
   A. Immediate return to the operating room for drainage
   B. Single attempt at aspiration with return to the operating room if it recurs
   C. Multiple attempts of aspiration with application of pressure dressings
   D. Observation

**Answer: C**
Seromas or lymphatic leaks may be difficult to manage at times. Depending on the volume and duration of leakage, control of a leak may take up to a few weeks to resolve with aspiration of seromas and the application of pressure dressings. If a seroma or leak does not resolve, it may be necessary to take the patient back to the operating room in order to place some form of closed suction drain into the wound. This usually is not necessary, and conservative management prevails. (See Schwartz 8th ed., p 341.)

3. Which of the following is the best test to predict successful extubation of a patient?
   A. Respiratory rate
   B. Negative inspiratory pressure
   C. Minute ventilation
   D. Tobin index

**Answer: D**
Unfortunately there is still no truly reliable way of predicting which patient will be successfully extubated after a weaning program, and the decision for extubation is based on a combination of clinical parameters and measured pulmonary mechanics. The Tobin Index (frequency:tidal volume ratio), also known as the rapid shallow breathing index (RSBI), is perhaps the best negative predictive instrument when performed as Yang and Tobin originally described. If the result equals <105, then there is nearly a 70% chance the patient will pass extubation. If the score is >105, the patient has an approximately 80% chance of failing extubation. (See Schwartz 8th ed., p 345.)

4.  The initial treatment of a patient with a suspected air embolism includes which of the following:
    A.  Place the patient in a right lateral decubitus position
    B.  Immediate angiographic aspiration of the air
    C.  Place the patient in a Trendelenburg position
    D.  Immediate thoracotomy with pump stand-by

**Answer: C**
Another error with central access lines involving either a venous line or a pulmonary artery line is that of air embolus. These are estimated to occur in 0.2 to 1% of patients. However, when an air embolism does occur, the results often can be dramatic and mortality can reach 50%. Treatment may prove futile if the diagnosis is ignored, especially if the air embolism bolus is larger than 50 mL. Clinical auscultation over the precordium often is nonspecific, so a portable chest X-ray may be required if the patient will tolerate the procedure. Nonetheless, aspiration via a central venous line accessing the heart may assist in decreasing the volume of gas in the right side of the heart, and minimize the amount traversing into the pulmonary circulation. Maneuvers to entrap the air in the right heart include placing the patient in the left lateral decubitus position and in Trendelenburg position, so the entrapped air can then be aspirated or anatomically stabilized within the right ventricle. If the patient survives these initial maneuvers, then consideration should be given as to whether the patient goes to the operating room for controlled surgical removal of the air, or if an angiographic approach is undertaken. The advantage of the operative approach is that the resources needed to salvage the patient are more readily available in the operating suite, should there be an acute deterioration in the patient's condition. (See Schwartz 8th ed., p 337.)

5.  Which of the following have been shown to decrease the time of postoperative ileus?
    A.  Erythromycin
    B.  Morphine patient-controlled analgesia
    C.  Nasogastric drainage until full return of bowel function
    D.  Cyclooxygenase-1 inhibitors

**Answer: A**
Pharmacologic agents commonly used to stimulate bowel function include metoclopramide and erythromycin. Metoclopramide's efficacy is limited to the stomach, and it may help primarily with gastroparesis. Erythromycin is a motilin-agonist that works throughout the stomach and bowel. Several studies demonstrate significant benefit from the administration of erythromycin in those suffering from an ileus. Several recent small studies have examined the role of cyclooxygenase-2 (COX-2) inhibitors and chewing gum, but larger controlled studies will be needed to support the findings that COX-2 inhibitors for analgesia and the use of chewing gum can lead to an earlier return of bowel function and decreased length of stay. (See Schwartz 8th ed., p 347.)

6.  The treatment of choice for a biloma after laparoscopic cholecystectomy is
    A.  Reoperation, closure of the leak, and drainage
    B.  Percutaneous drainage
    C.  Biliary stent
    D.  Observation

**Answer: C**
Patients with a biloma may present with diffuse abdominal pain that may be severe or moderate, with or without peritonitis. Liver function tests usually demonstrate hyperbilirubinemia, and the diagnosis of a biliary leak can be confirmed with a combination of computed tomography (CT) scan, endoscopic retrograde cholangiopancreatography (ERCP), or dimethyl iminodiacetic acid (HIDA) scan. Once a leak is confirmed, then a retrograde biliary stent and external drainage is the treatment of choice and surgery is not required. The leak may take several weeks to stop, and repeat laparotomy is only needed if the patient develops sepsis or peritonitis. (See Schwartz 8th ed., p 348.)

7. The first step in treating a 70-kg patient with a platelet count of 12,000 due to heparin-induced thrombocytopenia is
   A. Transfusion of 4 units of platelets
   B. Transfusion of 8 units of platelets
   C. Transfusion of 12 units of platelets
   D. Anticoagulation

**Answer: D**
Patients who are thrombocytopenic rarely need to be transfused with platelets. It is most important to delineate why the patient has a low platelet count. Usually there is a self-limiting or reversible condition such as sepsis. Rarely it is due to heparin-induced thrombocytopenia (HIT I and HIT II). Complications secondary to HIT II can be extremely morbid because of the thrombogenic nature of the complication. Simple precautions to limit this hypercoagulable state are to use saline solution flushes instead of heparin solutions, and to limit the use of heparin-coated catheters. The treatment is anticoagulation with synthetic agents such as argatroban. Thrombocytopenia actually develops in about 10% of patients treated with heparin. Transfusion of platelets during this diathesis only stimulates further degranulation of the platelets and promotes thrombosis. (See Schwartz 8th ed., p 350.)

8. Which of the following is a common nephrotoxic agent used in surgical patients?
   A. Cefuroxime
   B. Digitalis
   C. Furosemide
   D. Erythromycin

**Answer: C**
Intrinsic renal failure and subsequent acute tubular necrosis (ATN) are often the result of direct renal toxins. Aminoglycosides, vancomycin, and furosemide are well known agents that contribute directly to nephrotoxicity. Contrast-induced nephropathy usually leads to a subtle or transient rise in creatinine. In patients who are not adequately resuscitated or have poor cardiac function, a contrast nephropathy may have permanent effects on renal function. (See Schwartz 8th ed., p 349.)

9. Which of the following is the only thing that has been shown to decrease wound infections in surgical patients with contaminated wounds?
   A. Use of iodophor-impregnated polyvinyl drapes
   B. Antibiotic irrigation of the peritoneum and wound
   C. Saline irrigation of the peritoneum and wound
   D. 24 h of appropriate antibiotics postoperatively (in addition to preoperative dose)

**Answer: C**
The indiscriminate use of antibiotics is a universal problem that continues to plague intensive care units and hospitals across the country. Beginning with prophylactic antibiotics, there exist no prospective, randomized, double-blind, controlled studies that demonstrate that antibiotics used beyond 24 h in the perioperative period prevent infections. There is a general trend toward providing a single preoperative dose, as antibiotic prophylaxis may not impart any benefit at all beyond the initial dosing. Serial irrigation of the operative field and the surgical wound with saline solution has shown benefit in controlling wound inoculum. Irrigation with an antibiotic-based solution has not demonstrated significant benefit in controlling postoperative infection. (See Schwartz 8th ed., p 351.)

10. A schizophrenic patient who is status post colon resection for diverticulitis develops fever, muscle rigidity, tachycardia, and hemodynamic lability on postoperative day 5. Which of the following is the most appropriate intervention?
    A. Stop his anti-psychotic medication and administer empiric amantadine
    B. Draw blood cultures and start empiric antibiotics for intra-abdominal sepsis
    C. Order spiral computed tomography of the chest and start empiric heparin for pulmonary embolism
    D. Draw serum cortisol and start empiric steroids for adrenal insufficiency

**Answer: A**
Neuroleptic malignant syndrome (NMS) is different than malignant hyperthermia (MH). All classes of neuroleptics [dopamine ($D_2$)-receptor antagonists] are associated with NMS, and dopamine receptor blockade is considered to be the cause of NMS. NMS is more likely to develop following initiation of neuroleptic therapy or an increase in the dose. The onset can be within hours, but on average it is 4 to 14 days after initiation of therapy. However, NMS can occur at any time during neuroleptic use, even years after initiating therapy. Symptoms include muscle rigidity, tachycardia, urinary incontinence, hemodynamic lability, respiratory distress, and changes in mental status. As with MH, treatment

begins with discontinuing the offending medication and initiation of active cooling measures. In retrospective studies, dopamine agonists appear to decrease mortality and shorten the course of NMS, so the administration of medications such as bromocriptine or amantadine is used to control the syndrome's manifestations. The use of dantrolene in this setting is controversial. Despite aggressive treatment, mortality reaches 5%. Patients should avoid future use of the same medications that caused the initial NMS episode. (See Schwartz 8th ed., p 357.)

11. Which of the following is a dominant cytokine in the pathogenesis of systemic inflammatory response syndrome (SIRS)?
    A. Interleukin-2 (IL-2)
    B. IL-5
    C. IL-6
    D. IL-7

**Answer: C**
The dominant cytokines currently implicated in the development of SIRS include interleukin (IL)-1, IL-6, and tissue necrosis factor (TNF). Other mediators include nitric oxide, inducible macrophage-type nitric oxide synthase (iNOS), and prostaglandin $I_2$ ($PGI_2$). The precise delineation of all the mediators involved and the interactions of these mediators is still under active research, and a complete understanding of the etiology for SIRS/MODS has yet to be elucidated. (See Schwartz 8th ed., p 354.)

12. Which of the following statements about hypothermia is true?
    A. Bradycardia is the predominant arrhythmia.
    B. Paradoxic polyuria can interfere with evaluation of fluid resuscitation.
    C. Shivering ceases at a core temperate of 28°C or lower.
    D. An increase of 1°C/h is adequate rewarming.

**Answer: B**
Anatomic and physiologic concerns in hypothermic patients are related to the cardiac, respiratory, and renal systems. The most common cardiac abnormality is the development of arrhythmias when body temperature drops below 35°C, and these are usually related to ventricular dysfunction with the abnormal acid-base environment. Bradycardia begins to occur with temperatures below 30°C. It is well known that hypothermia may induce carbon dioxide retention until the body's production of $CO_2$ decreases significantly from the hypothermia, resulting in respiratory acidosis. Renal dysfunction of hypothermia manifests itself as a paradoxic polyuria, and is related to an increased glomerular filtration rate, as peripheral vascular constriction creates central shunting of blood. This is potentially perplexing for patients that are undergoing resuscitation for hemodynamic instability, because the brisk urine output provides a false sense of an adequate intravascular fluid volume. (See Schwartz 8th ed., p 356.)

13. Which of the following is most likely to be effective in the treatment of contrast-induced nephropathy?
    A. N-acetylcysteine
    B. Furosemide
    C. Mannitol
    D. Diazide diuretics

**Answer: A**
Renal-related complications of angiography occur in approximately 1 to 2% of patients. Contrast nephropathy often is a temporary and possibly a preventable complication of radiologic work-ups utilizing contrast dye for computed tomography (CT), angiography, and/or venography. The research results have been mixed regarding the prevention of acute tubular necrosis from intravenous contrast with administration of N-acetylcysteine. There are some studies that suggest an overall improvement of renal function with N-acetylcysteine use, and other studies that report that its use has no overall benefit. If N-acetylcysteine is to provide benefit, twice-daily dosing 24 h before and on the day of the radiographic study is suggested. It also is suggested that the

greatest benefit with n-acetylcysteine is derived from improved intravenous hydration before and after the procedure. Nonionic contrast also may be of benefit in higher-risk patients. The contemporary literature does not support the use of other adjuncts such as administration of furosemide or mannitol prior to angiography, and these practices may add to overall morbidity rather than salvage renal function. As a current minimum, improved intravenous hydration before and after the procedure is still likely the simplest and most efficient method for providing renal protection from dye contrast. (See Schwartz 8th ed., p 341.)

14. The Centers for Disease Control and Prevention definition of a central line infection is
    A. >25 colony forming units (CFUs) on agar roll plate
    B. >50 CFUs on agar roll plate
    C. >10 CFUs on sonification
    D. $>10^3$ CFUs on sonification

**Answer: D**

Nearly 15% of hospitalized patients will acquire central venous line sepsis (defined as >15 colony-forming units (CFU) on an agar roll plate, or $>10^3$ CFU on sonication). In many instances, once an infection is recognized as central line sepsis, removing the line is adequate. *Staphylococcus aureus* infections, however, present a unique problem because of the potential for metastatic seeding of bacterial emboli. The treatment for this situation is 4 to 6 weeks of tailored antibiotic therapy. (See Schwartz 8th ed., p 337.)

15. Laryngoscopic findings after a superior laryngeal nerve injury include
    A. Ipsilateral vocal cord in a paramedian position
    B. Ipsilateral vocal cord in a middling position
    C. Asymmetry of the glottic opening
    D. Normal examination

**Answer: C**

Superior laryngeal nerve injury is less debilitating, providing the patient's profession is not related to their vocal performance, as the common symptom is loss of projection of the voice. The glottic aperture is asymmetrical on direct laryngoscopy and management is based on clinical observation. (See Schwartz 8th ed., p 343.)

16. The risk of ventilator-acquired pneumonia after 30 days of intubation is approximately
    A. 20%
    B. 35%
    C. 55%
    D. 70%

**Answer: D**

Ventilator-associated pneumonia (VAP) occurs in 15 to 40% of ventilated ICU patients, and accrues at a daily probability rate of 5% per day, up to 70% at 30 days. In fact, transporting the ventilated patient out of the ICU to radiology or other hospital areas increases the risk of VAP by 15%. The 30-day mortality rate of nosocomial pneumonia can be as high as 40%, and depends on the microorganisms involved and the timeliness of initiating appropriate treatment. (See Schwartz 8th ed., p 344.)

17. The respiratory quotient when fat is metabolized is
    A. 0.5
    B. 0.7
    C. 0.8
    D. 1.0

**Answer: B**

The respiratory quotient (RQ), or respiratory exchange ratio (RER), is the ratio of the rate of carbon dioxide produced to the rate of oxygen uptake ($RQ = V_{CO_2}/V_{O_2}$). Briefly, lipids, carbohydrates, and protein, when used as fuel, have differing effects on energy. Patients consuming a diet consisting mostly of carbohydrates would have an RQ of 1 or greater. A diet mostly of lipids would be closer to 0.7, and a diet of mostly protein would be closer to 0.8. Ideally, an RQ of 0.75 to 0.85 would suggest that a patient's nutritional intake was of adequate balance and composition. An excess of carbohydrate in nutritional therapy occasionally may negatively affect ventilator weaning because of the abnormal RQ and altered pulmonary gas exchange. (See Schwartz 8th ed., p 345.)

18. All of the following are associated with an increased incidence of abdominal wound dehiscence EXCEPT
    A. Bringing a stoma through the incision
    B. Closure of the wound with a continuous suture
    C. Presence of jaundice
    D. Use of braided sutures

**Answer: B**
The incidence of wound dehiscence is no higher with a continuous suture closure than with an interrupted suture closure. Bringing a stoma through the incision significantly increases the possibility of dehiscence. The presence of jaundice or other evidence of liver failure is associated with an increased probability of wound dehiscence. Ascites is another associated factor. A monofilament suture closure is safer than a closure with a braided suture. Closure under tension and closure of a wound without adequate hemostasis are technical factors, which increase the possibility of dehiscence. (See Schwartz 7th ed.)

19. Which of the following agents may produce interstitial nephritis?
    A. Amphotericin B
    B. Gentamicin
    C. Lithium
    D. Methicillin

**Answer: D**
Methicillin produces an interstitial nephritis. The other three agents also may be nephrotoxic, but their site of toxicity is either the proximal tubule for gentamicin or the distal tubule for lithium. Amphotericin B has toxic effects in both proximal and distal tubules. (See Schwartz 7th ed.)

20. Which of the following values indicates an adult with a significant risk for pulmonary problems after an abdominal operation?
    A. Forced expiratory volume in 1 second ($FEV_1$) 2.5 L
    B. Forced vital capacity (FVC) 80% of predicted value
    C. Maximum breathing capacity (MBC) 70% of predicted value
    D. $Paco_2$ 50 mm Hg

**Answer: D**
$Paco_2$ of 50 mm Hg indicates a serious diffusion defect. Although $Pao_2$ of 70 mm Hg is low, it is more readily correctable by appropriate pulmonary measures. $FEV_1$ of under 2 liters would be a troublesome finding in an adult as would an FVC of <70% of predicted value or an MBC of <50% of predicted value. It is worth noting that significant information can be obtained by a simple physical examination. An adult who cannot walk up a flight of stairs without dyspnea or blow out a match with unpursed lips at 8 inches has significant pulmonary problems. (See Schwartz 7th ed.)

21. A 70-year-old man who has undergone a sigmoid resection for diverticulitis reaches the recovery room with a pulse rate of 86/min and a blood pressure of 130/70. Twenty minutes later, he has an abrupt onset of tachycardia. His pulse rate is 180/min, and his blood pressure is 60/0. The first step in management should be
    A. Cardioversion
    B. Insertion of a pacemaker
    C. Intravenous lidocaine
    D. Intravenous propranolol

**Answer: A**
An acute tachyarrhythmia of this degree requires rapid correction, and electrical cardioversion is the proper approach. The drugs all slow cardiac rate but not rapidly enough in an acute emergency. Pacemaker insertion would be an appropriate elective approach to a bradyarrhythmia. (See Schwartz 7th ed.)

22. Which of the following statements about acute suppurative parotitis is NOT correct?
    A. Decreased oral intake is a causative factor
    B. Most patients are older than 70 years of age
    C. Parotitis usually develops during the postoperative period
    D. Poor oral hygiene is a contributing factor

**Answer: C**
These infections develop in elderly individuals with poor oral hygiene and limited oral intake. The majority of infections are caused by staphylococci which invade Stensen's duct where there is minimal parotid secretion. Although these infections can occur in the postoperative period, the majority of cases are not related to an operation. (See Schwartz 7th ed.)

1. The point of critical oxygen delivery is defined as
   A. $Pa_{O_2}$ <50
   B. Arterial oxygen saturation <88%
   C. $\dot{D}_{O_2}$ (oxygen delivery) <400 mL/min/m$^2$
   D. $\dot{D}_{O_2} = \dot{V}_{O_2}$

**Answer: D**

Under normal conditions when the supply of oxygen is plentiful, aerobic metabolism is determined by factors other than the availability of oxygen. These factors include the hormonal milieu and mechanical workload of contractile tissue. However, in pathologic circumstances when oxygen availability is inadequate, oxygen utilization ($\dot{V}_{O_2}$) becomes dependent upon oxygen delivery ($\dot{D}_{O_2}$). The relationship of $\dot{V}_{O_2}$ to $\dot{D}_{O_2}$ over a broad range of $\dot{D}_{O_2}$ values is commonly represented as two intersecting straight lines. In the region of higher $\dot{D}_{O_2}$ values, the slope of the line is approximately equal to zero, indicating that $\dot{V}_{O_2}$ is largely independent of $\dot{D}_{O_2}$. In contrast, in the region of low $\dot{D}_{O_2}$ values, the slope of the line is nonzero and positive, indicating that $\dot{V}_{O_2}$ is supply-dependent. The region where the two lines intersect is called the point of critical oxygen delivery ($\dot{D}_{O_2crit}$), and represents the transition from supply-independent to supply-dependent oxygen uptake. (See Schwartz 8th ed., p 362.)

2. Cardiac preload is determined by
   A. End-diastolic volume
   B. End-diastolic pressure
   C. End-systolic volume
   D. End-systolic pressure

**Answer: A**

Starling's law of the heart states that the force of muscle contraction depends on the initial length of the cardiac fibers. Using terminology that derives from early experiments using isolated cardiac muscle preparations, preload is the stretch of ventricular myocardial tissue just prior to the next contraction. Preload is determined by end-diastolic volume (EDV). For the right ventricle, central venous pressure (CVP) approximates right ventricular end-diastolic pressure (EDP). For the left ventricle, pulmonary artery occlusion pressure (PAOP), which is measured by transiently inflating a balloon at the end of a pressure monitoring catheter positioned in a small branch of the pulmonary artery, approximates left ventricular end-diastolic pressure. The presence of atrioventricular valvular stenosis will alter this relationship. (See Schwartz 8th ed., p 364.)

3. The diagnosis of abdominal compartment syndrome is made with a bladder pressure greater than
   A. 20 mm Hg
   B. 40 mm Hg
   C. 60 mm Hg
   D. 80 mm Hg

**Answer: A**

The triad of oliguria, elevated peak airway pressures, and elevated intra-abdominal pressure is known as the abdominal compartment syndrome (ACS). This syndrome, first described in patients after repair of ruptured abdominal aortic aneurysm, is associated with interstitial edema of the abdominal organs, resulting in elevated intra-abdominal pressure. When intra-abdominal pressure exceeds venous or capillary pressures, perfusion of the kidneys and other intra-abdominal viscera is impaired. Oliguria is a cardinal sign. While the diagnosis of ACS is a clinical one, measuring intra-abdominal pressure is useful to confirm the diagnosis. Ideally, a catheter inserted into the peritoneal cavity could measure intra-abdominal pressure to substantiate the diagnosis. In practice, transurethral bladder pressure measurement reflects intra-abdominal pressure and is most often used to confirm the presence of ACS. After instilling 50 to 100 mL of sterile saline into the bladder via a Foley catheter, the tubing is connected to a transducing system to measure bladder pressure. Most authorities recommend that a bladder pressure greater than 20 to 25 mm Hg confirms the diagnosis of ACS. Less commonly, gastric or inferior vena cava pressures can be monitored with appropriate catheters to detect elevated intra-abdominal pressures. (See Schwartz 8th ed., p 374.)

4. Intracranial pressure monitoring is indicated for which of the following patients with severe traumatic brain injury?
   A. Glasgow Coma Score of 10 with an abnormal computed tomography (CT) scan
   B. Glasgow Coma Score of 8 with a normal CT scan
   C. Age >40 years, systolic blood pressure <90, normal CT scan
   D. Unilateral motor posturing, normal CT scan

**Answer: C**
Because the brain is rigidly confined within the bony skull, cerebral edema or mass lesions increase intracranial pressure (ICP). Monitoring of ICP is currently recommended in patients with severe traumatic brain injury (TBI), defined as a Glasgow Coma Scale (GCS) score less than or equal to 8 with an abnormal CT scan, and in patients with severe TBI and a normal CT scan if two or more of the following are present: age greater than 40 years, unilateral or bilateral motor posturing, or systolic blood pressure less than 90 mm Hg. ICP monitoring also is indicated in patients with acute subarachnoid hemorrhage with coma or neurologic deterioration, intracranial hemorrhage with intraventricular blood, ischemic middle cerebral artery stroke, fulminant hepatic failure with coma and cerebral edema on CT scan, and global cerebral ischemia or anoxia with cerebral edema on CT scan. The goal of ICP monitoring is to ensure that cerebral perfusion pressure (CPP) is adequate to support perfusion of the brain. CPP is equal to the difference between mean arterial pressure (MAP) and ICP: CPP = MAP – ICP. (See Schwartz 8th ed., p 374.)

5. The appropriately sized blood pressure cuff for an individual patient can be determined by
   A. Width approximately 40% of circumference
   B. Length equal to distance from elbow to wrist
   C. The patient's weight
   D. The patient's body surface area

**Answer: A**
Both manual and automated means for the noninvasive determination of blood pressure use an inflatable cuff to increase pressure around an extremity. If the cuff is too narrow (relative to the extremity), the measured pressure will be artifactually elevated. Therefore, the width of the cuff should be approximately 40% of its circumference. (See Schwartz 8th ed., p 362.)

6. The risk of distal ischemia from a radial arterial line can be reduced by
   A. Leaving the catheter in place less than 6 days
   B. Using a 20-gauge (or smaller) catheter
   C. Performing an arteriogram to document ulnar flow
   D. Performing a distal puncture in the artery

**Answer: B**
Distal ischemia is an uncommon complication of intra-arterial catheterization. The incidence of thrombosis is increased when larger-caliber catheters are employed and when catheters are left in place for an extended period of time. The incidence of thrombosis can be minimized by using a 20-gauge (or smaller) catheter in the radial position and leaving the catheter in place for as short a duration as feasible, preferably

less than 4 days. The risk of distal ischemic injury can be minimized by ensuring that adequate collateral flow is present. At the wrist, adequate collateral flow can be documented by performing a modified version of the Allen test, wherein the artery to be cannulated is digitally compressed while using a Doppler stethoscope to listen for perfusion in the palmar arch vessels. (See Schwartz 8th ed., p 363.)

7. Mean arterial blood pressure
   A. Is higher in the peripheral vessels than in the aorta
   B. Is higher in an overdamped arterial line
   C. Is lower in an overdamped arterial line
   D. Is the same regardless of location or damping

**Answer: D**
The fidelity of the catheter-tubing-transducer system is determined by numerous factors, including the compliance of the tubing, the surface area of the transducer diaphragm, and the compliance of the diaphragm. If the system is underdamped, then the inertia of the system, which is a function of the mass of the fluid in the tubing and the mass of the diaphragm, causes overshoot of the points of maximum positive and negative displacement of the diaphragm during systole and diastole, respectively. Thus in an underdamped system, systolic pressure will be overestimated and diastolic pressure will be underestimated. In an overdamped system, displacement of the diaphragm fails to track the rapidly changing pressure waveform, and systolic pressure will be underestimated and diastolic pressure will be overestimated. It is important to note that even in an underdamped or overdamped system, mean pressure will be accurately recorded, provided the system has been properly calibrated. When using direct measurement of intra-arterial pressure to monitor patients, physicians and nurses should be in the habit of using mean pressure for making clinical decisions. (See Schwartz 8th ed., p 363.)

8. What is the approximate mean arterial pressure (MAP) in a patient with an arterial pressure of 90/40?
   A. 45
   B. 55
   C. 65
   D. 75

**Answer: B**

$$MAP = [(2 \times diastolic) + systolic] / 3$$
$$(2 \times 40) + 90/3 = 56.6$$

9. Which of the following complications is LEAST likely during a 3-day period of monitoring with an arterial catheter?
   A. Arterial thrombosis
   B. Hemorrhage
   C. Infection at the catheter site
   D. Septicemia

**Answer: D**
Arterial monitoring is useful in the management of a severely ill or injured patient. However, the technique has some risk, and any of the listed complications may occur. Thrombosis is frequent with catheterization of the radial artery or other vessels of similar size. Continuous heparin flow reduces this problem but increases the risk of wound hematoma. Hemorrhage may occur if the catheter becomes disconnected. When the femoral artery is used, hemorrhage into the pelvis may be significant, and it may escape detection. Wound infection is unusual when careful wound care is maintained. Septicemia is rarely a problem unless the catheter is maintained for longer than 4 days. (See Schwartz 7th ed.)

10. The artery LEAST appropriate for catheterization studies in an adult is the
    A. Axillary artery
    B. Brachial artery
    C. Dorsalis pedis artery
    D. Femoral artery

**Answer: B**
There are possible problems with any arterial catheterization. However, the use of the brachial artery poses several specific problems. If collateral circulation is inadequate, brachial artery obstruction may lead to loss of the forearm and hand. In an awake patient, maintaining the site may be difficult because of movement, and hematoma formation presents a problem. If hematoma expands, nerve compression and Volkmann's ischemia contracture may result. (See Schwartz 7th ed.)

11. Catheterization of the subclavian vein is appropriate for all of the following uses EXCEPT
    A. Central venous pressure monitoring
    B. Drug infusion
    C. Total parenteral nutrition
    D. Trauma resuscitation

**Answer: D**
A large-bore peripheral line is an indication for trauma resuscitation when significant volumes must be administered in a short period. A subclavian catheter is appropriate for the other listed uses as well as for placement of cardiac pacemakers or pulmonary artery catheters. (See Schwartz 7th ed.)

12. Conditions necessary for pulmonary artery pressure to equal left atrial pressure include all of the following EXCEPT
    A. High levels of positive end-expiratory pressure are being delivered.
    B. Pulmonary artery pressure is greater than alveolar pressure.
    C. Pulmonary venous pressure is greater than alveolar pressure.
    D. The catheter is in the occluded (wedge) position.

**Answer: A**
High levels of positive end-expiratory pressure increase the alveolar pressure, and, under these circumstances, even a wedged pulmonary artery catheter measures alveolar pressure rather than left atrial pressure. If attention is paid to careful catheter placement and balloon inflation and if the alveolar pressure is appropriately controlled, the pulmonary artery pressure equals the left atrial pressure. (See Schwartz 7th ed.)

13. Before accurate pressure can be obtained with a pulmonary artery catheter, the pressure transducer must be calibrated and zeroed to the level of the
    A. Right atrium
    B. Right ventricle
    C. Main pulmonary artery
    D. Left atrium

**Answer: D**
Because measurements obtained are representative of left atrial pressure, the system must be equilibrated with the left atrium to assure accurate results. (See Schwartz 7th ed.)

14. The most common complication associated with the passage of a pulmonary artery catheter is
    A. Development of a dysrhythmia
    B. Hematoma at the entry site
    C. Knotting in the right ventricle
    D. Pneumothorax

**Answer: A**
Please see Answer text for Question 13.

15. All of the following values can be derived from direct measurement during blood-gas analysis EXCEPT
    A. Arterial blood oxygen tension ($PaO_2$)
    B. Arterial hemoglobin oxygen saturation ($SaO_2$)
    C. Mixed venous blood oxygen tension ($PvO_2$)
    D. Mixed venous hemoglobin oxygen saturation ($SvO_2$)
    E. Cerebral oxygen consumption ($CvO_2$)

**Answer: E**
$CvO_2$ is calculated using values obtained for $SvO_2$, $PvO_2$, and hemoglobin concentration. The other values are obtained freely from blood-gas analysis. The normal range of $CvO_2$ is 12–17 mL $O_2$/dL blood. (See Schwartz 7th ed.)

16. The oxyhemoglobin dissociation curve is shifted to the left by
    A. Decreased blood pH
    B. Increased erythrocyte 2,3-diphosphoglycerate (DPG) concentration
    C. Increased body temperature
    D. Methemoglobinemia

**Answer: D**

When the oxyhemoglobin curve is shifted to the left, less oxygen is available for use by the tissues. Conditions such as methemoglobinemia and carboxyhemoglobinemia shift the curve to the left, interfering with peripheral oxygen availability. Decreased pH (increase in hydrogen ion concentration), increased erythrocyte 2,3-DPG, increased body temperature, and a rising $P_{CO_2}$ all push the curve to the right, increasing available oxygen. (See Schwartz 7th ed.)

17. Positive end-expiratory pressure (PEEP) ventilation is widely used in the treatment of acute pulmonary failure. The beneficial effects of PEEP include all of the following EXCEPT
    A. Decreased pulmonary shunting
    B. Decreased extravascular lung water
    C. Increased resting volume of the lung
    D. Increased oxygenation

**Answer: B**

The mechanism of action of PEEP ventilation has not been completely elucidated. However, the beneficial effects of PEEP include (1) an increase in oxygenation ($Pa_{O_2}$); (2) an increase in resting volume (i.e., functional residual capacity, of the lung); (3) an increase in pulmonary compliance; (4) an increase in the ratio of ventilation to perfusion when the ratio is initially low; and (5) decreased pulmonary shunting (venous admixture). There has been no good experimental evidence that PEEP leads to a direct decrease in lung water. (See Schwartz 7th ed.)

18. All of the following findings would indicate that a patient requires mechanical ventilatory support EXCEPT
    A. Respiratory rate greater than 30 breaths per minute
    B. Vital capacity less than 15 mL/kg
    C. Maximal inspiratory force of 40 cm $H_2O$
    D. Alveolar-arterial oxygen gradient greater than 350 torr

**Answer: C**

The treatment of acute respiratory insufficiency is based primarily on ventilatory support. Endotracheal intubation, preferably through the nose, is considered the technique of choice. A maximal inspiratory force of –40 cm $H_2O$ is *not* a criterion for ventilatory support. On the other hand, a patient who has stable vital signs and who (1) exhibits adequate oxygenation on an inspired oxygen concentration of 0.4 or less, (2) has a resting minute ventilation less than 10 L/min, (3) has a vital capacity greater than 15 mL/kg, and (4) has a tidal volume greater than 5 mL/kg almost certainly will tolerate withdrawal of ventilatory support. A maximal inspiratory force of –30 cm $H_2O$ or less (i.e., more negative), however, generally is necessary to maintain spontaneous ventilation. Consideration of all of these parameters together would greatly assist in a decision whether or not to withdraw mechanical ventilation. (See Schwartz 7th ed.)

# CHAPTER 13

# Minimally Invasive Surgery

1. Nitrous oxide pneumoperitoneum
   A. Is more painful than carbon dioxide peritoneum
   B. Decreases end-tidal $CO_2$
   C. Is contraindicated because it is flammable
   D. Is slowly absorbed from the peritoneal cavity

**Answer: B**

The unique feature of endoscopic surgery in the peritoneal cavity is the need to lift the abdominal wall from the abdominal organs. Two methods have been devised for achieving this. The first, used by most surgeons, is the induction of a pneumoperitoneum. Throughout the early twentieth century intraperitoneal visualization was achieved by inflating the abdominal cavity with air, using a sphygmomanometer bulb. The problem with using air insufflation is that nitrogen is poorly soluble in blood and is slowly absorbed across the peritoneal surfaces. Air pneumoperitoneum was believed to be more painful than nitrous oxide pneumoperitoneum but less painful than carbon dioxide pneumoperitoneum. Subsequently, carbon dioxide and nitrous oxide were used for inflating the abdomen. $N_2O$ had the advantage of being physiologically inert and rapidly absorbed. It also provided better analgesia for laparoscopy performed under local anesthesia when compared with $CO_2$ or air. Despite initial concerns that $N_2O$ would not suppress combustion, controlled clinical trials have established its safety within the peritoneal cavity. In addition, nitrous oxide has recently been shown to reduce the intraoperative end-tidal $CO_2$ and minute ventilation required to maintain homeostasis when compared to $CO_2$ pneumoperitoneum. The effect of $N_2O$ on tumor biology and the development of port site metastasis are unknown. As such, caution should be exercised when performing laparoscopic cancer surgery with this agent. Finally, the safety of $N_2O$ pneumoperitoneum in pregnancy has yet to be elucidated. (See Schwartz 8th ed., p 381.)

2. The most common arrhythmia seen during laparoscopy is
   A. Sinus bradycardia
   B. Sinus tachycardia
   C. Premature ventricular contractions
   D. Atrial fibrillation

**Answer: A**

The pressure effects of the pneumoperitoneum on cardiovascular physiology also have been studied. In the hypovolemic individual, excessive pressure on the inferior vena cava and a reverse Trendelenburg position with loss of lower extremity muscle tone may cause decreased venous return and cardiac output. This is not seen in the normovolemic patient. The most common arrhythmia created by laparoscopy is bradycardia. A rapid stretch of the peritoneal membrane often causes a vagovagal response with bradycardia and occasionally hypotension. The appropriate management of this event is desufflation of the abdomen, administration of vagolytic agents (e.g., atropine), and adequate volume replacement. (See Schwartz 8th ed., p 382.)

3. Gas embolism during laparoscopy
   A. Is less likely when using helium for insufflation
   B. Occurs most commonly during difficult dissections of vascular pedicles
   C. Is treated by positioning the patient in a right lateral decubitus position
   D. Can be diagnosed by a characteristic murmur

**Answer: D**
The hemodynamic and metabolic consequences of pneumoperitoneum are well tolerated by healthy individuals for a prolonged period and by most individuals for at least a short period. Difficulties can occur when a patient with compromised cardiovascular function is subjected to a long laparoscopic procedure. It is during these procedures that alternative approaches should be considered or insufflation pressure reduced. Alternative gases that have been suggested for laparoscopy include the inert gases helium, neon, and argon. These gases are appealing because they cause no metabolic effects, but are poorly soluble in blood (unlike $CO_2$ and $N_2O$) and are prone to create gas emboli if the gas has direct access to the venous system. Gas emboli are rare but serious complications of laparoscopic surgery. They should be suspected if hypotension develops during insufflation. Diagnosis may be made by listening (with an esophageal stethoscope) for the characteristic "mill wheel" murmur. The treatment of gas embolism is to place the patient in a left lateral decubitus position with the head down to trap the gas in the apex of the right ventricle. A rapidly placed central venous catheter then can be used to aspirate the gas out of the right ventricle. (See Schwartz 8th ed., p 382.)

4. Which of the following occurs more commonly after laparoscopic surgery when compared to the equivalent open procedure?
   A. Decreased serum cortisol
   B. Increased immune suppression
   C. Faster equilibration of stress mediated hormones such as cytokines
   D. Increased urine output

**Answer: C**
Early it was predicted that the surgical stress response would be significantly lessened with laparoscopic surgery, but this is not always the case. Serum cortisol levels after laparoscopic operations are often higher than after the equivalent operation performed through an open incision. In terms of endocrine balance, the greatest difference between open and laparoscopic surgery is the more rapid equilibration of most stress-mediated hormone levels after laparoscopic surgery. Immune suppression also is less after laparoscopy than after open surgery. There is a trend toward more rapid normalization of cytokine levels after a laparoscopic procedure than after the equivalent procedure performed by celiotomy. (See Schwartz 8th ed., p 382.)

5. Capacitive coupling
   A. Results when energy bleeds from a port sleeve or laparoscope into adjacent (but not touching) bowel
   B. Is always recognized at the time of surgery
   C. Can result in malfunction of the electrocardiogram monitor
   D. Can result in inaccurate image transmission to the digital monitor

**Answer: A**
In order to avoid thermal injury to adjacent structures, the laparoscopic field of view must include all uninsulated portions of the electrosurgical electrode. In addition, the integrity of the insulation must be maintained and assured. Capacitive coupling occurs when a plastic trocar insulates the abdominal wall from the current; in turn the current is bled off of a metal sleeve or laparoscope into the viscera (Fig. 13-13A). This may result in thermal necrosis and a delayed fecal fistula. Another potential mechanism for unrecognized visceral injury may occur with the direct coupling of current to the laparoscope and adjacent bowel (Fig. 13-13B). (See Schwartz 8th ed., p 388.)

6. Laparoscopic surgery in pregnancy
    A. Is contraindicated due to the risk of premature labor
    B. Is safe if there is no maternal respiratory acidosis during surgery
    C. Should not be performed during the second trimester
    D. Should not be performed with intra-abdominal pressures >1 mm cm $H_2O$ pressure

**Answer: B**

Concerns about the safety of laparoscopic cholecystectomy or appendectomy in the pregnant patient have been eliminated. The pH of the fetus follows the pH of the mother linearly, and therefore fetal acidosis may be prevented by avoiding a respiratory acidosis in the mother. A second concern was that of increased intra-abdominal pressure, but it has been proved that midpregnancy uterine contractions provide a much greater pressure in utero than a pneumoperitoneum. Experience in well over 100 cases of laparoscopic cholecystectomy in pregnancy have been reported with uniformly good results. The operation should be performed during the second trimester if possible. Protection of the fetus against intraoperative X-rays is imperative. Some believe it advisable to track fetal pulse rates with a transvaginal ultrasound probe. Access to the abdomen in the pregnant patient should take into consideration the height of the uterine fundus, which reaches the umbilicus at 20 weeks. In order not to damage the uterus or its blood supply, most surgeons feel that the open (Hasson) approach should be used in favor of direct puncture laparoscopy. The patient should be positioned slightly on the left side in order to avoid compression of the vena cava by the uterus. Because pregnancy poses a risk for thromboembolism, sequential compression devices are essential for all procedures. (See Schwartz 8th ed., p 393.)

7. Argon beam electrocoagulation during laparoscopy
    A. Is less effective than spray electrocoagulation with a standard cautery
    B. Can decrease intra-abdominal pressure
    C. Increases the risk of gas embolism
    D. Is more effective than standard cautery for coagulating a single, large vessel that is bleeding

**Answer: C**

Another method of delivering radiofrequency electrosurgery is argon beam coagulation. This is a type of monopolar electrosurgery in which a uniform field of electrons is distributed across a tissue surface by the use of a jet of argon gas. The argon gas jet distributes electrons more evenly across the surface than does spray electrofulguration. This technology has its greatest application for coagulation of diffusely bleeding surfaces such as the cut edge of liver or spleen. It is of less use in laparoscopic procedures because the increased intra-abdominal pressures created by the argon gas jet can increase the chances of a gas embolus. It is paramount to vent the ports and closely monitor insufflation pressure when using this source of energy within the context of laparoscopy. (See Schwartz 8th ed., p 389.)

# CHAPTER 14

# Cell, Genomics, and Molecular Surgery

1. Which of the following is used to analyze RNA?
   A. Southern blot hybridization
   B. Northern blot hybridization
   C. Polymerase chain reaction (PCR)
   D. Immunoblotting

**Answer: B**
Northern blotting refers to the technique of size fractionation of RNA in a gel and the transferring of an RNA sample to a solid support (membrane) in such a manner that the relative positions of the RNA molecules are maintained. The resulting membrane is then hybridized with a labeled probe complementary to the messenger RNA (mRNA) of interest. Signals generated from detection of the membrane can be used to determine the size and abundance of the target RNA. In principle, Northern blot hybridization is similar to Southern blot hybridization (and hence its name), with the exception that RNA, not DNA, is on the membrane. Although reverse transcriptase-PCR (RT-PCR) has been used in many applications, Northern analysis is the only method that provides information regarding mRNA size and has remained a standard method for detection and quantitation of mRNA. The process of Northern hybridization involves several steps, as does Southern hybridization, including electrophoresis of RNA samples in an agarose-formaldehyde gel, transfer to a membrane support, and hybridization to a radioactively labeled DNA probe. Data from hybridization allows quantification of steady-state mRNA levels, and at the same time, provides information related to the presence, size, and integrity of discrete mRNA species. Thus, Northern blot analysis, also termed RNA gel blot analysis, is commonly used in molecular biology studies relating to gene expression. (See Schwartz 8th ed., p 417.)

2. Which of the following statements concerning the human genome is true?
   A. Approximately 88% of the genome is identical in all people.
   B. There are approximately 25,000 genes in the human genome.
   C. Fifteen million single-base DNA differences have been defined (single gene polymorphism).
   D. The human genome project was completed in 1995.

**Answer: B**
Genome is a collective term for all genes present in one organism. The human genome contains DNA sequences of 3 billion base pairs, carried by 23 pairs of chromosomes. The human genome has an estimated 25,000 to 30,000 genes, and overall it is 99.9% identical in all people. Approximately 3 million locations where single-base DNA differences exist have been identified and termed single nucleotide polymorphisms (SNPs). SNPs may be critical determinants of human variation in disease susceptibility and responses to environmental factors. (See Schwartz 8th ed., p 408.)

3. The translation of DNA to RNA is called
   A. Transcription
   B. Translation
   C. Replication
   D. Signaling

**Answer: A**

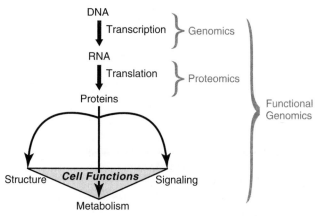

**FIG. 14-1.** The flow of genetic information from DNA to protein to cell functions. The process of transmission of genetic information from DNA to RNA is called *transcription*, and the process of transmission from RNA to protein is called *translation*. Proteins are the essential controlling components for cell structure, cell signaling, and metabolism. *Genomics* and *proteomics* are the study of the genetic composition of a living organism at the DNA and protein level, respectively. The study of the relationship between genes and their cellular functions is called *functional genomics*. (See Schwartz 8th ed., p 404.)

4. All of the following are involved in gene regulation EXCEPT
   A. Introns
   B. Control of messenger RNA (mRNA) stability
   C. Lack of modification of mRNA
   D. Control of export of mRNA from the nucleus to the cytoplasm

**Answer: C**
However, gene regulation is far more complex, particularly in eukaryotic organisms. For example, many gene transcripts must be spliced to remove the intervening sequences. The sequences that are spliced off are called *introns*, which appear to be useless, but in fact may carry some regulatory information. The sequences that are joined together, and are eventually translated into protein, are called *exons*. Additional regulation of gene expression includes modification of mRNA, control of mRNA stability, and its nuclear export into cytoplasm (where it is assembled into ribosomes for translation). After mRNA is translated into protein, the levels and functions of the proteins can be further regulated posttranslationally. (See Schwartz 8th ed., p 405.)

5. Translation takes place in
   A. The nucleus
   B. The cytoplasm
   C. The ribosome
   D. The mitochondria

**Answer: C**
DNA directs the synthesis of RNA; RNA in turn directs the synthesis of proteins. Proteins are variable-length polypeptide polymers composed of various combinations of 20 different amino acids and are the working molecules of the cell. The process of decoding information on messenger RNA (mRNA) to synthesize proteins is called *translation*. Translation takes place in ribosomes composed of ribosomal RNA (rRNA) and ribosomal proteins. (See Schwartz 8th ed., p 407.)

6. Which of the following is NOT one of the phases of the cell cycle?
   A. $G_1$
   B. $G_2$
   C. S
   D. $S_1$

**Answer: D**

All growing cells have the ability to duplicate their genomic DNA and pass along identical copies of this genetic information to every daughter cell. Thus the cell cycle is the fundamental mechanism to maintain tissue homeostasis. A cell cycle comprises four periods: $G_1$ (first gap phase before DNA synthesis), S (synthesis phase when DNA replication occurs), $G_2$ (the gap phase before mitosis), and M (mitosis, the phase when two daughter cells with identical DNA are generated). (See Schwartz 8th ed., p 409.)

7. Which of the following is a regulator of the cell cycle?
   A. Cyclin-dependent kinase
   B. Tyrosine kinase
   C. Pol II holoenzyme
   D. Caspase

**Answer: A**

The machinery that drives cell cycle progression is made up of a group of enzymes called cyclin-dependent kinases (CDK). Cyclin expression fluctuates during the cell cycle, and cyclins are essential for CDK activities and form complexes with CDK. The cyclin A/CDK1 and cyclin B/CDK1 drive the progression for the M phase, while cyclin A/CDK2 is the primary S phase complex. Early $G_1$ cyclin D/CDK4/6 or late $G_1$ cyclin E/CDK2 controls the $G_1$-S transition. There also are negative regulators for CDK termed *CDK inhibitors* (CKIs), which inhibit the assembly or activity of the cyclin-CDK complex. Expression of cyclins and CKIs often are regulated by developmental and environmental factors. (See Schwartz 8th ed., p 409.)

8. Which of the following is NOT a class of cell-surface receptor?
   A. Transmitter-gated ion channels
   B. Adhesive receptor
   C. Seven-transmembrane (G-protein coupled) receptor
   D. Enzyme-linked receptor

**Answer: B**

There are three major classes of cell-surface receptors: *transmitter-gated ion channels*, *seven-transmembrane (G-protein coupled) receptors (7TM/GPCRs)*, and *enzyme-linked receptors*. The superfamily of 7TM/GPCRs is one of the largest families of proteins, representing over 800 genes of the human genome. Members of this superfamily share a characteristic seven-transmembrane configuration. The ligands for these receptors are diverse and include hormones, chemokines, neurotransmitters, proteinases, inflammatory mediators, and even sensory signals such as odorants and photons. (See Schwartz 8th ed., p 411.)

9. SMAD proteins are
   A. Oncogenes
   B. Tumor suppressors
   C. Regulators of transcription
   D. Regulators of translation

**Answer: B**

Resistance to transforming growth factor-β's (TGF-β's) anticancer action is one hallmark of human cancer cells. TGF-β receptors and SMADs are identified as tumor suppressors. The TGF-β signaling circuit can be disrupted in a variety of ways and in different types of human tumors. Some lose TGF-β responsiveness through downregulation or mutations of their TGF-β receptors. The cytoplasmic SMAD4 protein, which transduces signals from ligand-activated TGF-β receptors to downstream targets, may be eliminated through mutation of its encoding gene. The locus encoding cell cycle inhibitor $p15^{INK4B}$ may be deleted. Alternatively, the immediate downstream target of its actions, cyclin-dependent kinase 4 (CDK4), may become unresponsive to the inhibitory actions of $p15^{INK4B}$ because of mutations that block p15 binding. The resulting cyclin D/CDK4 complexes constitutively inactivate tumor suppressor pRb by hyperphosphorylation. Finally, functional pRb, the end target of this pathway, may be lost through mutation of its gene. For example, in pancreatic and colorectal cancers 100% of cells derived from these cancers carry genetic defects in the TGF-β signaling pathway. Therefore, the antiproliferative pathway converging onto pRb and the cell division cycle is, in one way or another, disrupted in a majority of human cancer cells. (See Schwartz 8th ed., p 413.)

10. Which of the following drugs is a monoclonal antibody to an oncogene?
    A. Trastuzumab
    B. Methotrexate
    C. Adriamycin
    D. Gleevec

**Answer: A**

Trastuzumab is a monoclonal antibody that neutralizes the mitogenic activity of cell-surface growth factor receptor HER-2. Approximately 25% of breast cancers overexpress HER-2. These tumors tend to grow faster and are generally more likely to recur than tumors that do not overproduce HER-2. Trastuzumab is designed to attack cancer cells that overexpress HER-2. Trastuzumab slows or stops the growth of these cells and increases the survival of HER-2-positive breast cancer patients.

STI571, also known as Gleevec, is one of the first molecularly targeted drugs based on the changes that cancer causes in cells. STI571 offers promise for the treatment of chronic myeloid leukemia (CML) and may soon surpass interferon-γ as the standard treatment for the disease. In CML, STI571 is targeted at the Bcr-Abl kinase, an activated oncogene product in CML (Fig. 14-13). Bcr-Abl is an overly activated protein kinase resulting from a specific genetic abnormality generated by chromosomal translocation that is found in the cells of patients with CML. STI571-mediated inhibition of Bcr-Abl-kinase activity not only prevents cell growth of Bcr-Abl-transformed leukemic cells, but also induces apoptosis. Clinically, the drug quickly corrects the blood cell abnormalities caused by the leukemia in a majority of patients, achieving a complete disappearance of the leukemic blood cells and the return of normal blood cells. Additionally, the drug appears to have some effect on other cancers including certain brain tumors and gastrointestinal stromal tumors (GISTs), a very rare type of stomach cancer. (See Schwartz 8th ed., p 414.)

# CHAPTER 15

# Skin and Subcutaneous Tissue

1. The treatment of a hydrofluoric acid skin burn is
   A. Injection of sodium bicarbonate
   B. Irrigation with sodium bicarbonate
   C. Application of calcium carbonate gel
   D. Local wound care only

**Answer: C**

Hydrofluoric and sulfuric acid are common agents that cause skin injury from acidic solution exposure. The effect an acid has on the skin is determined by the concentration, duration of contact, amount, and penetrability. Hydrofluoric acid is a colorless, fuming liquid that has a highly corrosive effect on skin, causing extensive liquefactive necrosis and severe pain. Deep tissue injury may result, damaging nerves, blood vessels, tendons, and bone. The initial treatment after contact with the skin is copious irrigation, which must be continued for at least 15 to 30 min with either water or normal saline. The second aspect of treatment aims to inactivate the free fluoride ion by promoting the formation of an insoluble fluoride salt. Many topical therapies have been advocated and their role in treatment largely anecdotal. Topical quaternary ammonium compounds are still widely used. Topical calcium carbonate gel has been shown to detoxify the fluoride ion and relieve pain. The treatment involves massage of a 2.5% calcium carbonate gel into the area of exposure for at least 30 min. Some investigators advocate continuing this treatment six times per day for 4 days. (See Schwartz 8th ed., p 432.)

2. Histologically identifiable injury to the skin occurs after 1 h of pressure at which of the following levels?
   A. 60 mm Hg
   B. 120 mm Hg
   C. 180 mm Hg
   D. 240 mm Hg

**Answer: A**

Pressure ulcers, as the name implies, are caused by excessive, unrelieved pressure. In animal studies, 60 mm Hg of pressure applied to the skin for 1 h produces histologically identifiable injuries such as venous thrombosis, muscle degeneration, and tissue necrosis. (See Schwartz 8th ed., p 432.)

3. Sacral pressure of a patient lying on a hospital mattress is approximately
   A. 60 mm Hg
   B. 120 mm Hg
   C. 180 mm Hg
   D. 240 mm Hg

**Answer: B**

Normal arteriole, capillary, and venule pressures are 32, 20, and 12 mm Hg, respectively. Pressure generated under the ischial tuberosities while a person is seated can reach 300 mm Hg, and sacral pressure can range from 100 to 150 mm Hg while a person lies on a standard hospital mattress. Healthy individuals regularly shift their body weight, even while asleep. Sitting in one position for extended periods of time causes pain via increased pressure in certain areas; this, in turn, stimulates the initiation of movement. Patients unable to sense pain or to shift their body weight, such as paraplegics or bedridden individuals, develop prolonged elevated tissue pressures, and, eventually, necrosis. Muscle tissue is more sensitive to ischemia than the overlying skin. Therefore, the necrotic area is usually wider and deeper than it appears on first inspection (Fig. 15-2 A&B). (See Schwartz 8th ed., pp 432–433.)

4. The presence of sulfur granules in a draining wound should lead to the use of which of the following antibiotics?
   A. Penicillin
   B. Gentamicin
   C. Rifampin
   D. Amphotericin

**Answer: A**

Actinomycosis is a granulomatous suppurative bacterial disease caused by actinomyces. Forty to 60% of the actinomycotic infections occur in the craniofacial skeleton, and the mandible is the site of predilection. Actinomycotic infection is usually caused by tooth extraction, odontogenic infection, or trauma. *Actinomyces* is an organism of the Actinomycetaceae family in the Actinomycetales order. Other actinomycetes, including *Nocardia*, *Actinomadura*, and *Streptomyces* cause mycetomas, which are deep cutaneous infections that present as nodules and spread to form draining tracts to the skin and surrounding soft tissue. Chronic disease causes fibrosis and contractures. The most common site for infection is the foot (Madura foot).

The anaerobic gram-positive bacteria that cause these infections were once believed to be fungi because they grow slowly as branched filaments and chains. Diagnosis depends on the presence of characteristic sulfur granules on microscopic examination. Special stains should be used to exclude fungal infection. Penicillin and sulfonamides are effective against these infections. Abscesses and areas of chronic scarring may require surgical therapy. (See Schwartz 8th ed., p 435.)

5. Lymphogranuloma venereum is caused by
   A. *Treponema pallidum*
   B. *Chlamydia trachomatis*
   C. *Neisseria gonorrhea*
   D. *Mycobacterium fortuitum*

**Answer: B**

*Chlamydia trachomatis* is a sexually transmitted, intracellular, gram-negative bacterium. After infection and a 2-week incubation period, an inconspicuous ulcer appears on the penis or labia, although in more than half of the cases, this lesion is not noticed or does not appear. A few weeks later, inguinal lymphadenopathy is apparent. The nodes become very large and painful (buboes) and are occasionally confused with an incarcerated inguinal hernia. Adenopathy can occur above and below the inguinal ligament, forming a characteristic groove. The matted nodes may suppurate, and occasionally rupture. Surgical drainage of unruptured abscesses is not recommended because a chronic draining sinus often develops. Active infection is treated with doxycycline for 1 week or azithromycin in one dose for uncomplicated disease and 14 days of treatment with doxycycline for complicated disease. Inflammation from infection can lead to lymphatic obstruction and chronic lower extremity edema. Rectal strictures also can occur. (See Schwartz 8th ed., p 435.)

6. A 3-mm basal cell carcinoma of the skin should be treated with
   A. Biopsy and gross total excision
   B. Excision with 2- to 4-mm normal margin
   C. Dermatologic laser vaporization
   D. Electrodesiccation

**Answer: B**

Basal cell carcinomas usually are slow growing, and patients often neglect these lesions for years. Metastasis and death from this disease are extremely rare, but these lesions can cause extensive local destruction. The majority of small (less than 2 mm), nodular lesions may be treated by dermatologists with curettage and electrodesiccation or laser vaporization. A drawback to these procedures is that no pathologic specimen is obtained to confirm the diagnosis or evaluate the tumor margins. Larger tumors, lesions that invade bone or surrounding structures, and more aggressive histologic types (morpheaform, infiltrative, and basosquamous) are best treated by surgical excision with a 2- to 4-mm margin of normal tissue. Histologic confirmation that the margins of resection do not contain tumor is required. Because nodular lesions are less likely to recur, the smaller margin may be used, whereas other types need a wider margin of resection. Alternative methods of treatment, such as radiation therapy and Mohs' surgery, are discussed later under "Alternative Therapy." (See Schwartz 8th ed., p 440.)

7. What percentage of melanomas are not pigmented?
    A. 1–2%
    B. 5–10%
    C. 12–15%
    D. 18–22%

**Answer: B**
The important clinical features of a melanoma include a pigmented lesion with an irregular, raised surface and irregular borders. Approximately 5 to 10% of melanomas are not pigmented. Lesions that change in color and size and ulcerate over a few months' time are considered suspicious and should be biopsied. (See Schwartz 8th ed., p 441.)

8. Which of the following is the most common type of melanoma?
    A. Acral lentiginous
    B. Superficial spreading
    C. Nodular
    D. Lentigo maligna

**Answer: B**
There are four common types of melanoma. These are, in order of decreasing frequency, superficial spreading, nodular, lentigo maligna, and acral lentiginous. Each has distinct characteristics and behaviors.

The most common type, representing up to 70% of melanomas, is the superficial spreading type. These lesions occur anywhere on the skin except the hands and feet. They are flat, commonly contain areas of regression, and measure 1 to 2 cm in diameter at the time of diagnosis (Fig. 15-9). There is a relatively long radial growth phase before vertical growth begins.

The nodular type accounts for 15 to 30% of melanomas. These lesions are darker and raised. The histologic criterion for a nodular melanoma is the lack of radial growth peripheral to the area of vertical growth; hence, all nodular melanomas are in the vertical growth phase at the time of diagnosis. Although it is an aggressive lesion, the prognosis for a patient with a nodular-type lesion is the same as that for a patient with a superficial spreading lesion of the same depth of invasion.

The lentigo maligna type, accounting for 4 to 15% of melanomas, occurs mostly on the neck, the face, and the back of the hands of elderly people. These lesions are always surrounded by dermis with heavy solar degeneration. They tend to become quite large before a diagnosis is made, but also have the best prognosis because invasive growth occurs late. Only 5 to 8% of lentigo malignas are estimated to evolve to invasive melanoma. (See Schwartz 8th ed., p 441.)

9. What is the most common melanoma in dark-skinned people?
    A. Acral lentiginous
    B. Superficial spreading
    C. Nodular
    D. Lentigo maligna

**Answer: A**
Acral lentiginous type is the least-common subtype, representing only 2 to 8% of melanoma in whites. It occurs on the palms and soles and in the subungual regions. Although melanoma among dark-skinned people is relatively rare, the acral lentiginous type accounts for 29 to 72% of all melano-

mas in dark-skinned people (African Americans, Asians, and Hispanics) than in people with less-pigmented skin. Subungual lesions appear as blue-black discolorations of the posterior nail fold and are most common on the great toe or thumb. The additional presence of pigmentation in the proximal or lateral nail folds (Hutchinson's sign) is diagnostic of subungual melanoma. (See Schwartz 8th ed., p 441.)

10. The tumor, node, metastases classification for melanoma uses the following in its classification EXCEPT
    A. Regional lymph nodes
    B. Serum protein level
    C. Vertical thickness of the primary tumor
    D. Depth of invasion
    E. Metastases

**Answer: B**

The original staging system classified melanoma into local (stage I), regional lymph node (stage II), and metastatic (stage III) disease. This staging system was not advantageous given that most patients were categorized into stage I disease, therefore limiting its usefulness in prognostic studies. The most current staging system, from the American Joint Committee on Cancer (AJCC), contains the best method of interpreting clinical information in regard to prognosis of this disease (Table 15-1). Historically, the vertical thickness of the primary tumor (Breslow thickness) and the anatomic depth of invasion (Clark level) have represented the dominant factors in the T classification the melanoma staging system. (See Schwartz 8th ed., p 442.)

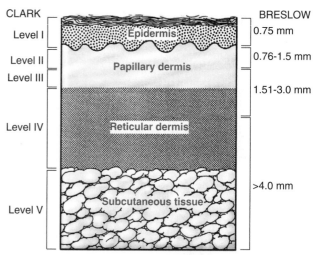

**FIG. 15-1.** *The primary melanoma is classified according to its depth of invasion in the skin. The criteria for Clark's and Breslow's levels are illustrated. The current T classification adopted by the AJCC is a modification of these classifications. See Schwartz 8th ed., p 442.*

11. Clark Level IV extends to which of the following structures?
    A. Epidermis
    B. Papillary dermis
    C. Reticular dermis
    D. Subcutaneous tissue

**Answer: C**

The T classification of lesions comes from the original observation by Clark that prognosis is directly related to the level of invasion of the skin by the melanoma. Clark used the histologic level: I, superficial to basement membrane (in situ); II, papillary dermis; III, papillary/reticular dermal junction; IV, reticular dermis; and V, subcutaneous fat. (See Schwartz 8th ed., p 442.)

12. A patient with a 3-mm deep melanoma of the face with a clinically positive jugular node should undergo what procedure in addition to resection of the primary?
    A. None
    B. Resection of grossly positive nodes
    C. Modified radical neck dissection
    D. Modified radical neck dissection and superficial parotidectomy

**Answer: C**
All clinically positive lymph nodes should be removed by regional nodal dissection. If possible, the lymphatics between the lesion and the regional nodes are removed in continuity. Leaving tumor behind results in recurrence of lesions that cause great morbidity. When groin lymph nodes are removed, the deep (iliac) nodes must be removed along with the superficial (inguinal) nodes, or disease will recur in that region. For axillary dissections the nodes medial to the pectoralis minor muscle must also be resected. For lesions on the face, anterior scalp, and ear, a superficial parotidectomy to remove parotid nodes and a modified neck dissection is recommended. Disruption of the lymphatic outflow does cause significant problems with chronic edema, especially of the lower extremity. (See Schwartz 8th ed., p 443.)

13. A patient with a 5-mm depth melanoma of the thigh and no clinically positive nodes should undergo what procedure in addition to resection of the primary?
    A. None
    B. Superficial femoral node resection
    C. Superficial and deep femoral node resection
    D. Resection of femoral and inguinal nodal basins

**Answer: A**
Treatment of regional lymph nodes that do not obviously contain tumor in patients without evidence of metastasis (stages I and II) is determined by considering the possible benefits of the procedure as weighed against the risks. In patients with thin lesions (less than 0.75 mm), the tumor cells are still localized in the surrounding tissue, and the cure rate is excellent with wide excision of the primary lesion; therefore treatment of regional lymph nodes is not beneficial. With very thick lesions (more than 4 mm), it is highly likely that the tumor cells have already spread to the regional lymph nodes and distant sites. Removal of the lymph nodes has no effect on survival. Most of these patients die of metastatic disease before developing problems in regional nodes. Because there are significant morbid effects of lymphadenectomy, most surgeons defer the procedure until clinically evident disease appears. Approximately 40% of these patients eventually develop disease in the lymph nodes and require a second palliative operation. Elective lymphadenectomy is sometimes performed in these patients as a staging procedure before entry into clinical trials. (See Schwartz 8th ed., p 443.)

14. The treatment of a Merkel cell carcinoma is
    A. Biopsy and observation
    B. Local excision only
    C. Resection with a 1-cm margin
    D. Resection with a 3-cm margin and prophylactic nodal resection

**Answer: D**
Originally thought to be a variant of squamous cell carcinoma, it was only recently demonstrated by immunohistochemical markers that Merkel cell carcinomas are of neuroepithelial differentiation. These tumors are associated with a synchronous or metasynchronous squamous cell carcinoma 25% of the time. These tumors are very aggressive, and wide local resection with 3-cm margins is recommended. Local recurrence rates are high, and distant metastases occur in one-third of patients. Prophylactic regional lymph node dissection and adjuvant radiation therapy are recommended. Overall, the prognosis is worse than for malignant melanoma. (See Schwartz 8th ed., p 445.)

15. The treatment of Kaposi's sarcoma is
    A. Local excision only
    B. Wide local excision and chemotherapy
    C. Wide local excision, chemotherapy, and radiation therapy
    D. Radiation therapy only

**Answer: D**
Kaposi's sarcoma (KS) appears as rubbery bluish nodules that occur primarily on the extremities but may appear anywhere on the skin and viscera. These lesions are usually multifocal rather than metastatic. Histologically the lesions are composed of capillaries lined by atypical endothelial cells.

Early lesions may resemble hemangiomas, while older lesions contain more spindle cells and resemble sarcomas.

Classic KS is seen in people of Eastern Europe or sub-Saharan Africa. The lesions are locally aggressive but undergo periods of remission. Visceral spread of the lesions is rare, but a subtype of the African variety has a predilection for spreading to lymph nodes. A different variety of KS has been described for people with acquired immunodeficiency syndrome (AIDS) or with immunosuppression from chemotherapy. For reasons not yet understood, AIDS-related KS occurs primarily in male homosexuals and not in intravenous drug abusers or hemophiliacs. In this form of the disease, the lesions spread rapidly to the nodes, and the gastrointestinal and respiratory tract often are involved. Development of AIDS-related KS may be associated with concurrent infection with a herpes-like virus.

Treatment for all types of KS consists of radiation to the lesions. Combination chemotherapy is effective in controlling the disease, although most patients develop an opportunistic infection during or shortly after treatment. Surgical treatment is reserved for lesions that interfere with vital functions, such as bowel obstruction or airway compromise. (See Schwartz 8th ed., p 446.)

16. All of the following statements about hidradenitis suppurativa are true EXCEPT
    A. Lesions are found in the axilla, the groin, and the perianal area.
    B. Plugged apocrine glands with secondary infection cause the problem.
    C. When chronic hydradenitis is present, wide surgical excision is the preferred treatment.
    D. When surgical procedures are done, the wound should be left open to granulate in by secondary intention.

**Answer: D**
Hydradenitis suppurativa occurs when apocrine gland ducts become plugged from grease or poor hygiene. Lesions occur in areas of the body with numerous apocrine glands such as the axilla, groin, and perianal region. When the process becomes chronic, wide surgical excision is the procedure of choice. Wounds in the affected area do not heal well by secondary intention, and immediate application of a split thickness skin graft is more appropriate. (See Schwartz 7th ed.)

17. Correct statements about toxic epidermal necrolysis (TEN) include all of the following EXCEPT
    A. Corticosteroid use is a primary part of therapy
    B. Lesions are similar in appearance to partial thickness burns
    C. The process develops at the dermoepidermal junction
    D. Toxic epidermal necrolysis is believed to be an immunologic problem

**Answer: A**
TEN can be an extension process, with skin sloughing over large areas of the body. The slough occurs at the dermoepidermal junction, and the skin rejuvenates spontaneously if secondary infection is avoided. The process appears to be an immunologic one secondary to certain drugs, such as the sulfamides and the barbiturates. Corticosteroids have not been effective therapy, and their use may lead to problems with infection. (See Schwartz 7th ed.)

18. Staphylococcal scalded skin syndrome
    A. Is caused by an exotoxin
    B. Is a toxic reaction to antibiotics used in treating staphylococcal abscesses
    C. Presents as a papillary rash in skin fold areas
    D. Usually begins around a neglected carbuncle

**Answer: A**
Staphylococcal scalded skin syndrome is caused by an exotoxin produced during a staphylococcal infection of the nasopharynx or middle ear. The process occurs in young children with wide areas of skin sloughing in the granular layer of the epidermis. (See Schwartz 7th ed.)

19. The best cosmetic results for large capillary (port wine) hemangiomas are achieved by
    A. Excision and split-thickness graft
    B. Tattooing
    C. Cryosurgery
    D. Laser destruction

**Answer: D**
The capillary (port wine) hemangioma is a lesion made up of closely packed, dilated, abnormal capillaries in the subpapillary, dermal, or subdermal layer of the skin. Growth of the hemangioma parallels that of the involved area. If the lesion is small, it may be treated by excision and closure, but larger lesions are difficult to manage because excision causes a contour defect and scar. Recently, the introduction of laser destruction of large lesions has provided the most effective and best cosmetic results. Achieving a good color match between normal skin and a hemangioma by tattooing has proved difficult, and because the tattoo pigment is absorbed, repeated procedures are necessary. (See Schwartz 7th ed.)

20. The cancer with the highest rise in incidence in the United States in the past decade is
    A. Basal cell carcinoma of the skin
    B. Cancer of the breast
    C. Cancer of the lung
    D. Malignant melanoma
    E. Cancer of the colon

**Answer: D**
The incidence of melanoma was 1 in 1500 persons in the United States in 1935. By 1987, this rate had changed to 1 in 135. Ultraviolet irradiation from sun exposure is considered the major reason for its dramatic rise. The incidences of lung and breast cancer have also increased significantly. Basal cell carcinomas, also secondary to sun exposure, have always been common lesions. The incidence rate of colon cancer has not changed significantly. (See Schwartz 7th ed.)

21. All of the following statements about Kaposi's sarcoma in patients with acquired immunodeficiency syndrome (AIDS) are correct EXCEPT
    A. The lesions are usually multifocal.
    B. Lesions are rubbery blue nodules that resemble hemangiomas.
    C. The gastrointestinal tract is often involved.
    D. Intravenous drug abusers are frequently affected.

**Answer: D**
Kaposi's sarcoma in young people was one of the first recognized manifestations of AIDS. The lesions, which are usually multifocal, are initially rubbery blue nodules that resemble hemangiomas. In the AIDS population, gastrointestinal involvement is frequent. Individual lesions are radiosensitive. For unclear reasons, Kaposi's sarcoma in AIDS patients has been found in male homosexuals but not in intravenous drug abusers or hemophiliacs who developed AIDS after receiving contaminated blood products. (See Schwartz 7th ed.)

22. A 65-year-old farmer presents with a 1.5-cm ulcerated lesion on the middle third of his lower lip. The lesion has been present for 4 months and is not painful. No lymph nodes are palpable in the patient's neck. The most likely diagnosis is
    A. Squamous cell carcinoma
    B. Herpes simplex
    C. Keratoacanthoma
    D. Lichen planus

**Answer: A**
The majority of cancers of the lip are squamous cell carcinomas, and 93% of these arise in the lower lip. The lesions grow slowly but relentlessly. Lymph node metastases occur late in the natural course of the tumors and most often involve the submental node on the side of the lesion. The prognosis for small squamous cell carcinomas of the lip is excellent, whereas that for large lesions with metastasis is significantly worse. Surgery and radiotherapy have been shown to be equally effective, and the choice between the two is often based on convenience and attendant morbidity. In most cases, the treatment of choice is surgical excision for small lesions, radiotherapy for medium lesions, and a combination of the two for very large lesions. Because carcinoma is related to prolonged exposure to sunlight and because radiotherapy increases sensitivity to such exposure, surgery is often preferable in patients such as farmers. (See Schwartz 7th ed.)

23. A 65-year-old patient who spends winters in Florida presents with a painless, ulcerated lesion on his right cheek. The lesion has been present for 1 year. Physical examination of the patient's neck reveals no lymph node enlargement. The most likely diagnosis is
    A. Melanoma
    B. Basal cell carcinoma
    C. Squamous cell carcinoma
    D. Sebaceous cyst

**Answer: B**
Basal cell carcinoma is the most common low-grade malignancy of skin found in the head and neck region. Regional lymph node metastases are rare in this condition compared with the incidence of regional node metastasis that occurs with squamous cell carcinoma or melanoma. Basal cell carcinoma tends to be less clearly defined and to grow more slowly than squamous cell carcinoma, and differential diagnosis between the two conditions usually can be made on the basis of site, appearance, history, type of skin, and the presence or absence of scars. Neglected basal cell lesions cause destruction by local invasion and erosion of contiguous structures, including the skull and brain. (See Schwartz 7th ed.)

1. The treatment of choice for a 1.8 cm in diameter, N0, M0 invasive breast cancer is
   A. Lumpectomy alone
   B. Lumpectomy, sentinel node biopsy, and radiation
   C. Mastectomy with sentinel node biopsy and radiation
   D. Mastectomy with axillary node dissection and radiation

**Answer: B**
Currently, mastectomy with assessment of axillary lymph node status and breast conservation (lumpectomy with assessment of axillary lymph node status and radiation therapy) are considered equivalent treatments for stages I and II breast cancer. Axillary lymphadenopathy or metastatic disease in a sentinel axillary lymph node necessitates an axillary lymph node dissection. Breast conservation is considered for all patients because of the important cosmetic advantages. Relative contraindications to breast conservation therapy include (1) prior radiation therapy to the breast or chest wall; (2) involved surgical margins or unknown margin status following re-excision; (3) multicentric disease; and (4) scleroderma or other connective-tissue disease. (See Schwartz 8th ed., p 482.)

2. Which of the following is associated with an increased risk of in situ carcinoma of the breast?
   A. Sclerosing adenosis
   B. Intraductal papilloma
   C. Fibroadenoma
   D. Atypical lobular hyperplasia

**Answer: D**

**Table 16-1.**
**Cancer Risk Associated with Benign Breast Disorders and In Situ Carcinoma of the Breast**

| Abnormality | Relative Risk |
| --- | --- |
| Nonproliferative lesions of the breast | No increased risk |
| Sclerosing adenosis | No increased risk |
| Intraductal papilloma | No increased risk |
| Florid hyperplasia | 1.5 to 2-fold |
| Atypical lobular hyperplasia | 4-fold |
| Atypical ductal hyperplasia | 4-fold |
| Ductal involvement by cells of atypical ductal hyperplasia | 7-fold |
| Lobular carcinoma in situ | 10-fold |
| Ductal carcinoma in situ | 10-fold |

Source: Modified with permission from Dupont WD, Page DL: Risk factors for breast cancer in women with proliferative breast disease *N Engl J Med* 312:146, 1985.
See Schwartz 8th ed., p 464.

3. The benign disorder most likely to mimic carcinoma of the breast is
   A. Fibroadenoma
   B. Papilloma
   C. Sclerosing adenosis
   D. Apocrine metaplasia

**Answer: C**
Proliferative breast disorders without atypia include sclerosing adenosis, radial scars, complex sclerosing lesions, ductal epithelial hyperplasia, and intraductal papillomas. Sclerosing adenosis is prevalent during the childbearing and perimenopausal years and has no malignant potential. Histologic changes are both proliferative (ductal proliferation)

and involutional (stromal fibrosis, epithelial regression) in nature. Sclerosing adenosis is characterized by distorted breast lobules and usually occurs in the context of multiple microcysts, but occasionally presents as a palpable mass. Benign calcifications are often associated with this disorder. The clinical significance of sclerosing adenosis lies in its mimicry of cancer. It may be confused with cancer on physical examination, by mammography, and at gross pathologic examination. Excisional biopsy and histologic examination are frequently necessary to exclude the diagnosis of cancer. The diagnostic work-up for radial scars and complex sclerosing lesions frequently involves stereoscopic biopsy. It is usually not possible to differentiate these lesions with certainty from cancer by mammography features, so biopsy is recommended. (See Schwartz 8th ed., p 465.)

4. Which of the following increases the risk of breast cancer?
   A. Multiple gestations
   B. Late menarche
   C. Late menopause
   D. Prolonged and multiple episodes of lactation

**Answer: C**
Increased exposure to estrogen is associated with an increased risk for developing breast cancer, whereas reducing exposure is thought to be protective. Correspondingly, factors that increase the number of menstrual cycles, such as early menarche, nulliparity, and late menopause, are associated with increased risk. Moderate levels of exercise and a longer lactation period, factors that decrease the total number of menstrual cycles, are protective. The terminal differentiation of breast epithelium associated with a full-term pregnancy is also protective, so older age at first live birth is associated with an increased risk of breast cancer. Finally, there is an association between obesity and increased breast cancer risk. Because the major source of estrogen in postmenopausal women is the conversion of androstenedione to estrone by adipose tissue, obesity is associated with a long-term increase in estrogen exposure. (See Schwartz 8th ed., p 466.)

5. The most appropriate treatment for a woman with lobular carcinoma in situ (LCIS) involving one quadrant is
   A. Observation
   B. Lumpectomy
   C. Lumpectomy with radiation therapy
   D. Mastectomy

**Answer: A**
LCIS originates from the terminal duct lobular units and only develops in the female breast. It is characterized by distention and distortion of the terminal duct lobular units by cancer cells, which are large but maintain a normal nuclear:cytoplasmic ratio. Cytoplasmic mucoid globules are a distinctive cellular feature. LCIS may be observed in breast tissues that contain microcalcifications, but the calcifications associated with LCIS typically occur in adjacent tissues. This neighborhood calcification is a feature that is unique to LCIS and contributes to its diagnosis. The frequency of LCIS in the general population cannot be reliably determined because it usually presents as an incidental finding. The age at diagnosis is 44 to 47 years, which is approximately 15 to 25 years younger than the age at diagnosis for invasive breast cancer. LCIS has a distinct racial predilection, occurring 12 times more frequently in white women than in African American women. Invasive breast cancer develops in 25 to 35% of women with LCIS. Invasive lobular cancer may develop in either breast, regardless of which breast harbored the initial focus of LCIS, and is detected synchronously with LCIS in 5% of cases. In women with a history of LCIS, up

to 65% of subsequent invasive cancers are ductal, not lobular in origin. For these reasons, LCIS is regarded as a marker of increased risk for invasive breast cancer rather than an anatomic precursor. (See Schwartz 8th ed., p 472.)

6. BRCA-1 gene mutations
   A. Result in cancers that are usually hormone receptor negative
   B. Have a high incidence in Sephardic Jews
   C. Are associated with an increased risk of cancer of the bile ducts
   D. Result in a lifetime risk of breast cancer of 20%

**Answer: A**

Five to 10% of breast cancers are caused by inheritance of germline mutations such as BRCA-1 and BRCA-2, which are inherited in an autosomal dominant fashion with varying penetrance (Table 16-8). BRCA-1 is located on chromosome 17q, spans a genomic region of about 100 kb of DNA, and contains 22 coding exons. The full-length messenger RNA (mRNA) is 7.8 kb and encodes a protein of 1863 amino acids. Both BRCA-1 and BRCA-2 function as tumor-suppressor genes, and for each gene, loss of both alleles is required for the initiation of cancer. Data accumulated since the isolation of the BRCA-1 gene suggest a role in transcription, cell-cycle control, and DNA damage repair pathways. More than 500 sequence variations in BRCA-1 have been identified. It now is known that germline mutations in BRCA-1 represent a predisposing genetic factor in as many as 45% of hereditary breast cancers and in at least 80% of hereditary ovarian cancers. Female mutation carriers have up to a 90% lifetime risk for developing breast cancer and up to a 40% lifetime risk for developing ovarian cancer. Breast cancer in these families appears as an autosomal dominant trait with high penetrance. Approximately 50% of children of carriers inherit the trait. In general, BRCA-1–associated breast cancers are invasive ductal carcinomas, are poorly differentiated, and are hormone receptor–negative. BRCA-1 associated breast cancers have a number of distinguishing clinical features, such as an early age of onset when compared with sporadic cases; a higher prevalence of bilateral breast cancer; and the presence of associated cancers in some affected individuals, specifically ovarian cancer and possibly colon and prostate cancers. (See Schwartz 8th ed., p 468.)

7. The most appropriate treatment for a woman with ductal carcinoma in situ (DCIS) involving 2 quadrants is
   A. Observation
   B. Lumpectomy
   C. Lumpectomy with radiation therapy
   D. Mastectomy

**Answer: D**

Women with DCIS and evidence of widespread disease (two or more quadrants) require mastectomy. For women with limited disease, lumpectomy and radiation therapy are recommended. Low-grade DCIS of the solid, cribriform, or papillary subtype, which is less than 0.5 cm in diameter, may be managed by lumpectomy alone. For nonpalpable DCIS, needle localization techniques are used to guide the surgical resection. Specimen mammography is performed to ensure that all visible evidence of cancer is excised. Adjuvant tamoxifen therapy is considered for all DCIS patients. The gold standard against which breast conservation therapy for DCIS is evaluated is mastectomy. Women treated with mastectomy have local recurrence and mortality rates of less than 2%. Women treated with lumpectomy and adjuvant radiation therapy have a similar mortality rate, but the local recurrence rate increases to 9%. Forty-five percent of these recurrences will be invasive cancer. Both Lagios and Gump noted that recurrence of DCIS was greatest when the cancers were more than 2.5 cm in size, the criteria for histologic

8. Lobular carcinoma in situ (LCIS)
   A. Can be diagnosed on mammogram by microcalcifications adjacent to a mass
   B. Can occur in men, although it is rare
   C. Is usually diagnosed in the sixth decade of life
   D. Progresses to lobular carcinoma in 50% of women

9. Paget's disease
   A. Is associated with underlying lobular carcinoma
   B. Can be differentiated from melanoma by carcinoembryonic antigen staining
   C. Is self-limiting and requires no treatment
   D. Is diagnosed by characteristic skin changes in the axilla

10. Medullary cancer of the breast
    A. Is associated with the BRCA-2 gene
    B. Often has enlarged lymph nodes in the axilla at presentation
    C. Has a worse prognosis than invasive ductal carcinoma
    D. Is rarely associated with ductal carcinoma in situ (DCIS)

confirmation of clear margins were not rigorously applied, and the DCIS was of the comedo type. They noted that recurrences frequently occurred within the original surgery site, indicating that inadequate clearance of DCIS, rather than the biology of the cancer, was responsible. (See Schwartz 8th ed., p 481.)

**Answer: A**

LCIS may be observed in breast tissues that contain microcalcifications, but the calcifications associated with LCIS typically occur in adjacent tissues. (See Schwartz 8th ed., p 472.)

**Answer: B**

Paget's disease of the nipple frequently presents as a chronic, eczematous eruption of the nipple, which may be subtle, but may progress to an ulcerated, weeping lesion. Paget's disease is usually associated with extensive ductal carcinoma in situ (DCIS) and may be associated with an invasive cancer. A palpable mass may or may not be present. Biopsy of the nipple will show a population of cells that are identical to the underlying DCIS cells (pagetoid features or pagetoid change). Pathognomonic of this cancer is the presence of large, pale, vacuolated cells (Paget's cells) in the rete pegs of the epithelium. Paget's disease may be confused with superficial spreading melanoma. Differentiation from pagetoid intraepithelial melanoma is based on S-100 antigen immunostaining in melanoma and carcinoembryonic antigen (CEA) immunostaining in Paget's disease. Surgical therapy for Paget's disease may involve lumpectomy, mastectomy, or modified radical mastectomy, depending on the extent of involvement and the presence of invasive cancer. (See Schwartz 8th ed., p 474.)

**Answer: B**

Medullary carcinoma is a special-type breast cancer; it accounts for 4% of all invasive breast cancers and is a frequent phenotype of BRCA-1 hereditary breast cancer. Grossly, the cancer is soft and hemorrhagic. A rapid increase in size may occur secondary to necrosis and hemorrhage. On physical examination, it is bulky and often positioned deep within the breast. Bilaterality is reported in 20% of cases. Medullary carcinoma is characterized microscopically by (1) a dense lymphoreticular infiltrate composed predominantly of lymphocytes and plasma cells; (2) large pleomorphic nuclei that are poorly differentiated and show active mitosis; and (3) a sheet-like growth pattern with minimal or absent ductal or alveolar differentiation (Fig. 16-19). Approximately 50% of these cancers are associated with DCIS, which is characteristically present at the periphery of the cancer, and fewer than 10% demonstrate hormone receptors. In rare circumstances, mesenchymal metaplasia or anaplasia is noted. Because of the intense lymphocyte response associated with the cancer, benign or hyperplastic enlargement of the lymph nodes of the axilla may contribute to erroneous clinical staging. Women with this cancer have a better 5-year survival rate than those with no special type (NST) or invasive lobular carcinoma. (See Schwartz 8th ed., p 474.)

11. Mondor's disease
    A. Is usually self-limiting and spontaneously resolves in 4–6 weeks
    B. Is indicative of an increased risk of breast cancer
    C. Requires surgical treatment for cure
    D. Is often bilateral

**Answer: A**

Mondor's disease is a variant of thrombophlebitis which involves the superficial veins of the anterior chest wall and breast. Frequently involved veins include the lateral thoracic vein, the thoracoepigastric vein, and, less frequently, the superficial epigastric vein. Typically, a woman presents with acute pain in the lateral aspect of the breast or the anterior chest wall. A tender, firm cord is found to follow the distribution of one of the major superficial veins. Rarely, the presentation is bilateral, and most women have no evidence of thrombophlebitis in other anatomic sites. This benign, self-limited disorder is not indicative of a cancer. When the diagnosis is uncertain, or when a mass is present near the tender cord, biopsy is indicated. Therapy for Mondor's disease includes the liberal use of anti-inflammatory medications and warm compresses that are applied along the symptomatic vein. Restriction of motion of the ipsilateral extremity and shoulder as well as brassiere support of the breast are important. The process usually resolves within 4 to 6 weeks. When symptoms persist or are refractory to therapy, excision of the involved vein segment is appropriate. (See Schwartz 8th ed., p 463.)

12. The false-positive rate for mammography in the diagnosis of breast cancer is
    A. <1%
    B. ~5%
    C. ~10%
    D. ~15%

**Answer: C**

An experienced radiologist can detect breast cancer with a false-positive rate of 10% and a false-negative rate of 7%. Specific mammography features that suggest a diagnosis of a breast cancer include a solid mass with or without stellate features, asymmetric thickening of breast tissues, and clustered microcalcifications. The presence of fine, stippled calcium in and around a suspicious lesion is suggestive of breast cancer and occurs in as many as 50% of nonpalpable cancers. These microcalcifications are an especially important sign of cancer in younger women, in whom it may be the only mammography abnormality. (See Schwartz 8th ed., p 476.)

13. Clinical determination of lymph node status in women with breast cancer has an accuracy of
    A. ~20%
    B. ~33%
    C. ~50%
    D. ~74%

**Answer: B**

The clinical stage of breast cancer is determined primarily through physical examination of the skin, breast tissue, and lymph nodes (axillary, supraclavicular, and cervical). However, clinical determination of axillary lymph node metastases has an accuracy of only 33%. Mammography, chest X-ray, and intraoperative findings (primary cancer size, chest wall invasion) also provide necessary staging information. Pathologic stage combines clinical stage data with findings from pathologic examination of the resected primary breast cancer and axillary lymph nodes. (See Schwartz 8th ed., p 477.)

14. Which of the following occurs in Poland's syndrome?
    A. Juvenile hypertrophy of the breast
    B. Hamartoma of the breast
    C. Polythelia
    D. Amastia

**Answer: D**

Absence of the breast (amastia) is rare and results from an arrest in mammary ridge development that occurs during the sixth fetal week. Poland's syndrome consists of hypoplasia or complete absence of the breast, costal cartilage and rib defects, hypoplasia of the subcutaneous tissues of the chest wall, and brachysyndactyly. Breast hypoplasia also may be iatrogenically induced prior to puberty by trauma, infection, or radiation therapy. (See Schwartz 8th ed., p 456.)

15. Symmastia is
    A. Duplication of the breast
    B. Ectopic breast tissue
    C. Ectopic nipples
    D. Webbing of the breast across the midline

**Answer: D**

Symmastia is a rare anomaly recognized as webbing between the breasts across the midline. (See Schwartz 8th ed., p 456.)

16. Which of the following is a benign disorder associated with stromal development of the breast?
    A. Fibroadenoma
    B. Adolescent hypertrophy
    C. Duct ectasia
    D. Epithelial hyperplasia

**Answer: B**

**Table 16-2.**
**ANDI Classification of Benign Breast Disorders**

| Normal → | Disorder→ | Disease |
|---|---|---|
| **Early reproductive years (age 15–25)** | | |
| Lobular development | Fibroadenoma | Giant fibroadenoma |
| Stromal development | Adolescent hypertrophy | Gigantomastia |
| Nipple eversion | Nipple inversion | Subareolar abscess Mammary duct fistula |
| **Later reproductive years (age 25–40)** | | |
| Cyclical changes of menstruation | Cyclical mastalgia Nodularity | Incapacitating mastalgia |
| Epithelial hyperplasia of pregnancy | Bloody nipple discharge | |
| **Involution (age 35–55)** | | |
| Lobular involution | Macrocysts Sclerosing lesions | |
| Duct involution –Dilatation –Sclerosis | Duct ectasia Nipple retraction | Periductal mastitis |
| Epithelial turnover | Epithelial hyperplasia | Epithelial hyperplasia with atypia |

ANDI = aberrations of normal development and involution.
Source: Modified with permission from Hughes LE: in Hughes LE, Mansel RE, Webster DJT (eds): Aberrations of normal development and involution (ANDI): A concept of benign breast disorders based on pathogenesis. *Benign Disorders and Diseases of the Breast: Concepts and Clinical Management*. London: WB Saunders, 2000, p 23.
See Schwartz 8th ed., p 463.

17. A breast cancer that is larger than 5 cm with no positive nodes or metastases is
    A. Stage I
    B. Stage II
    C. Stage III
    D. Stage IV

**Answer: C**
(See Table 16-4 on pp 121–122.)

18. Level II axillary nodes
    A. Are located around the axillary vein
    B. Are medial to or above the pectoralis minor muscle
    C. Are made up of the central and interpectoral nodes
    D. Are made up of the external mammary and scapular nodes

**Answer: C**

Lymph node groups are assigned levels according to their relationship to the pectoralis minor muscle. Lymph nodes located lateral to or below the lower border of the pectoralis minor muscle are referred to as level I lymph nodes, which include the axillary vein, external mammary, and scapular groups. Lymph nodes located superficial or deep to the pectoralis minor muscle are referred to as level II lymph nodes, which include the central and interpectoral groups. Lymph nodes located medial to or above the upper border of the pectoralis minor muscle are referred to as level III lymph nodes, which consist of the subclavicular group. (See Schwartz 8th ed., p 458.)

19. The use of screening mammography in women older than 50 years decreases the mortality from breast cancer by
    A. ~15%
    B. ~18%
    C. ~25%
    D. ~33%

**Answer: D**

Routine use of screening mammography in women age 50 years and older reduces mortality from breast cancer by 33%. This reduction comes without substantial risks and at an acceptable economic cost. However, the use of screening mammography is more controversial in women younger than age 50 years for several reasons: (1) breast density is greater and screening mammography is less likely to detect early breast cancer; (2) screening mammography results in more false-positive tests, resulting in unnecessary biopsies; and (3) younger women are less likely to have breast cancer so fewer young women will benefit from screening. However, on a population basis, the benefits of screening mammography in women between the ages of 40 and 49 years still appear to outweigh the risks. Targeting mammography to women at higher risk of breast cancer may also improve the balance of risks and benefits. In one study of women ages 40 to 49 years, an abnormal mammography finding was three times as likely to be cancer in a woman with a family history of breast cancer. (See Schwartz 8th ed., p 468.)

20. Mucinous carcinoma (colloid carcinoma) of the breast
    A. Occurs most commonly in young women
    B. Is associated with the BRCA-1 gene
    C. Has a good prognosis with a 5-year survival of >70%
    D. Is usually hormone receptor negative

**Answer: C**

Mucinous carcinoma (colloid carcinoma), another special-type breast cancer, accounts for 2% of all invasive breast cancers and typically presents in the elderly population as a bulky tumor. This cancer is defined by extracellular pools of mucin, which surround aggregates of low-grade cancer cells. The cut surface of this cancer is glistening and gelatinous in quality. Fibrosis is variable, and when abundant it imparts a firm consistency to the cancer. Approximately 66% of mucinous carcinomas display hormone receptors. Lymph node metastases occur in 33% of cases and 5- and 10-year survival rates are 73 and 59%, respectively. Because of the mucinous component, cancer cells may not be evident in all microscopy sections and analysis of multiple sections is essential to confirm the diagnosis of a mucinous carcinoma. (See Schwartz 8th ed., p 474.)

21. Tubular carcinoma of the breast
    A. Occurs most commonly in elderly women
    B. Has a poor prognosis if there are any axillary nodal metastases
    C. Is related to cribriform carcinoma
    D. Is rarely diagnosed by mammography

**Answer: C**

Tubular carcinoma is another special-type breast cancer and accounts for 2% of all invasive breast cancers. It is reported in as many as 20% of women whose cancers are diagnosed by mammography screening and is usually diagnosed in the perimenopausal or early menopausal periods. Under low-power magnification, a haphazard array of small, randomly arranged tubular elements is seen. Approximately 10% of women with tubular carcinoma or with invasive cribriform carcinoma, a special-type cancer closely related to tubular carcinoma, will develop axillary lymph node metastases, which are usually confined to the lowest axillary lymph nodes (level I). However, the presence of metastatic disease in one or two axillary lymph nodes does not adversely affect survival. Distant metastases are rare in tubular carcinoma and invasive cribriform carcinoma. Long-term survival approaches 100%. (See Schwartz 8th ed., p 475.)

22. What percentage of breast cancers are caused by a mutation in the BRCA gene?
    A. <3%
    B. 5–10%
    C. 15–20%
    D. 25–30%

**Answer: B**
Five to 10% of breast cancers are caused by inheritance of germline mutations such as BRCA-1 and BRCA-2, which are inherited in an autosomal dominant fashion with varying penetrance. (See Schwartz 8th ed., p 468.)

23. The BRCA genes are
    A. Tumor suppressor genes
    B. Proto-oncogenes
    C. Regulators of RNA transcription
    D. Regulators of protein modification

**Answer: A**
Both BRCA-1 and BRCA-2 function as tumor-suppressor genes, and for each gene, loss of both alleles is required for the initiation of cancer. Data accumulated since the isolation of the BRCA-1 gene suggest a role in transcription, cell-cycle control, and DNA damage repair pathways. (See Schwartz 8th ed., p 468.)

24. The histological characteristic that defines in situ (as opposed to invasive) ductal carcinoma is
    A. Fewer than three cell layers protruding into the lumen of the duct
    B. Fewer than five cell layers protruding into the lumen of the duct
    C. No invasion through the basement membrane
    D. Invasion into a blood vessel

**Answer: C**
Cancer cells are in situ or invasive depending on whether or not they invade through the basement membrane. Broder's original description of in situ breast cancer stressed the absence of invasion of cells into the surrounding stroma and their confinement within natural ductal and alveolar boundaries. As areas of invasion may be minute, the accurate diagnosis of in situ cancer necessitates the analysis of multiple microscopy sections to exclude invasion. (See Schwartz 8th ed., p 472.)

25. Mild ductal hyperplasia is characterized by
    A. Three to four cell layers above the basement membrane
    B. Five or more cell layers above the basement membrane
    C. Obstruction of 10–30% of the ductal lumen
    D. Obstruction of 70% or more of the ductal lumen

**Answer: A**
Mild ductal hyperplasia is characterized by the presence of three or four cell layers above the basement membrane. Moderate ductal hyperplasia is characterized by the presence of five or more cell layers above the basement membrane. Florid ductal epithelial hyperplasia occupies at least 70% of a minor duct lumen. It is found in more than 20% of breast tissue specimens, is either solid or papillary, and carries an increased cancer risk. (See Schwartz 8th ed., p 465.)

26. The risk of invasive ductal carcinoma in women with ductal carcinoma in situ (DCIS) is increased
    A. 5-fold
    B. 15-fold
    C. 30-fold
    D. 50-fold

**Answer: A**
The risk for invasive breast cancer is increased nearly five-fold in women with DCIS. The invasive cancers are observed in the ipsilateral breast, usually in the same quadrant as the DCIS that was originally detected, suggesting that DCIS is an anatomic precursor of invasive ductal carcinoma. (See Schwartz 8th ed., p 473.)

27. The average lifetime risk for breast cancer in American women is
    A. 3%
    B. 8%
    C. 12%
    D. 20%

**Answer: C**

The average lifetime risk of breast cancer for newborn U.S. females is 12%. The longer a woman lives without cancer, the lower her risk of developing breast cancer. Thus, a woman age 50 years has an 11% lifetime risk of developing breast cancer, and a woman age 70 years has a 7% lifetime risk of developing breast cancer. (See Schwartz 8th ed., p 467.)

28. Antibodies in colostrum are produced by
    A. Duct epithelium
    B. Lactiferous sinus epithelium
    C. Lymphocytes
    D. Myoepithelial cells

**Answer: C**

Colostrum produced during the first few days after delivery is low in lipid content. Colostrum contains a considerable quantity of preformed antibodies that are transferred to the fetus. Lymphocytes and plasma cells that infiltrate the breast during pregnancy are the source of these antibodies. (See Schwartz 7th ed.)

29. Which statement best describes lymphatic drainage from the breast?
    A. All quadrants of the breast drain into both the axillary and the parasternal nodes
    B. The areolar area of the breast drains into retrosternal internal mammary nodes
    C. The lateral area of the breast drains into axillary nodes
    D. The medial area of the breast drains into parasternal nodes

**Answer: A**

Vital dye flow studies report that both the axillary and the parasternal lymphatic groups receive lymph from all quadrants of the breast. (See Schwartz 7th ed.)

30. Maintenance of lactation requires all of the following EXCEPT
    A. Estradiol secretion
    B. Intact hypothalamic pituitary axis
    C. Oxytocin release
    D. Prolactin release

**Answer: A**

Regular sucking sets up a neural reflex arc. In these circumstances, an intact hypothalamic pituitary axis leads to prolactin release that stimulates milk production and oxytocin release that initiates smooth muscle contraction of myoepithelial cells around the alveoli, leading to expansion of milk under pressure into the lactiferous sinuses. Estradiol and progesterone, elevated during pregnancy, inhibit prolactin activity. (See Schwartz 7th ed.)

31. Drugs that may produce gynecomastia include all of the following EXCEPT
    A. Cimetidine
    B. Diazepam
    C. Furosemide
    D. Tamoxifen

**Answer: D**

Tamoxifen is occasionally used to treat benign disease such as gynecomastia. Cimetidine and diazepam are among the drugs that inhibit the synthesis of testosterone. Furosemide and verapamil induce gynecomastia, although the mechanism is not clear. Gynecomastia also is produced by digitalis and marijuana, which have estrogenic-related activity. (See Schwartz 7th ed.)

32. Mammography is indicated for evaluation of a 40-year-old woman in all of the following situations EXCEPT
    A. Breast pain and discomfort in large fatty breasts without palpable nodules
    B. Breasts with multiple nodules but no dominant area
    C. Follow-up of the opposite breast after contralateral mastectomy for carcinoma
    D. Presence of a small, smooth, solitary lesion as a substitute for biopsy

**Answer: D**

Mammography is not a substitute for biopsy, and a 40-year-old patient with an isolated breast lesion should undergo biopsy regardless of mammographic findings. Mammography is particularly useful in evaluation of a patient with multiple nodules throughout both breasts; it is easy to miss a small carcinoma in these circumstances. Evaluation after surgical treatment for cancer is important to evaluate recurrence or for early detection of a cancer in the opposite breast. In a symptomatic patient, the study may offer reassurance to both patient and physician that no occult cancer is present. (See Schwartz 7th ed.)

33. A 40-year-old woman is found to have a 3-cm, firm, smooth mass in the upper outer quadrant of the breast. The mass is aspirated, and 10 mL of cloudy green fluid is removed. The appropriate management at this time is
    A. Administration of estrogen
    B. Cytologic evaluation of the aspirated fluid
    C. Excision of the cyst
    D. Observation only

**Answer: D**
A cyst containing clear or cloudy green fluid is appropriately managed by cyst aspiration. Unless the fluid is bloody, cytology is not required. There is no need to remove a solitary cyst. Hormone manipulation is not required in this situation. (See Schwartz 7th ed.)

34. A smooth, rubbery, 3-cm lesion is removed from the breast of a 35-year-old woman with a preoperative diagnosis of fibroadenoma. Histologically, this lesion is found to be a phyllode tumor. Appropriate management at this time is
    A. Observation only
    B. Reexcision of the area with a 1-cm margin
    C. Total (simple) mastectomy
    D. Total mastectomy with axillary dissection

**Answer: B**
Although most small phyllode tumors are benign, re-excision of the biopsy scar should be done on this patient to make certain that complete removal has been achieved. More radical observation or hormone therapy is not required. (See Schwartz 7th ed.)

35. Which of the following biopsy findings has the greatest relative risk for later carcinoma?
    A. Apocrine metaplasia
    B. Atypical lobular hyperplasia
    C. Ductal ectasia
    D. Sclerosing adenosis

**Answer: B**
Apocrine metaplasia and ductal ectasia have no increased risk. Intraductal papilloma and sclerosing adenosis have a slightly increased risk (1.5 to 2 times). Atypical lobular hyperplasia has a moderately increased risk (4 to 5 times) of later cancer. (See Schwartz 7th ed.)

36. A breast cancer that is 3 cm in diameter with positive, moveable, ipsilateral nodes is
    A. Stage I
    B. Stage II
    C. Stage III
    D. Stage IV

**Answer: B**
See Table 16-4 on pp 121–122.

**Table 16-3.**
**Tumor (T), Node (N), Metastases (M) Stage Groupings**

| Stage 0 | Tis | N0 | M0 |
|---|---|---|---|
| Stage I | T1[a] | N0 | M0 |
| Stage IIA | T0 | N1 | M0 |
| | T1[a] | N1 | M0 |
| | T2 | N0 | M0 |
| Stage IIB | T2 | N1 | M0 |
| | T3 | N0 | M0 |
| Stage IIIA | T0 | N2 | M0 |
| | T1[a] | N2 | M0 |
| | T2 | N2 | M0 |
| | T3 | N1 | M0 |
| | T3 | N2 | M0 |
| Stage IIIB | T4 | N0 | M0 |
| | T4 | N1 | M0 |
| | T4 | N2 | M0 |
| Stage IIIC | Any T | N3 | M0 |
| Stage IV | Any T | Any N | M1 |

[a]T1 includes T1 mic.
Source: Modified with permission from American Joint Committee on Cancer: AJCC Cancer Staging Manual, 6th ed. New York: Springer, 2002, p 228.
See Schwartz 8th ed., p 484.

**Table 16-4.**
**Tumor (T), Node (N), Metastases (M) Staging System for Breast Cancer**

*Primary tumor (T) definitions for classifying the primary tumor (T) are the same for clinical and for pathologic classification. If the measurement is made by physical examination, the examiner will use the major headings (T1, T2, or T3); if other measurements, such as mammographic or pathologic measurements, are used, the subsets of T1 can be used. Tumors should be measured to the nearest 0.1-cm increment*

| | |
|---|---|
| TX | Primary tumor cannot be assessed |
| T0 | No evidence of primary tumor |
| Tis | Carcinoma in situ |
| Tis(DCIS) | Ductal carcinoma in situ |
| Tis (LCIS) | Lobular carcinoma in situ |
| Tis(Paget's) | Paget's disease of the nipple with no tumor (Note: Paget's disease associated with a tumor is classified according to the size of the tumor) |
| T1 | Tumor 2 cm or less in greatest dimension |
| T1mic | Microinvasion 0.1 cm or less in greatest dimension |
| T1a | Tumor more than 0.1 cm but not more than 0.5 cm in greatest dimension |
| T1b | Tumor more than 0.5 cm but not more than 1 cm in greatest dimension |
| T1c | Tumor more than 1 cm but not more than 2 cm in greatest dimension |
| T2 | Tumor more than 2 cm but not more than 5 cm in greatest dimension |
| T3 | Tumor more than 5 cm in greatest dimension |
| T4 | Tumor of any size with direct extension to (a) chest wall or (b) skin, only as described below |
| T4a | Extension to chest wall, not including pectoralis muscle |
| T4b | Edema (including peau d'orange), or ulceration of the skin of the breast, or satellite skin nodules confined to the same breast |
| T4c | Both T4a and T4b |
| T4d | Inflammatory carcinoma |

**Regional lymph nodes—Clinical (N)**

| | |
|---|---|
| NX | Regional lymph nodes cannot be assessed (e.g., previously removed) |
| N0 | No regional lymph node metastasis |
| N1 | Metastasis to movable ipsilateral axillary lymph node(s) |
| N2 | Metastases in ipsilateral axillary lymph nodes fixed or matted, or in clinically apparent[a] ipsilateral internal mammary nodes in the absence of clinically evident axillary lymph node metastasis |
| N2a | Metastasis in ipsilateral axillary lymph nodes fixed to one another (matted) or to other structures |
| N2b | Metastasis only in clinically apparent[a] ipsilateral internal mammary nodes and in the absence of clinically evident axillary lymph node metastasis |
| N3 | Metastasis in ipsilateral infraclavicular lymph node(s) with or without axillary lymph node involvement, or in clinically apparent[a] ipsilateral internal mammary lymph node(s) and in the presence of clinically evident axillary lymph node metastasis; or metastasis in ipsilateral supraclavicular lymph node(s) with or without axillary or internal mammary lymph node involvement |
| N3a | Metastasis in ipsilateral infraclavicular lymph node(s) |
| N3b | Metastasis in ipsilateral internal mammary lymph nodes(s) and axillary lymph node(s) |
| N3c | Metastasis in ipsilateral supraclavicular lymph node(s) |

**Regional lymph nodes—Pathologic (pN)**

| | |
|---|---|
| PNx | Regional lymph nodes cannot be assessed (e.g., previously removed, or not removed for pathologic study) |
| pN0[b] | No regional lymph node metastasis histologically, no additional examination for isolated tumor cells (Note: Isolated tumor cells [ITC] are defined as single tumor cells or small cell clusters not greater than 0.2 mm, usually detected only by immunohistochemical [IHC] or molecular methods but which may be verified on H&E stains; ITCs do not usually show evidence of malignant activity [e.g., proliferation or stromal reaction]) |
| pN0(i–) | No regional lymph node metastasis histologically, negative IHC |
| pN0(i+) | No regional lymph node metastasis histologically, positive IHC, no IHC cluster greater than 0.2 mm |
| pN0(mol–) | No regional lymph node metastasis histologically, negative molecular findings (RT-PCR) |
| pN0(mol+) | No regional lymph node metastasis histologically, positive molecular findings (RT-PCR) |
| pN1 | Metastasis in 1 to 3 axillary lymph nodes, and/or in internal mammary nodes with microscopic disease detected by sentinel lymph nodes dissection, not clinically apparent[c] |
| pN1mi | Micrometastasis (greater than 0.2 mm, none greater than 2.0 mm) |
| pN1a | Metastasis in 1 to 3 axillary lymph nodes |
| pN1b | Metastasis in internal mammary nodes with microscopic disease detected by sentinel lymph node dissection, not clinically apparent[c] |

*(continued)*

**Table 16-4.**
**Tumor (T), Node (N), Metastases (M) Staging System for Breast Cancer  (Continued)**

| | |
|---|---|
| pN1c | Metastasis in 1 to 3 axillary lymph nodes and in internal mammary lymph nodes with microscopic disease detected by sentinel lymph node dissection but not clinically apparent[c] (if associated with greater than 3 positive axillary lymph nodes, the internal mammary nodes are classified as pN3b to reflect increased tumor burden) |
| pN2 | Metastasis in 4 to 9 axillary lymph nodes, or in clinically apparent[a] internal mammary lymph nodes in the absence of axillary lymph node metastasis |
| pN2a | Metastasis in 4 to 9 axillary lymph nodes (at least one tumor deposit greater than 2.0 mm) |
| pN2b | Metastasis in clinically apparent[a] internal mammary lymph nodes in the absence of axillary lymph node metastasis |
| pN3 | Metastasis in ≥10 axillary lymph nodes, or in infraclavicular lymph nodes, or in clinically apparent[a] ipsilateral internal mammary lymph nodes in the presence of 1 or more positive axillary lymph nodes; or in more than 3 axillary lymph nodes with clinically negative microscopic metastasis in internal mammary lymph nodes; or in ipsilateral supraclavicular lymph nodes |
| pN3a | Metastasis in 10 or more axillary lymph nodes (at least one tumor deposit greater than 2.0 mm), or metastasis to the infraclavicular lymph nodes |
| pN3b | Metastasis in clinically apparent[a] ipsilateral internal mammary lymph nodes in the presence of 1 or more positive axillary lymph nodes; or in more than 3 axillary lymph nodes and in internal mammary lymph nodes with microscopic disease detected by sentinel lymph node dissection, not clinically apparent[c] |
| pN3c | Metastasis in ipsilateral supraclavicular lymph nodes |
| **Distant metastasis (M)** | |
| MX | Distant metastasis cannot be assessed |
| M0 | No distant metastasis |
| M1 | Distant metastasis |

[a]Clinically apparent is defined as detected by imaging studies (excluding lymphoscintigraphy) or by clinical examination or grossly visible pathologically.

[b]Classification is based on axillary lymph node dissection with or without sentinel lymph node dissection. Classification based solely on sentinel lymph node dissection without subsequent axillary lymph node dissection is designated (sn) for "sentinel node" e.g., pN-(l+) (sn).

[c]Not clinically apparent is defined as not detected by imaging studies (excluding lymphoscintigraphy) or by clinical examination.

RT-PCR = reverse transcriptase polymerase chain reaction.

Source: Modified with permission from American Joint Committee on Cancer: AJCC Cancer Staging Manual, 6th ed. New York: Springer, 2002, pp 227–228.

See Schwartz 8th ed., p 483.

# CHAPTER 17

# Disorders of the Head and Neck

1. Which of the following statements about choleste-
   atoma is true?
   A. It is a malignant tumor.
   B. The primary symptom is tinnitus.
   C. It is caused from eustachian tube dysfunction.
   D. It is a disease of the inner ear.

**Answer: C**
Cholesteatoma is an epidermoid cyst of the middle ear and/or
mastoid, which causes bone destruction secondary to its expansile nature and through enzymatic destruction. Cholesteatoma develops as a consequence of eustachian tube dysfunction and chronic otitis media secondary to retraction of
squamous elements of the tympanic membrane into the middle ear space. Squamous epithelium may also migrate into the
middle ear via a perforation. Chronic mastoiditis that fails
medical management or is associated with cholesteatoma is
treated by mastoidectomy. (See Schwartz 8th ed., p 503.)

2. Diagnosis of chronic sinusitis is best made by
   A. Computed tomography scan
   B. Magnetic resonance imaging
   C. Nuclear medicine scanning
   D. History, physical, and nasal endoscopy

**Answer: D**
Nasal endoscopy is a critical element of the diagnosis of
chronic sinusitis. Anatomic abnormalities, such as septal deviation, nasal polyps, and purulence may be observed. The
finding of purulence by nasal endoscopy is diagnostic of sinusitis, regardless of whether other criteria are met. In a setting in which symptoms persist for at least 12 weeks, purulence on nasal exam represents an acute exacerbation of
chronic sinusitis. Pus found on endoscopic exam may be cultured, and subsequent antibiotic therapy can be directed accordingly. The spectrum of bacteria found in chronic sinusitis
is highly variable and includes higher prevalences of polymi-
crobial infections and antibiotic-resistant organisms. Overall,
*S. aureus*, coagulase-negative staphylococci, gram-negative
bacilli, and streptococci are isolated, in addition to the typical
pathogens of acute sinusitis. (See Schwartz 8th ed., p 504.)

3. Which of the following is an indication for tonsillec-
   tomy?
   A. Patient's request
   B. Chronic middle ear infection
   C. Three or more infections per year
   D. Missing more than one week of school per year

**Answer: C**
Tonsillectomy and adenoidectomy are indicated for chronic
or recurrent acute infection and for obstructive hypertrophy.
The American Academy of Otolaryngology–Head and Neck
Surgery Clinical Indicators Compendium (2000) suggests
tonsillectomy after three or more infections per year despite
adequate medical therapy. Some feel that tonsillectomy is
indicated in children who miss 2 or more weeks of school
annually secondary to tonsil infections. Multiple techniques
have been described, including electrocautery, sharp dissection, laser, and radiofrequency ablation. There is no consensus as to the best method. In cases of chronic or recurrent infection, surgery is considered only after failure of medical
therapy. (See Schwartz 8th ed., p 507.)

4. Which of the following statements concerning surgery for sleep apnea is true?
   A. Surgery is indicated in all patients.
   B. Most patients improve with time, and surgery is therefore not indicated.
   C. The majority of patients are treated with tracheostomy alone.
   D. The most common procedure performed is correction of soft palate collapse.

**Answer: D**

Sleep disorders represent a continuum from simple snoring to upper airway resistance syndrome (UARS) to obstructive sleep apnea (OSA). UARS and OSA are associated with excessive daytime somnolence and frequent sleep arousals. In OSA, polysomnogram demonstrates at least 10 episodes of apnea or hypopnea per hour of sleep. The average number of apneas and hypopneas per hour can be used to calculate a respiratory disturbance index (RDI), which, along with oxygen saturation, can be used to grade the severity of OSA. These episodes occur as a result of collapse of the pharyngeal soft tissues during sleep. In adults, it should be noted that in addition to tonsil size, factors such as tongue size and body mass index are significant predictors of OSA. Other anatomic findings associated with OSA include obese neck, retrognathia, low hyoid bone, and enlarged soft palate. Surgery should be considered after failure of more conservative measures, such as weight loss, elimination of alcohol use, and continuous positive airway pressure, and should be tailored to the particular patient's pattern of obstruction. In children, surgical management typically involves tonsillectomy and/or adenoidectomy, because the disorder is usually caused by hypertrophy of these structures. In adults, uvulopalatoplasty is frequently performed to alleviate soft-palate collapse and is the most common operation performed for sleep-disordered breathing. Multiple techniques have been described for this. Tongue base reduction, tongue advancement, hyoid suspension, and a variety of maxillomandibular advancement procedures also have been described with varying success. Adults with significant nasal obstruction may benefit from septoplasty or sinus surgery. Patients with severe OSA (RDI >40, lowest nocturnal oxygen saturation <70%) and unfavorable anatomy or comorbid pulmonary disease may require tracheotomy. (See Schwartz 8th ed., p 508.)

5. Hemangioma of the face in children
   A. Should be resected in the newborn period
   B. Should be resected only if it persists past 10 years of age
   C. Will involute by 3 years of age in most children
   D. Can be treated by laser ablation

**Answer: D**

Hemangiomas are the most common vascular lesions present in infancy and childhood. These lesions are present at birth in up to 30% of cases, but usually become apparent in the first few weeks of life. The lesions proliferate in size over the first year before beginning involution, which subsequently occurs over the next 2 to 12 years. Forty percent of cases will resolve completely, while the remainder requires intervention. Once the proliferative phase has ended, the lesion should be observed every 3 months for involution, and surgery should be considered for those that have not significantly involuted by 3 to 4 years of age. Surgical treatment of proliferating hemangiomas is reserved for lesions associated with severe functional or cosmetic problems, such as those involving the nasal tip or periorbital region. Treatment is performed with either the flashlamp-pumped pulsed-dye laser (FPDL), the potassium titanyl phosphate (KTP) laser, or the neodymium yttrium-aluminum garnet (Nd:YAG) laser, repeated every 4 to 6 weeks until the lesion disappears. Systemic steroids may be employed to arrest rapidly proliferating lesions until the child reaches 12 to 18 months, after which growth should stabilize or involution begin. Subcutaneous interferon-α 2a may also be used for this purpose. This treatment, however, is associated with neurologic side effects and should be used with caution. (See Schwartz 8th ed., p 510.)

6. Trauma of the auricle of the ear with hematoma formation
   A. Requires transcartilage sutures for approximation
   B. Requires bolstering for most injuries
   C. Can be treated conservatively with dressings only
   D. Aggressive débridement is essential

**Answer: B**

With laceration of the auricle, key structures such as the helical rim and antihelix must be carefully aligned. These injuries must be repaired such that the cartilage is covered. The principles of auricular repair are predicated on the fact that the cartilage has no intrinsic blood supply and is thus susceptible to ischemic necrosis following trauma. The suture should be passed through the perichondrium, while placement though the cartilage itself should be avoided. Auricular hematomas should be drained promptly, with placement of a bolster as a pressure dressing. A pressure dressing is frequently advocated after closure of an ear laceration. It also deserves note that the surgeon must avoid the temptation to perform aggressive débridement after injuries to the eyelid or auricle. Given the rich vascular supply to the face and neck, many soft-tissue components that appear devitalized will indeed survive. (See Schwartz 8th ed., p 512.)

7. Le Fort II fracture entails injuries to all of the following EXCEPT
   A. Medial wall of the orbit
   B. Alveolus
   C. Zygomaticomaxillary articulation
   D. Nasofrontal buttress
   E. Mandible

**Answer: E**

Le Fort I fractures occur transversely across the alveolus, above the level of the teeth apices. In a pure Le Fort I fracture, the palatal vault is mobile while the nasal pyramid and orbital rims are stable. The Le Fort II fracture extends through the nasofrontal buttress, medial wall of the orbit, across the infraorbital rim, and through the zygomaticomaxillary articulation. The nasal dorsum, palate, and medial part of the infraorbital rim are mobile. The Le Fort III fracture is also known as craniofacial disjunction. The frontozygomaticomaxillary, frontomaxillary, and frontonasal suture lines are disrupted. The entire face is mobile from the cranium. It is convenient to conceptualize complex midface fractures according to these patterns; however, in reality, fractures reflect a combination of these three types. (See Schwartz 8th ed., p 513.)

8. The most common site of Kaposi's sarcoma in the head and neck is
   A. Buccal mucosa
   B. Palate
   C. Tongue
   D. Floor of mouth

**Answer: B**

Squamous cell carcinoma and minor salivary gland tumors are the most common malignancies of the palate. The latter include adenoid cystic carcinoma, mucoepidermoid carcinoma, adenocarcinoma, and polymorphous low-grade adenocarcinoma. Mucosal melanoma may occur on the palate and presents as a nonulcerated, pigmented plaque. Kaposi's sarcoma of the palate is the most common intraoral site for this tumor. Tumors may present as either an ulcer or an exophytic or submucosal mass. Minor salivary gland tumors tend to arise at the junction of the hard and soft palate. (See Schwartz 8th ed., p 523.)

9. Lymph node metastases from oropharyngeal cancers most commonly occur at
   A. Level I
   B. Level II
   C. Level III
   D. Level IV
   E. Level V

**Answer: B**

Lymph node metastasis from oropharyngeal cancer most commonly occurs in the subdigastric area of level II. Metastases also are found in levels III, IV, and V, in addition to the retropharyngeal and parapharyngeal lymph nodes. Forty to 50% of patients have metastases at the time of presentation. Bilateral metastases are common from tumors arising in the tongue base and soft palate. (See Schwartz 8th ed., p 524.)

10. Prognostic factors for patients with laryngeal cancers include all of the following EXCEPT
    A. Tumor size
    B. Tumor grade
    C. Nodal metastasis
    D. Perineural invasions

**Answer: B**

Prognostic factors for patients with cancer of the larynx are tumor size, nodal metastasis, perineural invasion, and extracapsular spread of disease in cervical lymph nodes. Prognosis and patient comorbidity are two important considerations when arriving at a treatment plan for patients with laryngeal cancer. (See Schwartz 8th ed., p 528.)

11. Which of the following are level III lymph nodes of the neck?
    A. Upper jugular chain nodes
    B. Middle jugular chain nodes
    C. Lower jugular chain nodes
    D. Posterior triangle nodes
    E. Submental nodes

**Answer: B**

Level III—middle jugular chain nodes; inferior to the hyoid, superior to the level of the hyoid, deep to sternocleidomastoid muscle (SCM) from posterior border of the muscle to the strap muscles medially. (See Schwartz 8th ed., p 535.)

12. A lymph node that is inferior to the cricoid, superior to the clavicle and deep to the sternocleidomastoid muscle (SCM) is in what level?
    A. I
    B. II
    C. III
    D. IV

**Answer: D**

Level IV—lower jugular chain nodes; inferior to the level of the cricoid, superior to the clavicle, deep to SCM from posterior border of the muscle to the strap muscles medially. (See Schwartz 8th ed., p 535.)

# CHAPTER 18

# Chest Wall, Lung, Mediastinum, and Pleura

1. Which of the following is the preferred treatment of tracheal stenosis after prolonged intubation?
   A. Observation
   B. Balloon dilatation
   C. Laser ablation of scar
   D. Resection and primary anastomosis

**Answer: D**
The treatment of tracheal stenosis is resection and primary anastomosis. In nearly all postintubation injuries the injury is transmural, and significant portions of the cartilaginous structural support are destroyed. Measures such as laser ablation are temporizing. In the early phase of evaluating patients, dilatation using a rigid bronchoscope is useful to gain immediate dyspnea relief and to fully assess the lesion as well as its length, position, and relation to the vocal cords. Rarely if ever is a tracheostomy necessary. For patients unable to tolerate general anesthesia because of comorbidities, internal stents, typically silicone T tubes, are useful. Wire mesh stents should not be used, given their known propensity to erode through the wall of the airway. (See Schwartz 8th ed., p 547.)

2. The modified Chamberlain procedure is used to biopsy
   A. Aortopulmonary window nodes
   B. Paraesophageal nodes
   C. Supradiaphragmatic periaortic nodes
   D. Subcarinal nodes

**Answer: A**
A modified Chamberlain procedure can be used for evaluation of aortopulmonary window lymph nodes. A 4- to 5-cm incision is made over the left second costal cartilage, which on occasion is excised. The internal mammary vessels can be ligated or preserved. The dissection proceeds into the mediastinum along the aortic arch. Biopsy of the aortopulmonary window lymph nodes can then be performed. This approach also is used frequently to biopsy anterior mediastinal lymphomas, which are usually located just beneath the second and third costal cartilages. This procedure is less frequently performed with improved techniques of computed tomography (CT)-guided biopsy and positron emission tomography (PET) scanning. (See Schwartz 8th ed., p 552.)

3. Which of the following is NOT a non-small-cell tumor of the lung?
   A. Squamous cell carcinoma
   B. Bronchoalveolar carcinoma
   C. Large-cell carcinoma
   D. Carcinoid tumor

**Answer: D**
The term non-small-cell lung carcinoma (NSCLC) is used to distinguish a group of tumors from small-cell carcinoma. Tumors in the NSCLC group include squamous cell carcinoma, adenocarcinoma (including bronchoalveolar carcinoma), and large-cell carcinoma. Although they differ in appearance histologically, their clinical behavior and treatment is similar. As such, they are usefully thought of as a uniform group. However, each type has unique features that affect their clinical presentation and findings. (See Schwartz 8th ed., p 560.)

4. The 5-year survival after complete resection of a stage I lung cancer is
   A. 92%
   B. 78%
   C. 65%
   D. 44%

**Answer: C**

The current standard of treatment is surgical resection, accomplished by lobectomy or pneumonectomy, depending on the tumor location. Despite the term "early-stage," surgery as a single treatment modality remains disappointing. After surgical resection of postoperative pathologic stage IA disease, 5-year survival is only 67% as reported by Mountain in 1997. The figures decline with higher stages. The overall 5-year survival rate for stage I disease as a group is about 65%; for stage II disease it is about 41%. (See Schwartz 8th ed., p 571.)

5. Which of the following is an indication for surgical drainage of a lung abscess?
   A. Abscess >3 cm in diameter
   B. Hemoptysis
   C. Failure to decrease in size after 1 week of antibiotic therapy
   D. Persistent fever

**Answer: B**

Surgical drainage of lung abscesses is uncommon since drainage usually occurs spontaneously via the tracheobronchial tree. Indications for intervention include failure of medical therapy; an abscess under tension; an abscess increasing in size during appropriate treatment; contralateral lung contamination; an abscess larger than 4 to 6 cm in diameter; necrotizing infection with multiple abscesses, hemoptysis, abscess rupture, or pyopneumothorax; and inability to exclude a cavitating carcinoma. External drainage may be accomplished with tube thoracostomy, percutaneous drainage, or surgical cavernostomy. The choice between thoracostomy and radiologically-placed catheter drainage depends on the treating physician's preference and the availability of interventional radiology. Surgical resection is required in fewer than 10% of lung abscess patients. Lobectomy is the preferred intervention for bleeding from a lung abscess or pyopneumothorax. An important intraoperative consideration is to protect the contralateral lung with a double-lumen tube, bronchial blocker, or contralateral main stem intubation. Surgical treatment has a 90% success rate, with an associated mortality of 1 to 13%. (See Schwartz 8th ed., p 575.)

6. Which of the following is NOT a typical clinical presentation of pulmonary cryptococcosis?
   A. Granulomas
   B. Granulomatous pneumonia
   C. Lobar pneumonia
   D. Diffuse interstitial infiltrate

**Answer: C**

Cryptococcosis is a subacute or chronic infection caused by *Cryptococcus neoformans*, a round, budding yeast (5 to 20 μm in diameter) that is sometimes surrounded by a characteristic wide gelatinous capsule. Cryptococci are typically present in soil and dust contaminated by pigeon droppings. When inhaled, such droppings can cause a nonfatal disease primarily affecting the pulmonary and central nervous systems. At present, cryptococcosis is the fourth most common opportunistic infection in patients with human immunodeficiency virus (HIV) infection, affecting 6 to 10% of that population. Four basic pathologic patterns are seen in the lungs of infected patients: granulomas; granulomatous pneumonia; diffuse alveolar or interstitial involvement; and proliferation of fungi in alveoli and lung vasculature. Symptoms are nonspecific, as are the radiographic findings. *Cryptococcus* may be isolated from sputum, bronchial washings, percutaneous needle aspiration of the lung, or cerebrospinal fluid. Multiple antifungal agents are effective against *C. neoformans*, including amphotericin B and the azoles. (See Schwartz 8th ed., p 578.)

7. What percentage of chest wall masses are malignant?
   A. 10–20%
   B. 20–30%
   C. 40–50%
   D. 50–80%

**Answer: D**

Pain from a chest wall mass is typically localized to the area of the tumor. Pain is more often present (and more intense) with malignant tumors, but it can also be present in up to one-third of patients with benign tumors. With Ewing's sarcoma, fever and malaise may also be present. Age can provide guidance as to the possibility of malignancy. Patients with benign chest wall tumors are on average 26 years old; the average age for patients with malignant tumors is 40 years old. Overall, the probability of a chest wall tumor being malignant is 50 to 80%. (See Schwartz 8th ed., p 585.)

8. Chylothorax in a patient who is n.p.o. is diagnosed by
   A. Cloudy appearance of the fluid
   B. Triglycerides >110 mg/mL in the pleural fluid
   C. Lymphocytosis in the pleural fluid
   D. Leucocytosis in the pleural fluid

**Answer: C**

The main function of the duct is to transport fat absorbed from the digestive system. The composition of normal chyle is fat, with variable amounts of protein and lymphatic material (Table 18-24). Given the high volumes of chyle that flow through the thoracic duct, significant injuries can cause leaks in excess of 2 L per day; if left untreated, protein, volume, and lymphocyte depletion can lead to serious metabolic effects and death. The diagnosis generally requires thoracentesis, which may be grossly suggestive; often the pleural fluid is milky and nonpurulent. However, if the patient is nil per os (n.p.o., nothing by mouth), the pleural fluid may not be grossly abnormal. Laboratory analysis of the pleural fluid shows a high lymphocyte count and high triglyceride levels. If the triglyceride level is greater than 110 mg/100 mL, a chylothorax is almost certainly present (a 99% accuracy rate). If the triglyceride level is less than 50 mg/mL, there is only a 5% chance of chylothorax. In many clinical situations, the accumulation of chyle may be slow, because of minimal digestive fat flowing through the gastrointestinal tract after major trauma or surgery, so the diagnosis may be more difficult to establish. (See Schwartz 8th ed., p 603.)

9. Desmoid tumors
   A. Arise from the periosteum of the rib
   B. Require chemotherapy to treat or prevent metastatic disease
   C. Require radical excision (sacrificing neurovascular structures) to obtain 4-cm margins
   D. Are treated with wide local excision with a 2- to 4-cm margin

**Answer: D**

Desmoid tumors are unusual soft tissue neoplasms that arise from fascial or musculoaponeurotic structures. Histologically, they consist of proliferations of benign-appearing fibroblastic cells, abundant collagen, and few mitoses. Accordingly, some authorities consider desmoid tumors to be a form of fibrosarcoma.

Although the cause is unknown, multiple associations with other diseases and conditions are well documented, such as familial polyposis (Gardner syndrome), states of increased estrogen (pregnancy), and trauma. Surgical incisions (abdominal and thorax) have been the site of desmoid development, either in or near the scar.

Desmoid tumors do not metastasize, but they have a significant propensity to recur locally, with local recurrence rates as high as 5 to 50%, sometimes despite complete initial resection with histologically negative margins. Such locally aggressive behavior is secondary to microscopic tumor infiltration of muscle and surrounding soft tissues.

Surgery consists of wide local excision with a margin of 2 to 4 cm, and with intraoperative assessment of resection margins by frozen section. Typically, a rib is removed above and below the tumor with a 4- to 5-cm margin of rib. A margin of less than 1 cm results in much higher local recurrence rates. If a major neurovascular structure would have to be sacrificed, leading to high morbidity, then a margin of less than 1 cm would have to suffice. Survival after wide local excision with negative margins is 90% at 10 years. (See Schwartz 8th ed., p 586.)

10. A patient with an anterior mediastinal mass and elevated serum alpha fetoprotein most likely has
    A. A teratoma
    B. A seminomatous germ-cell tumor
    C. A non-seminomatous germ-cell tumor
    D. Metastatic hepatocellular carcinoma

**Answer: C**

The use of serum markers to evaluate a mediastinal mass can be invaluable in some patients. For example, seminomatous and nonseminomatous germ cell tumors can frequently be diagnosed and often distinguished from one another by the levels of alpha-fetoprotein (AFP) and human chorionic gonadotropin (hCG). In over 90% of nonseminomatous germ cell tumors, either the AFP or the hCG level will be elevated. Results are close to 100% specific if the level of either AFP or hCG is greater than 500 ng/mL. Some centers institute chemotherapy based on this result alone, without a biopsy. In contrast, the AFP level is always normal in patients with mediastinal seminomas; only 10% will have an elevated hCG, which is usually less than 100 ng/mL. Other serum markers, such as intact parathyroid hormone level for ectopic parathyroid adenomas, may be useful for diagnosing and also for intraoperatively confirming complete resection. After successful resection of a parathyroid adenoma, this hormone level should rapidly normalize. (See Schwartz 8th ed., p 592.)

11. The most appropriate biopsy to perform for a presumed osteosarcoma of the chest wall is
    A. Fine-needle biopsy
    B. Incisional biopsy
    C. Excisional biopsy
    D. Resection with 2-cm margin

**Answer: A**

When the diagnosis cannot be made by radiographic evaluation, a needle biopsy (fine-needle aspiration [FNA] or core) should be done. Pathologists experienced with sarcomas can accurately diagnose approximately 90% of patients using FNA techniques. A needle biopsy (FNA or core) has the advantage of avoiding wound and body cavity contamination (a potential complication with an incisional biopsy). (See Schwartz 8th ed., p 585.)

12. The most appropriate treatment of a 2-cm chondroma of the chest wall is
    A. Observation
    B. Gross total excision
    C. Resection with a 2-cm margin
    D. Resection with a 5-cm margin

**Answer: C**

Chondromas are one of the more common benign tumors of the chest wall. They are primarily seen in children and young adults. Chondromas usually occur at the costochondral junction anteriorly. Given their typical location and the young age of most patients, chondromas may be confused with costochondritis. Clinically, a mass (usually without pain) is present in the case of chondromas. Radiographically, the lesion is lobulated and radiodense; it may have diffuse or focal calcifications, and may displace the bony cortex without penetration. Chondromas may grow to huge sizes if left untreated. Treatment is surgical resection with a 2-cm margin. One must be certain, however, that the lesion is not a well-differentiated chondrosarcoma. In this case, a wider 4-cm margin is required to prevent local recurrence. Therefore, large chondromas should be treated surgically as low-grade chondrosarcomas. (See Schwartz 8th ed., p 585.)

13. What percentage of patients with myasthenia gravis has improvement in their symptoms after resection of a thymoma (by thymectomy)?
    A. 25%
    B. 50%
    C. 75%
    D. 95%

**Answer: A**

Thymoma is the most frequently encountered neoplasm of the anterior mediastinum in adults (seen most frequently between 40 and 60 years of age). They are rare in children. Most patients with thymomas are asymptomatic, but depending on the institutional referral patterns, between 10 and 50% have symptoms suggestive of myasthenia gravis or have circulating antibodies to acetylcholine receptor. However, less than 10% of patients with myasthenia gravis are found to have a thymoma on computed tomography (CT). Thymectomy leads to improvement or resolution of symptoms of myasthenia gravis in only about 25% of patients with thymomas. In contrast, in patients with myasthenia gravis and no thymoma, thymectomy results are superior: up to 50% of patients have a complete remission and 90% improve. In 5% of patients with thymomas, other paraneoplastic syndromes, including red cell aplasia, hypogammaglobulinemia, systemic lupus erythematosus, Cushing's syndrome, or syndrome of inappropriate antidiuretic hormone (SIADH) may be present. Large thymic tumors may present with symptoms related to a mass effect, which may include cough, chest pain, dyspnea, or superior vena cava syndrome. (See Schwartz 8th ed., pp 593–594.)

14. An "onion-peel" appearance of a rib on computed tomography is suggestive of
    A. Chondroma
    B. Osteosarcoma
    C. Plasmacytoma
    D. Ewing's sarcoma

**Answer: D**

Ewing's sarcomas occur in adolescents and young adults who present with progressive chest wall pain, but without the presence of a mass. Systemic symptoms of malaise and fever are often present. Laboratory studies reveal an elevated erythrocyte sedimentation rate and mild white blood cell elevation. Radiographically, the characteristic onion-peel appearance is produced by multiple layers of periosteum in the bone formation. Evidence of bony destruction is also common. The diagnosis can be made by a percutaneous needle biopsy or an incisional biopsy. (See Schwartz 8th ed., p 587.)

15. The appropriate treatment for a 4-cm incidentally discovered pericardial cyst is
    A. Observation
    B. Percutaneous image–guided drainage
    C. Thoracoscopic resection
    D. Open resection

**Answer: A**

Pericardial cysts, the most common type of mediastinal cysts, are usually asymptomatic and detected incidentally. Typically they contain a clear fluid and appear in the right costophrenic angle. The cyst wall lining is a single layer of mesothelial cells. For most simple, asymptomatic pericardial cysts, observation alone is recommended. Surgical resection or aspiration may be indicated for complex cysts or large symptomatic cysts. (See Schwartz 8th ed., p 597.)

16. Increased pleural adenosine deaminase is diagnostic for
    A. Adenocarcinoma
    B. Tuberculosis
    C. Bacterial infection
    D. Mesothelioma

**Answer: B**

If an exudative effusion is suggested, further diagnostic studies may be helpful. If total and differential cell counts reveal a predominance of neutrophils (>50% of cells), the effusion is likely to be associated with an acute inflammatory process (such as a parapneumonic effusion or empyema, pulmonary embolus, or pancreatitis). A predominance of mononuclear cells suggests a more chronic inflammatory process (such as cancer or tuberculosis). Gram's stains and cultures should be obtained, if possible with inoculation into culture bottles at the bedside. Pleural fluid glucose levels are frequently decreased (<60 mg/dL) with complex parapneumonic effusions or malignant effusions. Cytologic testing should be done on exudative effusions to rule out an associated malignancy. Cytologic diagnosis is accurate in diagnosing over 70% of malignant effusions associated with adenocarcinomas, but is less sensitive for mesotheliomas (<10%), squamous cell carcinomas (20%), or lymphomas (25 to 50%). If the diagnosis remains uncertain after drainage and fluid analysis, thoracoscopy and direct biopsies are indicated. Tuberculous effusions can now be diagnosed accurately by increased levels of pleural fluid adenosine deaminase (above 40 U per L). (See Schwartz 8th ed., p 599.)

17. Parapneumonic effusions should be drained if the pH is less than
    A. 7.4
    B. 7.3
    C. 7.2
    D. 7.1

**Answer: C**
Thoracic empyema is defined by a purulent pleural effusion. The most common causes are parapneumonic, but postsurgical or posttraumatic empyema is also common (Table 18-22). Grossly purulent, foul-smelling pleural fluid makes the diagnosis of empyema obvious on visual examination at the bedside. In the early stage, small to moderate turbid pleural effusions in the setting of a pneumonic process may require further pleural fluid analysis. Close clinical follow-up is also imperative to determine if progression to empyema is occurring. A deteriorating clinical course or a pleural pH of less than 7.20 and a glucose level of less than 40 mg/dL indicates the need to drain the fluid. (See Schwartz 8th ed., p 601.)

18. Mesotheliomas
    A. Occur only in the pleural space
    B. Are usually diagnosed by cytology on pleural fluid
    C. Have a better outcome with a mixed cell type
    D. Are treated by pleurectomy for early stage disease

**Answer: D**
The authors' current approach to malignant mesotheliomas is based on tumor stage and pulmonary performance status. For patients with early-stage mesotheliomas and good pulmonary function, extrapleural pneumonectomy is recommended, especially for epithelial mesotheliomas. Patients are referred for clinical trials of multimodality therapy, if available. For more advanced disease, or if patients have less-than-optimal pulmonary function or performance status, talc pleurodesis or supportive therapy is recommended. (See Schwartz 8th ed., p 607.)

19. The most appropriate treatment of a 2-cm fibrous dysplasia of the rib is
    A. Observation
    B. Gross total excision
    C. Resection with a 2-cm margin
    D. Resection with a 5-cm margin

**Answer: C**
The ribs are a frequent site of origin of fibrous dysplasia. As with chondromas, fibrous dysplasia most frequently occurs in young adults. However, pain is infrequent, and the location is more often in the posterolateral aspect of the rib cage. Fibrous dysplasia may be associated with trauma. Radiographically, an expansile mass is present, with cortical thinning and no calcification. Local excision with a 2-cm margin is curative. (See Schwartz 8th ed., p 585.)

20. Treatment of a malignant pleural effusion
    A. Should only be done if the lung can be expanded
    B. Requires at least two chest tubes to be placed
    C. Is successful in only 20–30% of patients
    D. Is indicated in all patients to improve quality of life

**Answer: A**

Malignant effusions are exudative and often tinged with blood. An effusion in the setting of a malignancy means a more advanced stage; it generally indicates an unresectable tumor, with a mean survival of 3 to 11 months. Occasionally, benign pleural effusions may be associated with a bronchogenic non-small-cell lung carcinoma (NSCLC), and surgical resection may still be indicated if the cytology of the effusions is negative for malignancy. An important issue is the size of the effusion and the degree of dyspnea that results. Symptomatic, moderate to large effusions should be drained by chest tube, pigtail catheter, or video-assisted thoracic surgery (VATS), followed by instillation of a sclerosing agent. Before sclerosing the pleural cavity, whether by chest tube or VATS, the lung should be nearly fully expanded. Poor expansion of the lung (because of entrapment by tumor or adhesions) generally predicts a poor result. The choice of sclerosant includes talc, bleomycin, or doxycycline. Success rates of controlling the effusion range from 60 to 90%, depending on the exact scope of the clinical study, the degree of lung expansion after the pleural fluid is drained, and the care with which the outcomes were reported. (See Schwartz 8th ed., p 600.)

21. The most common benign tumor of the rib is
    A. Osteochondroma
    B. Fibrous dysplasia
    C. Chondroma
    D. Eosinophilic granuloma

**Answer: A**

Osteochondromas are overall the most common benign bone tumor. Many are detected as incidental radiographic findings. Most are solitary; however, patients with multiple osteochondromas have a higher incidence of malignancy. Osteochondromas occur in the first 2 decades of life and they arise at or near the growth plate of bones. The lesions are benign during youth or adolescence. Osteochondromas that enlarge after completion of skeletal growth have the potential to develop into chondrosarcomas. When seen in the thorax they usually arise from the rib cortex and are often part of the autosomal dominant syndrome hereditary multiple exostoses. Key features in this circumstance are the known potential to degenerate into chondrosarcomas, which may be heralded by new onset of pain or gradual enlargement of the mass over time. Patients with multiple osteochondromatosis may have benign osteochondromas scattered throughout their rib cage. Thus, the presence of new or increasing localized pain would warrant excisional biopsy of the offending osteochondroma. Local excision of a benign osteochondroma is sufficient. If malignancy is determined, wide excision is performed with a 4-cm margin. (See Schwartz 8th ed., p 585.)

22. Which of the following is associated with a chest wall plasmacytoma?
    A. Elevation of alkaline phosphatase
    B. Elevation of serum immunoglobulins
    C. Elevation of erythrocyte sedimentation rate
    D. Elevation of serum calcium

**Answer: B**

Laboratory evaluations are usually of little help in assessing chest wall masses. In plasmacytoma, there may be monoclonality of one of the immunoglobulins with normal levels of other immunoglobulins. Another exception is osteosarcoma, in which alkaline phosphatase levels may be elevated. Still another exception is Ewing's sarcoma, in which the erythrocyte sedimentation rate may be elevated. (See Schwartz 8th ed., p 585.)

23. Eosinophilic granulomas are associated with
    A. Crohn's disease
    B. Parasitic infections
    C. Langerhans cell histiocytosis
    D. Gardner's syndrome

**Answer: C**

Eosinophilic granulomas are benign osteolytic lesions. They were originally thought to be destructive lesions with large numbers of eosinophilic cells. Yet eosinophilic granulomas of the ribs can also occur as solitary lesions or as part of a more generalized disease process of the lymphoreticular system termed Langerhans cell histiocytosis (LCH). In LCH, the involved tissue is infiltrated with large numbers of histiocytes (similar to Langerhans cells seen in skin and other epithelia), which are often organized as granulomas. The cause is unknown. Of all LCH bone lesions, 79% are solitary eosinophilic granulomas, 7% involve multiple eosinophilic granulomas, and 14% belong to other forms of more systemic LCH. (See Schwartz 8th ed., p 586.)

24. Osteosarcoma of the rib
    A. Is considered non-operable if pulmonary metastases are present
    B. Is treated with adjuvant chemotherapy before resection
    C. Is treated with radiation therapy before resection
    D. Requires excision with a 6-cm margin

**Answer: B**

Osteosarcomas are potentially sensitive to chemotherapy. Currently, preoperative chemotherapy before surgical resection is common. After chemotherapy, complete resection is performed with wide (4-cm) margins, followed by reconstruction. In patients presenting with lung metastases that are potentially amenable to surgical resection, induction chemotherapy may be given, followed by surgical resection of the primary tumor and of the pulmonary metastases. Following surgical treatment of known disease, additional maintenance chemotherapy is usually recommended. (See Schwartz 8th ed., p 587.)

25. Askin's tumor
    A. Is a tumor of neural crest origin
    B. Is associated with trisomy 11
    C. Expresses *n*-myc
    D. Occurs in all bones of the body

**Answer: A**

Primitive neuroectodermal tumors (PNETs) derive from primordial neural crest cells that migrate from the mantle layer of the developing spinal cord. This group of tumors includes neuroblastomas, ganglioneuroblastomas, and ganglioneuromas. Ewing's sarcomas and Askin's tumors are closely related to PNETs; together they are referred to as the Ewing's sarcoma/PNET family of tumors. Askin's tumors were originally described by Askin in 1979 as a "malignant, small-cell, round tumor of the thoracopulmonary region," and are now known to be members of the Ewing's sarcoma/PNET family. Ewing's sarcomas and PNETs have a common site: a genetic abnormality, a translocation between the long arms of chromosomes 11 and 22. They also share a consistent pattern of proto-oncogene expression and have been found to express the product of the MIC2 gene. Histologically, they are small-round cell tumors. (See Schwartz 8th ed., p 587.)

1. The most common form of atrial septal defect (ASD) is
   A. Sinus venosus defect
   B. Ostium primum defect
   C. Ostium secundum defect
   D. Combined primum and secundum defect

**Answer: C**

ASDs can be classified into three different types: (1) sinus venosus defects, comprising approximately 5 to 10% of all ASDs; (2) ostium primum defects, which are more correctly described as partial atrioventricular canal defects; and (3) ostium secundum defects, which are the most prevalent subtype, comprising 80% of all ASDs. (See Schwartz 8th ed., p 612.)

2. The most common age to close asymptomatic atrial septal defects (ASDs) is
   A. In the immediate newborn period
   B. After the child reaches 10 kg in weight
   C. Age 4–5 years
   D. During puberty

**Answer: C**

ASDs are closed when patients are between 4 and 5 years of age. Children of this size can usually be operated on without the use of blood transfusion and generally have excellent outcomes. Patients who are symptomatic may require repair earlier, even in infancy. Some surgeons, however, advocate routine repair in infants and children, as even smaller defects are associated with the risk of paradoxical embolism, particularly during pregnancy. In a recent review by Reddy and colleagues, 116 neonates weighing less than 2500 g who underwent repair of simple and complex cardiac defects with the use of cardiopulmonary bypass were found to have no intracerebral hemorrhages, no long-term neurologic sequelae, and a low operative-mortality rate (10%). These results correlated with the length of cardiopulmonary bypass and the complexity of repair. These investigators also found an 80% actuarial survival at 1 year and, more importantly, that growth following complete repair was equivalent to weight-matched neonates free from cardiac defects. (See Schwartz 8th ed., p 613.)

3. Which of the following is the most acceptable treatment for isolated aortic valvular stenosis?
   A. Balloon valvotomy
   B. Surgical valvotomy/revision
   C. Aortic valve replacement in childhood
   D. Conservative management with aortic valve replacement in adolescence

**Answer: A**

Balloon valvotomy performed in the cath lab has gained widespread acceptance as the procedure of choice for reduction of transvalvular gradients in symptomatic infants and children. This procedure is an ideal palliative option because mortality from surgical valvotomy can be high due to the critical nature of these patients' condition. Furthermore, balloon valvotomy provides relief of the valvular gradient by opening the valve leaflets without the trauma created by open surgery, and allows future surgical intervention to be performed on an unscarred chest. In general, most surgical groups have abandoned open surgical valvotomy and favor catheter-based balloon valvotomy. The decision regarding the most appropriate method to use depends on several crucial factors including the available medical expertise, the patient's overall status and hemodynamics, and the presence of associated cardiac defects requiring repair. (See Schwartz 8th ed., p 615.)

4. The most common location for a coarctation of the aorta is
   A. Aortic arch
   B. Distal to the left subclavian artery
   C. At the diaphragm
   D. At the level of the renal arteries

**Answer: B**
Coarctation of the aorta (COA) is defined as a luminal narrowing in the aorta that causes an obstruction to blood flow. This narrowing is most commonly located distal to the left subclavian artery. The embryologic origin of COA is a subject of some controversy. One theory holds that the obstructing shelf, which is largely composed of tissue found within the ductus, forms as the ductus involutes. The other theory holds that a diminished aortic isthmus develops secondary to decreased aortic flow in infants with enhanced ductal circulation. (See Schwartz 8th ed., pp 618–619.)

5. The treatment of choice for coarctation of the aorta (COA) in the newborn period is
   A. Resection and primary anastomosis
   B. Resection with interposition graft
   C. Balloon dilatation alone
   D. Balloon dilatation with stenting

**Answer: A**
The routine management of hemodynamically significant COA in all age groups has traditionally been surgical. The most common technique in current use is resection with end-to-end anastomosis or extended end-to-end anastomosis, taking care to remove all residual ductal tissue. The subclavian flap aortoplasty is another frequently used repair. In this method, the left subclavian artery is transected and brought down over the coarcted segment as a vascularized patch. The main benefit of these techniques is that they do not involve the use of prosthetic materials.

In summary, children younger than age 6 months with native COA should be treated with surgical repair, while those requiring intervention at later ages may be ideal candidates for balloon dilatation or primary stent implantation. Additionally, catheter-based therapy should be employed for those cases of restenosis following either surgical or primary endovascular management. (See Schwartz 8th ed., pp 619–620.)

6. Which of the following is a true surgical emergency in a newborn?
   A. Tetralogy of Fallot
   B. Truncus arteriosus
   C. Total anomalous pulmonary venous connection
   D. Coarctation of the aorta

**Answer: C**
Total anomalous pulmonary venous connection (TAPVC) occurs in 1 to 2% of all cardiac malformations and is characterized by abnormal drainage of the pulmonary veins into the right heart, whether through connections into the right atrium or into its tributaries. Accordingly, the only mechanism by which oxygenated blood can return to the left heart is through an atrial septal defect (ASD), which is almost uniformly present with TAPVC.

Unique to this lesion is the absence of a definitive form of palliation. Thus, TAPVC represents one of the only true surgical emergencies across the entire spectrum of congenital heart surgery. (See Schwartz 8th ed., p 622.)

7. The Fontan procedure is used to correct
   A. Tricuspid atresia
   B. Aortic stenosis
   C. Truncus arteriosus
   D. Total anomalous pulmonary venous connection

**Answer: A**
Recognizing the inadequacies of the initial repairs for tricuspid atresia, Glenn described the first successful cavopulmonary anastomosis, an end-to-side right pulmonary artery (RPA)-to-superior vena cava (SVC) shunt in 1958, and later modified this to allow flow to both pulmonary arteries. This end-to-side RPA-to-SVC anastomosis was known as the bidirectional

Glenn, and is the first stage to final Fontan repair in widespread use today. The Fontan repair was a major advancement in the treatment of congenital heart disease, as it essentially bypassed the right heart, and allowed separation of the pulmonary and systemic circulations. (See Schwartz 8th ed., p 627.)

8. Hypoplastic left heart syndrome is surgically treated with the
   A. Fontan procedure
   B. Norwood procedure
   C. Catheter balloon septoplasty
   D. Nothing, there is no effective treatment

**Answer: B**
In 1983, Norwood and colleagues described a two-stage palliative surgical procedure for relief of hypoplastic left heart syndrome that was later modified to the currently used three-stage method of palliation. Stage 1 palliation, also known as the modified Norwood procedure, bypasses the left ventricle by creating a single outflow vessel, the neoaorta, which arises from the right ventricle. (See Schwartz 8th ed., p 629.)

9. The arterial switch operation for transposition of the great vessels is best performed
   A. Within 2 weeks of births
   B. At 1 year of age
   C. At 10 kg of weight
   D. In adolescence

**Answer: A**
The most important consideration is the timing of surgical repair, because arterial switch should be performed within 2 weeks after birth, before the left ventricle loses its ability to pump against systemic afterload. In patients presenting later than 2 weeks, the left ventricle can be retrained with preliminary pulmonary artery banding and aortopulmonary shunt followed by definitive repair. Alternatively, the unprepared left ventricle can be supported following arterial switch with a mechanical assist device for a few days while it recovers ability to manage systemic pressures. Echocardiography can be used to assess left ventricular performance and guide operative planning in these circumstances. (See Schwartz 8th ed., p 634.)

10. Which of the following is NOT one of the components of the tetralogy of Fallot?
    A. Atrial septal defect
    B. Ventricular septal defect
    C. Right ventricular hypertrophy
    D. Right ventricular outflow obstruction

**Answer: A**
The four features of tetralogy of Fallot (TOF) are (1) malalignment ventricular septal defect, (2) dextroposition of the aorta, (3) right ventricular outflow tract obstruction, and (4) right ventricular hypertrophy. This combination of defects arises as a result of underdevelopment and anteroleftward malalignment of the infundibular septum. (See Schwartz 8th ed., p 636.)

11. The most commonly recommended age for correction of a tetralogy of Fallot (TOF) is
    A. Newborn period
    B. 6 months of age
    C. 1 year of age
    D. 4–5 years of age

**Answer: A**
The optimal age and surgical approach of repair of TOF have been debated for several decades. Currently, most centers favor primary elective repair in infancy, as contemporary perioperative techniques have improved outcomes substantially in this population. In addition, definitive repair protects the heart and other organs from the pathophysiology inherent in the defect, as well as its palliated state. (See Schwartz 8th ed., p 636.)

12. Which of the following is NOT a type of ventricular septal defect (VSD)?
    A. Perimembranous
    B. Atrioventricular canal
    C. Supracristal
    D. Sinus venosal

**Answer: D**
VSD refers to a hole between the left and right ventricles. These defects are common, comprising 20 to 30% of all cases of congenital heart disease, and may occur as an isolated lesion or as part of a more complex malformation. VSDs vary in size from 3 to 4 mm to more than 3 cm, and are classified into four types based on their location in the ventricular septum: perimembranous, atrioventricular canal, outlet or supracristal, and muscular. (See Schwartz 8th ed., p 637.)

13. Which of the following is the most common type of ventricular septal defect (VSD)?
    A. Ostium primum
    B. Ostium secundum
    C. Muscular
    D. Outlet

**Answer: C**

Muscular VSDs are the most common type, and may lie in four locations: anterior, midventricular, posterior, or apical. These are surrounded by muscle, and can occur anywhere along the trabecular portion of the septum. The rare "Swiss-cheese" type of muscular VSD consists of multiple communications between the right and left ventricles, complicating operative repair. (See Schwartz 8th ed., p 637.)

14. What is the best predictor of spontaneous closure of a ventricular septal defect (VSD)?
    A. Size
    B. Age at diagnosis
    C. Gestational age
    D. Lack of electrocardiogram changes

**Answer: B**

VSDs may close or narrow spontaneously, and the probability of closure is inversely related to the age at which the defect is observed. Thus, infants at 1 month of age have an 80% incidence of spontaneous closure, whereas a child at 12 months of age has only a 25% chance of closure. This has an important impact on operative decision making, because a small or moderate-size VSD may be observed for a period of time in the absence of symptoms. Large defects and those in severely symptomatic neonates should be repaired during infancy to relieve symptoms and because irreversible changes in pulmonary vascular resistance may develop during the first year of life. (See Schwartz 8th ed., p 638.)

15. Deletions in the 22q11 regions are associated with
    A. Atrial septal defect
    B. Mitral valve insufficiency
    C. Tricuspid valve stenosis
    D. Truncus arteriosus

**Answer: D**

There is growing interest in the genetic basis of cardiac abnormalities. A deletion in the 22q11 region is associated with a variety of aortic anomalies, including truncus arteriosus, interrupted aortic arch, and tetralogy of Fallot. (See Schwartz 7th ed.)

16. Which of the following cardiac abnormalities, all of them well-tolerated during fetal life, becomes a serious problem at birth?
    A. Aortic arch
    B. Ductus arteriosus
    C. Foramen ovale
    D. Pulmonary valve stenosis

**Answer: D**

In fetal life, blood reaching the right atrium has been oxygenated by the placenta. This blood bypasses the high-resistance pulmonary circulation to enter the systemic circulation through septal defects and the ductus arteriosus. When the child is born, the pulmonary circulation becomes important. Septal defects and the ductus arteriosus can be tolerated by the newborn child, but pulmonic valve stenosis or right ventricular outflow obstruction forces a right-to-left shunt, with development of cyanotic heart disease. (See Schwartz 7th ed.)

17. Sudden death in infants with critical aortic stenosis is most frequently caused by
    A. Increasing pulmonary vascular resistance
    B. Ventricular arrhythmia
    C. Left ventricular failure
    D. Systemic hypotension

**Answer: B**

Ventricular arrhythmia, especially during exercise, is frequently lethal in young babies with aortic stenosis. Newborns with critical aortic stenosis or coarctation of the aorta develop increasing left ventricular hypertrophy, which is associated with severe heart failure. Surgical intervention should be timed before ventricular dysfunction becomes too severe. (See Schwartz 7th ed.)

18. An infant with a large ventricular septal defect and no other cardiac lesion can be expected to develop all of the following EXCEPT
    A. Cyanosis
    B. Failure to thrive
    C. Increased basal energy expenditure
    D. Increased susceptibility to lower respiratory tract infection

**Answer: A**

A ventricular septal defect produces a left-to-right shunt because systemic vascular resistance is greater than pulmonary vascular resistance. The extra work required by the shunt leads to increased basal energy expenditure and a failure to thrive. The shunt into the pulmonary circulation produces congestion and an associated increased susceptibility to lower respiratory tract infection. (See Schwartz 7th ed.)

19. Beyond early childhood, high pulmonary blood flow is most apt to produce
    A. Cyanosis on exercise
    B. Diminished exercise tolerance
    C. Periodic episodes of hemoptysis
    D. Right ventricular hypertrophy

**Answer: B**

High pulmonary blood flow beyond infancy may produce surprisingly little disability for a period of time, and the diminished exercise tolerance may be subtle. Cyanosis, hemoptysis, and pneumonia are not anticipated. With the volume overloading in the right ventricle, ventricular dilatation is more common than ventricular hypertrophy. (See Schwartz 7th ed.)

20. The most important diagnostic assessment modality for evaluating infants and children with congenital heart disease is
    A. Cardiac catheterization
    B. Chest X-ray
    C. Transesophageal echocardiogram
    D. Transthoracic echocardiogram

**Answer: D**

Although chest X-ray may define heart size and electrocardiograms indicate cardiac rhythm, transthoracic and subcostal echocardiograms provide information on cardiac structure and function. Transesophageal echocardiogram, often very important in adults, is not required in children because children have excellent acoustic windows for the conventional studies. Cardiac catheterization is currently used most frequently for therapeutic reasons such as balloon dilatation of an uncomplicated isolated valvular pulmonic stenosis or coil occlusion of a patent ductus arteriosus. (See Schwartz 7th ed.)

21. The major determinant of operability in patients who have a ventricular septal defect is
    A. The size of the defect
    B. The location of the defect
    C. The pulmonary vascular resistance
    D. The age of the patient

**Answer: C**

The specific anatomy of a ventricular defect, its size, and the age of the affected patient are not much hindrance to closure of the defect, and the major determinant of operability is the degree of pulmonary vascular resistance that is present. It is important to differentiate between pulmonary artery pressure and vascular resistance. The pressure may be elevated by a large increase in blood flow, and yet the resistance may be normal; conversely, the pressure may be markedly elevated in the presence of an almost normal blood flow if the resistance is increased. When pulmonary vascular resistance exceeds one-half the systemic resistance, the defect generally is considered inoperable. Those patients who have severe pulmonary vascular resistance increase their cardiac output by right-to-left shunting across the defect because they cannot increase their pulmonary blood flow. If the defect is closed, they have no mechanism to increase cardiac output with exercise. Most cases of ventricular septal defect are detected today and the affected patient successfully operated on within the first years of life before pulmonary vascular resistance has become severely elevated. (See Schwartz 7th ed.)

22. On the second day after repair of coarctation of the aorta, a patient develops abdominal pain with some tenderness. Correct management for the patient's problem is most likely to include
    A. Antibiotic agents
    B. Antacids
    C. Steroids
    D. Antihypertensive drugs

**Answer: D**

Hypertension may rebound paradoxically in the postoperative stage after repair of coarctation of the aorta, with diastolic pressures exceeding 110 mm Hg. Apparently, the hypertension is related to sudden perfusion of visceral arteries that previously were functioning with a lower perfusion pressure. If untreated, the hypertension can produce significant abdominal pain or even intestinal necrosis, which is probably attributable to a mesenteric arteritis. The condition will almost always resolve with the use of antihypertensive medication, usually reserpine, and if the condition is treated promptly, serious complications virtually are unknown. (See Schwartz 7th ed.)

23. A patient's cardiac catheterization data are given below:

    Pulmonary artery pressure: 20/10 mm Hg
    Pulmonary artery mean pressure: 8 mm Hg
    Right ventricular pressure: 120/8 mm Hg
    Left ventricular pressure: 95/6 mm Hg
    Peripheral oxygen saturation: 96%

    The data are characteristic of
    A. Patent ductus arteriosus
    B. Complete endocardial cushion defect
    C. Ventricular septal defect after pulmonary artery banding
    D. Pulmonic valvular stenosis

**Answer: D**

In pulmonic valvular stenosis, the basic physiologic disturbance is obstruction to flow of blood from the right ventricle. Right ventricular pressures of 75 to 100 mm Hg are found with moderate pulmonic stenosis, whereas severe obstruction results in right ventricular pressures of 100 to 200 mm Hg, and levels as high as 270 mm Hg have been recorded. The cardiac catheterization values given in the question show a right ventricular pressure of 120 mm Hg and a systolic pressure gradient from the right ventricle to the pulmonary artery of 100 mm Hg, which indicates significant valvular obstruction. The fact that the right ventricular pressure obtained exceeds the left ventricular pressure rules out a diagnosis of ventricular septal defect and hence tetralogy of Fallot. (See Schwartz 7th ed.)

24. A premature infant is discovered at birth to have a patent ductus arteriosus with moderate respiratory distress. The infant does not improve after 48 h of medical management with fluid restriction, diuretics, and respiratory support. The next step in management is
    A. Acetylsalicylic acid
    B. Indomethacin
    C. Surgical correction of the ductus
    D. Transvenous occlusion of the ductus

**Answer: B**

Prostaglandins oppose contraction of the smooth muscle that obliterates the ductus. Indomethacin is a prostaglandin inhibitor and, given intravenously, leads to closure of the ductus in the premature infant. A national cooperative study found that indomethacin effected closure in 79% of 3,559 patients studied. Although surgical closure of the ductus is surprisingly well-tolerated in these infants, operation should not be done unless this therapy does not close the ductus and symptoms are poorly controlled. (See Schwartz 7th ed.)

25. A newborn infant has cyanosis with signs of pulmonic stenosis. Except for the cyanosis, the infant looks well. During the next 24 h, the cyanosis and hypoxemia markedly worsen. The reason for this change is
    A. Closure of the ductus arteriosus
    B. Pulmonary vascular hypertension
    C. Right ventricular failure
    D. Stasis in the pulmonary circulation

**Answer: A**

The cyanotic newborn with pulmonic stenosis depends on a patent ductus and a patent interatrial septum to supply blood to the lung. This child's condition worsens as the ductus closes, and prostaglandin E should be started immediately to maintain ductal patency. (See Schwartz 7th ed.)

26. Brain abscesses and paradoxical cerebral emboli are complications that occur with an increased frequency in patients who have
   A. Aortic stenosis
   B. Tetralogy of Fallot
   C. A sinus venosus type of atrial septal defect
   D. Corrected transposition of the great vessels with a ventricular septal defect

**Answer: B**

Cardiac anomalies that permit systemic venous blood and its contents (e.g., bacteria and thrombi) to pass directly into the systemic arterial circulation without being filtered by the lungs are associated with an increased susceptibility to brain abscesses and paradoxical cerebral emboli. Tetralogy of Fallot is associated with a higher incidence of brain abscess than any other conditions involving a right-to-left shunt; however, the reason for this phenomenon is not completely understood. Permanent neurologic injury that results from paradoxical emboli and most often manifests as hemiplegia is not uncommon in children who have chronic severe cyanosis, and early surgical therapy therefore should be considered for these children. (See Schwartz 7th ed.)

# CHAPTER 20

# Acquired Heart Disease

1. Which of the following is true about angina pectoris?
   A. The midscapular region is an unusual but known location for angina.
   B. "Typical" angina occurs in approximately 50% of patients with coronary disease.
   C. "Atypical" angina occurs more commonly in men.
   D. Angina is a typical symptom for mitral stenosis.

**Answer: A**

Angina pectoris is the hallmark of myocardial ischemia secondary to coronary artery disease, although a variety of other conditions can produce chest pain, and it is up to the clinician to distinguish between chest pain of cardiac and noncardiac origin. Classic angina is precordial pain described as squeezing, heavy, or burning in nature, lasting from 2 to 10 minutes. The pain is usually substernal, often radiating into the left shoulder and arm, but occasionally occurring in the midepigastrium, jaw, right arm, or midscapular region. Angina is usually provoked by exercise, emotion, sexual activity, or eating, and is relieved by rest or nitroglycerin. Angina is present in its classic form in 75% of patients with coronary disease, while atypical symptoms occur in 25% of patients and more frequently in women. A small but significant number of patients have "silent" ischemia, most typically occurring in diabetics. Angina also is a classic symptom of aortic stenosis, occurring secondary to a combination of left ventricular hypertrophy, increased intracardiac pressure, increased ventricular wall tension (leading to higher oxygen requirements), and decreased cardiac output. This combination results in a myocardial oxygen supply-demand mismatch with resultant ischemia and angina. (See Schwartz 8th ed., p 646.)

2. A patient who develops angina after climbing one flight of stairs at a normal pace is
   A. Canadian Cardiovascular Society Class I
   B. Canadian Cardiovascular Society Class II
   C. Canadian Cardiovascular Society Class III
   D. Canadian Cardiovascular Society Class IV

**Answer: C**

Canadian Cardiovascular Society (CCS)

- Class I: Angina may occur with strenuous, rapid or prolonged exertion
- Class II: Slight limitation of ordinary activity. Angina may occur with walking stairs rapidly, walking uphill after meals or in the cold, climbing more than 1 flight of stairs at a normal pace, walking more than 2 level blocks
- Class III: Limitation of ordinary activity. Angina may occur after walking one level block or climbing one flight of stairs
- Class IV: Inability to carry out any physical activity without discomfort.

(See Schwartz 8th ed., p 647.)

3. Dobutamine stress echocardiography
   A. If negative, is 93–100% predictive of no cardiac event after surgery
   B. If positive, predicts a 20% risk of myocardial infarction (MI) or death from a non-cardiac event after surgery
   C. If positive, predicts a 50% risk of some cardiac event after surgery
   D. Is the most common and most accurate predictive test of coronary insufficiency

4. Which of the following statements about coronary artery bypass grafting is true?
   A. Being male is a risk factor for a poor outcome.
   B. Angina is relieved in ~75% of patients.
   C. Reintervention is required in <10% of patients in the first 5 years.
   D. 10-year survival after coronary artery bypass graft is ~60%.

**Answer: A**

Dobutamine stress echocardiography has evolved as an important noninvasive provocative study. This study is used to assess cardiac wall motion in response to inotropic stimulation, as wall motion abnormalities reflect underlying ischemia. Several reports have documented the accuracy of dobutamine stress echocardiography in identifying patients with significant coronary artery disease. The predictive value of a positive test for MI or death after noncardiac surgery is approximately 10%, while 20 to 40% will have some cardiac event. A negative test is 93 to 100% predictive that no cardiac event will occur. (See Schwartz 8th ed., p 648.)

**Answer: C**

The operative mortality for coronary artery bypass is 1 to 3%, depending on the number of risk factors present. Both the Society of Thoracic Surgeons (STS) and New York State have established large databases to establish risk factors and report outcomes. Variables that have been identified as influencing operative risk according to STS risk modeling include: female gender, age, race, body surface area, New York Heart Association (NYHA) class IV status, low ejection fraction, hypertension, peripheral vascular disease, prior stroke, diabetes, renal failure, chronic obstructive pulmonary disease, immunosuppressive therapy, prior cardiac surgery, recent myocardial infarction (MI), urgent or emergent presentation, cardiogenic shock, left main disease, and concomitant valvular disease. Perioperative complications include MI, bleeding, stroke, arrhythmias, tamponade, wound infection, aortic dissection, pneumonia, respiratory failure, renal failure, gastrointestinal complications, and multiorgan failure.

Late results demonstrate that relief of angina is striking after CABG. Angina is completely relieved or markedly decreased in over 98% of patients, and recurrent angina is rare in the first 5 to 7 years. Reintervention is required in less than 10% of patients within 5 years. Symptoms begin to recur more frequently between 8 and 15 years due to progression of disease or late graft occlusion. However, tight control of risk factors can minimize the risk of recurrence. Cessation of smoking and control of hypercholesterolemia are especially important, as late graft occlusion is five to seven times higher in patients who continue to smoke or have persistent hypercholesterolemia. If recurrent angina develops, angiography should be performed promptly, followed by repeat revascularization as indicated.

Exercise capacity generally improves significantly after CABG, with most patients demonstrating a markedly improved functional response to exercise secondary to improved blood flow. This functional improvement lasts up to 10 years, with longer improvement in patients receiving inferior mesenteric artery (IMA) grafts.

Late survival is similarly excellent after CABG, with a 5-year survival of over 90% and a 10-year survival of 75 to 90%, depending on the number of comorbidities present. Late survival is influenced by age, diabetes, left ventricular function, NYHA class, congestive heart failure, associated valvular insufficiency, completeness of revascularization, and nonuse of an IMA graft. Intense medical therapy for control of diabetes, hypercholesterolemia, and hypertension, and cessation of smoking significantly improves late survival. (See Schwartz 8th ed., p 655.)

5. The operation of choice for ventricular aneurysm after an acute myocardial infarction is
   A. Primary excision of the aneurysm with primary repair alone
   B. Primary excision of the aneurysm with coronary artery bypass
   C. Coronary artery bypass with "reefing" of the aneurysm
   D. Endoventricular patch reconstruction with coronary artery bypass

**Answer: D**
Operative treatment requires excision or exclusion of the aneurysm and bypass grafting of diseased coronary arteries. The classic repair was performed by excision of the aneurysm and linear closure of the ventricle. However, this technique had a geometrically deforming effect on the remaining left ventricle, and did not address aneurysmal deformity of the septum. Therefore, a more physiologic technique of intracavitary endoventricular patch reconstruction, or left ventricular restoration, was proposed by Jatene, Cooley, and Dor. (See Schwartz 8th ed., pp 657–658.)

6. Mitral insufficiency
   A. Is most commonly caused by rheumatic disease
   B. Is suggested by an apical holosystolic murmur
   C. Is best diagnosed by coronary catheterization
   D. Is always treated with mitral valve replacement in symptomatic patients

**Answer: B**
Degenerative disease is the most common cause of mitral insufficiency in the United States, accounting for 50 to 60% of the patients requiring surgery.

On physical examination the characteristic findings of mitral insufficiency are an apical holosystolic murmur and a forceful apical impulse. The apical murmur usually is harsh and transmitted to the axilla (in cases of anterior leaflet pathology), or to the left sternal border (typically in cases of posterior leaflet pathology), although this is variable. However, the severity of the insufficiency may not correlate with the intensity of the murmur.

The severity of mitral insufficiency can be determined accurately with echocardiography, along with the site of valvular prolapse or restriction, and the level of left ventricular function.

Once the commissure has been accurately identified and the chordae noted, a right-angle clamp is introduced beneath the fused commissure, stretching the adjacent chordae and leaflets, after which the commissure is carefully incised. The incision is made 2 to 3 mm at a time, serially confirming that the separated margins of the commissural leaflet remain attached to chordae tendineae. The usual commissurotomy curves slightly anteriorly and does not go directly laterally. (See Schwartz 8th ed., p 665.)

7. What valvular lesion is most commonly found in a patient with Ehlers-Danlos syndrome?
   A. Mitral stenosis
   B. Mitral insufficiency
   C. Aortic stenosis
   D. Aortic insufficiency

**Answer: D**
Degenerative valvular disease is a manifestation of fibroelastic deficiency or myxomatous degeneration that produces thin and elongated valvular tissue. The aortic valve leaflets sag into the ventricular lumen, often with no other tissue abnormality, producing central aortic insufficiency. The gross and histologic appearances suggest that this is a variant of the more common mitral valve prolapse. (See Schwartz 8th ed., p 672.)

8. The most common etiology of chronic constrictive pericarditis is
   A. Viral infection
   B. Syphilis
   C. Tuberculosis
   D. Bacterial infection

**Answer: A**

In the majority of patients, the cause of chronic constrictive pericarditis is unknown and probably is the end stage of an undiagnosed viral pericarditis. Tuberculosis is a rarity. Intensive radiation is a significant cause in some series. Constrictive pericarditis may develop after an open-heart operation. (See Schwartz 8th ed., p 678.)

9. Mitral valve stenosis
   A. Is caused by rheumatic disease in ~40% of patients
   B. Usually presents with substernal chest pain
   C. May present initially with an ischemic leg
   D. Is suggested by an axillary diastolic murmur

**Answer: C**

The main symptoms of mitral stenosis are exertional dyspnea and decreased exercise capacity. Dyspnea occurs when the left atrial pressure becomes elevated due to the stenotic valve, resulting in pulmonary congestion. Orthopnea and paroxysmal nocturnal dyspnea may also occur, or in advanced cases, hemoptysis. The most serious development is pulmonary edema. When the stenosis is chronic, with pulmonary hypertension, the patient may develop right-sided heart failure, manifest as jugular venous distention, hepatomegaly, ascites, or ankle edema.

Atrial fibrillation develops in a significant number of patients with chronic mitral stenosis, and in some patients arterial embolization is the initial presenting symptom. Atrial thrombi result from dilation and stasis of the left atrium, with the left atrial appendage being especially susceptible to clot formation. Angina is a rare symptom that may result from coronary embolization. (See Schwartz 8th ed., p 663.)

10. The most common cardiac tumor is
    A. Papillary fibroelastoma
    B. Lymphangioma
    C. Myxoma
    D. Metastatic tumor

**Answer: D**

Primary cardiac neoplasms are rare, reported to occur with incidences ranging from 0.001 to 0.3% in autopsy series. Benign tumors account for 75% of primary neoplasms and malignant tumors account for 25%. The most frequent primary cardiac neoplasm is myxoma, comprising 30 to 50%. Other benign neoplasms, in decreasing order of occurrence, include lipoma, papillary fibroelastoma, rhabdomyoma, fibroma, hemangioma, teratoma, lymphangioma, and others. Most primary malignant neoplasms are sarcomas (angiosarcoma, rhabdomyosarcoma, fibrosarcoma, leiomyosarcoma, and liposarcoma), with malignant lymphomas accounting for 1 to 2%.

Metastatic cardiac neoplasms are more common than primary neoplasms, occurring in 4 to 12% of patients dying of cancer. Symptoms include dyspnea, fever, malaise, weight loss, arthralgias, and dizziness. Clinical findings may include murmurs of mitral stenosis or insufficiency, heart failure, pulmonary hypertension, and systemic embolization. (See Schwartz 8th ed., p 679.)

11. An absolute contraindication to a coronary artery bypass operation is
    A. Acute coronary artery insufficiency with persistent or progressive angina despite optimal medical therapy
    B. Acute subendocardial infarction with multivessel coronary artery disease
    C. Cardiogenic shock after myocardial infarction
    D. Chronic congestive failure and ischemic cardiomyopathy with no signs of angina

**Answer: D**

Ischemic cardiomyopathy with chronic congestive failure but no signs of angina indicates that the majority of the left ventricular muscle is already necrotic. The only therapy that might help this patient is cardiac transplantation. The other listed situations are indicative of high mortality, but a few of the individuals may be rescued by emergency coronary artery bypass. (See Schwartz 7th ed.)

12. The most important preoperative study in evaluating a patient for coronary artery bypass grafting is
   A. Cardiac catheterization
   B. Electrocardiogram
   C. Exercise thallium scan
   D. Positron emission tomographic scan

**Answer: A**
All of the listed tests provide useful information, but cardiac catheterization allows the measurement of cardiac output, localization of intracardiac shunts, determination of cardiac wall motion by cineradiography, and determination of coronary anatomy by coronary angiography. Exercise thallium scan is the best test to diagnose myocardial ischemia, provided the patient can exercise on the treadmill. Positron emission tomographic scan assesses myocardial viability in underperfused areas of the heart. Transesophageal echocardiography is most useful for evaluating myocardial thickness, cardiac wall motion, and valvular infarction. (See Schwartz 7th ed.)

13. Each of the following is a risk factor for the development of coronary artery disease EXCEPT
   A. Alcoholism
   B. Hypertension
   C. Obesity
   D. Sedentary lifestyle

**Answer: A**
Alcoholism is not a risk factor for coronary artery disease, but each of the other items is a recognized risk factor. Additional risk factors include diabetes, hypercholesterolemia, hyperlipidemia, male gender, and type A personality. (See Schwartz 7th ed.)

14. Which of the following is the greatest risk for an adverse cardiac event during a noncardiac operation?
   A. Advanced age
   B. Decompensated heart failure
   C. Hypertension
   D. Old myocardial infarction

**Answer: B**
All of the listed items are cardiac risk factors for a patient undergoing an operation. However, only decompensated heart failure, recent myocardial infarction, significant arrhythmia, and severe valvular disease are considered major risk factors. (See Schwartz 7th ed.)

15. Treatment for unstable angina includes all of the following EXCEPT
   A. Aspirin
   B. Heparin
   C. Lidocaine
   D. Propranolol

**Answer: C**
Unstable angina requires vigorous medical management. Operation in the acute situation is considered if medical management fails. All of the listed agents except lidocaine have a place in this therapy. In addition, a calcium antagonist or a long-acting nitrate may be used. Lidocaine is useful for managing ventricular arrhythmias. (See Schwartz 7th ed.)

16. A 20-year-old woman complains of exertional dyspnea and fatigue. On examination, she is in atrial fibrillation. On auscultation, she has an increased first heart sound, an opening gallop, and a diastolic rumble. The diagnostic method of choice in evaluating this patient's cardiac diagnosis is
   A. Cardiac catheterization
   B. Electrocardiogram
   C. Positron-emission tomographic scan
   D. Transesophageal echocardiogram

**Answer: D**
This patient has mitral stenosis, and some information could be obtained from each of the listed studies. For instance, cardiac catheterization would provide information about cardiac output, and chest X-ray would show the cardiac silhouette and the extent of pulmonary congestion. Electrocardiogram would confirm the clinical impression of atrial fibrillation. A positron-emission tomographic scan is more appropriate when myocardial viability is in question. Transesophageal echocardiogram provides an accurate measurement of the cross-section area of the mitral valve and allows assessment of leaflet mobility and calcification. It also allows visualization of the left atrium and the atrial appendage. (See Schwartz 7th ed.)

17. Characteristics of a patient with aortic stenosis include all of the following EXCEPT
   A. Angina
   B. Exertional dyspnea
   C. Prolonged asymptomatic latent period
   D. Widened pulse pressure

**Answer: D**
Widened pulse pressure is characteristic of aortic insufficiency rather than aortic stenosis. It is typical for a patient with aortic stenosis to live for a long time without symptoms. When symptoms begin, angina and exertional dyspnea are usually rapidly progressive. Syncope and sudden

18. Which of the following is the best predictor of a significantly increased operative risk for coronary artery bypass surgery?
    A. Electrocardiography
    B. The degree of proximal arterial stenosis
    C. The ventricular ejection fraction
    D. A history of multiple myocardial infarcts

19. Indications for surgical ablation of cardiac conduction pathways include each of the following EXCEPT
    A. Paroxysmal supraventricular tachycardia
    B. Sustained ventricular tachycardia
    C. Third-degree heart block
    D. Wolff-Parkinson-White syndrome

20. A patient presents with a history of fatigue and dyspnea. He is found to have hepatomegaly, ascites, and an elevated jugular venous pulse. Heart sounds are normal, no murmurs are present, and the heart is of normal size. The pulse pressure is decreased by palpation. Electrocardiography is normal except for low voltage. The most likely diagnosis is
    A. Constrictive pericarditis
    B. Tricuspid valve disease
    C. Right atrial myxoma
    D. Primary pulmonary artery hypertension

death become a threat, and operative correction is indicated on an urgent basis. (See Schwartz 7th ed.)

**Answer: C**
When a patient is being considered for coronary artery bypass surgery, assessment of ventricular function is a crucial part of preoperative evaluation because it indicates the degree of previous cardiac muscle injury. In patients who have normal ventricular function, operative risk is less than 3%, and the likelihood of improvement is high; in patients who have severely impaired ventricular function and congestive failure, the operative risk is as high as 20–25%, and the chance of improvement is similarly impaired. Reduction of the ventricular ejection fraction to a point at which the percentage of blood in the ventricles that is ejected during systole is less than 15–20% indicates a serious operative risk. The ejection fraction seems to correlate better with operative mortality and to be a better predictor of surgical outcome than the left ventricular end-diastolic pressure, which tends to be a measure of wall stiffness. Although elevation of the end-diastolic pressure above 20–25 mm Hg is believed to indicate a poor prognosis, when more than 100 patients who had values in this range were operated on at New York University, the operative risk was only near 10%, and the 5-year survival rate was 83%. (See Schwartz 7th ed.)

**Answer: C**
Ablation of conduction pathways began with the management of Wolff-Parkinson-White syndrome. It has been extended to paroxysmal supraventricular tachycardia with atrioventricular node reentry or concealed atrioventricular pathways, and it is now the preferred method of treating sustained ventricular tachycardia unresponsive to medical therapy. The maze procedure, in which a number of atrial incisions are made to interfere with most pathways from the SA node to the AV node, is being used for the treatment of chronic atrial fibrillation. Heart block results from interference with intracardiac conduction and would not be helped by surgical ablation procedures. (See Schwartz 7th ed.)

**Answer: A**
Once the diagnosis of constrictive pericarditis is suspected on the basis of a patient's clinical presentation, it usually can be confirmed on the basis of electrocardiographic findings, chest X-rays, and cardiac catheterization data. In fact, most diagnostic errors in this condition arise from a failure to even consider constrictive pericarditis as a diagnosis because of its relatively rare occurrence. The condition is most frequently misdiagnosed as cirrhosis of the liver or congestive heart failure from another cause. The findings of a normal heart size, an absence of cardiac murmurs, and a low voltage on electrocardiography are the principal diagnostic points that distinguish constrictive pericarditis from other forms of heart disease. The electrocardiogram also may show inverted T waves, and chest X-ray will show calcifica-

tion in the pericardium in approximately 50% of cases. Cardiac catheterization may reveal almost identical pressure in the right atrium as in the right ventricle and pulmonary artery during diastole. (See Schwartz 7th ed.)

21. Each of the following effects is anticipated after insertion of an intraaortic balloon pump EXCEPT
    A. Afterload decrease
    B. Coronary blood flow increase
    C. Improvement in cardiac index
    D. Increased total myocardial oxygen consumption

**Answer: D**
The intraaortic balloon pump, inserted through the femoral artery, is the most common effective clinical technique for improved circulation. With electronic synchronization, the device increases coronary blood flow and reduces both preload and afterload. The cardiac index improves. Because the cardiac muscle is being supported, myocardial oxygen consumption decreases. (See Schwartz 7th ed.)

22. The adequacy of the perfusion supplied by a heart-lung machine to meet the metabolic needs of a patient may be monitored best by measuring
    A. Arterial pH
    B. Arterial oxygen saturation
    C. Venous oxygen saturation
    D. Urine output

**Answer: C**
In judging the adequacy of perfusion supplied by a heart-lung machine, the finding of a greatly reduced venous oxygen saturation would suggest that oxygen was being extracted maximally from the perfused blood at the tissue level and hence that the perfusion was less than adequate in terms of either flow rate or arterial oxygen saturation. Extracorporeal circulatory perfusion usually is done at a flow rate of approximately 2.5 L/m$^2$/min, which provides a flow rate of between 4 and 5 L/min for adults of normal size. With flow rates in this range and a venous oxygen saturation of greater than 50%, the oxygen requirements of the body tissues should be met, and metabolic acidosis should not occur. Serial determination of the oxygen saturation of mixed venous blood in a critically ill patient can also be used to make a judgment as to the adequacy of tissue perfusion. (See Schwartz 7th ed.)

23. The most frequent benefit from coronary bypass surgery is
    A. Improved longevity
    B. Relief of angina
    C. Prevention of myocardial infarction
    D. Prevention of sudden death

**Answer: B**
Although in some selected patients improved longevity has been achieved with coronary bypass surgery, the most frequent benefit is relief of angina. Decrease in cardiac arrhythmia has not been a frequent benefit, and, indeed, cardiac arrhythmia may increase after coronary bypass surgery. Although coronary bypass surgery can prevent myocardial infarction, this is not the most frequent benefit. In a small percentage of patients, the risk of sudden death can be decreased after coronary bypass surgery. (See Schwartz 7th ed.)

# CHAPTER 21

# Thoracic Aneurysms and Aortic Dissection

1. Which of the following is the most common cause of thoracic aortic aneurysms?
   A. Nonspecific medial degeneration
   B. Marfan syndrome
   C. Takayasu's arteritis
   D. Atherosclerosis

**Answer: A**
Nonspecific medial degeneration is the most common cause of thoracic aortic disease. Histologic findings of mild medial degeneration, including fragmentation of elastic fibers and loss of smooth muscle cells, are expected in the aging aorta. However, an advanced, accelerated form of medial degeneration leads to progressive weakening of the aortic wall, aneurysm formation, and eventual rupture and/or dissection. The underlying causes of medial degenerative disease remain unknown. (See Schwartz 8th ed., p 692.)

**Table 21-1.**
**Causes of Thoracic Aortic Aneurysms**

| |
|---|
| Nonspecific medial degeneration |
| Aortic dissection |
| Genetic disorders |
|    Marfan syndrome |
|    Ehlers-Danlos syndrome |
|    Familial aortic aneurysms |
|    Bicuspid aortic valves |
| Poststenotic dilatation |
| Infection |
| Aortitis |
|    Takayasu's arteritis |
|    Giant cell arteritis |
|    Rheumatoid aortitis |
| Trauma |

See Schwartz 8th ed., p 692.

2. Marfan syndrome is caused by an abnormality in which of the following proteins?
   A. Elastin
   B. Metalloproteinase
   C. Collagen
   D. Fibrillin

**Answer: D**
Marfan syndrome is an autosomal dominant genetic disorder characterized by a specific connective tissue defect that leads to aneurysm formation. The phenotype of patients with Marfan syndrome typically includes a tall stature, high palate, joint hypermobility, lens disorders, mitral valve prolapse, and aortic aneurysms. The aortic wall is weakened by fragmentation of elastic fibers and deposition of extensive amounts of mucopolysaccharides (cystic medial degeneration). Patients with Marfan syndrome have a mutation involving the fibrillin gene located on the long arm of the chromosome 15. Abnormal fibrillin in the extracellular matrix decreases connective tissue strength in the aortic wall and produces abnormal elastic properties that predispose the

aorta to dilatation from wall tension resulting from left ventricular ejection impulses. Seventy-five to 85% of patients with Marfan syndrome exhibit dilation of the ascending aorta with annuloaortic ectasia (dilation of the aortic sinuses and annulus). (See Schwartz 8th ed., p 693.)

3. The most common cause of death in patients with type IV Ehlers-Danlos syndrome is
   A. Myocardial infarction
   B. Aortic dissection
   C. Ruptured visceral artery
   D. Pulmonary emboli

**Answer: C**
Ehlers-Danlos syndrome includes a spectrum of inherited connective tissue disorders of collagen synthesis; the subtypes represent differing defective steps of collagen production. Type IV Ehlers-Danlos syndrome is characterized by an autosomal dominant defect in type III collagen synthesis, and may produce life-threatening cardiovascular manifestations. Spontaneous arterial rupture, usually involving the mesenteric vessels, is the most common cause of death in these patients. Thoracic aortic aneurysms and dissections represent less common entities associated with Ehlers-Danlos syndrome, but nonetheless are reported and require challenging surgical management secondary to altered tissue integrity. (See Schwartz 8th ed., p 693.)

4. Worldwide, the most common cause of mycotic aneurysm is
   A. *Salmonella*
   B. *Staphylococcus*
   C. *Treponema*
   D. *Actinomyces*

**Answer: C**
While once the most common cause of ascending aortic aneurysms, the advent of effective antibiotic therapy has made syphilitic aneurysms a rarity in developed nations. In other parts of the world, however, syphilitic aneurysms remain a major cause of morbidity and mortality. The spirochete *Treponema pallidum* causes an obliterative endarteritis of the vasa vasorum, resulting in medial ischemia and loss of the elastic and muscular elements of the aortic wall. The ascending aorta and arch are the most common areas of involvement. The emergence of the human immunodeficiency virus (HIV) in the 1980s has been associated with a substantial increase in the incidence of syphilis in both HIV-infected and non–HIV-infected patients. Because syphilitic aortitis often presents 10 to 30 years after the primary infection, the incidence of associated aneurysms may increase in the near future. (See Schwartz 8th ed., p 693.)

5. The most common presenting symptom in patients with an ascending thoracic aneurysm is
   A. Anterior chest pain
   B. Posterior chest pain
   C. Aortic valve insufficiency
   D. Sudden death

**Answer: A**
The most common symptom in patients with ascending aortic aneurysms is anterior chest discomfort; the pain is frequently precordial in location, but may radiate to the neck and jaw, mimicking angina. Aneurysms of the ascending aorta and transverse aortic arch can cause symptoms related to compression of the superior vena cava, the pulmonary artery, the airway, or the sternum. Although unusual, erosion can occur into the superior vena cava or right atrium, causing acute high-output failure. Expansion of the distal aortic arch can stretch the recurrent laryngeal nerve, resulting in left vocal cord paralysis and hoarseness. Descending thoracic and thoracoabdominal aneurysms frequently cause back pain localized between the scapulae. When the aneurysm is largest in the region of the aortic hiatus, middle back and epigastric pain may occur. Thoracic or lumbar vertebral body erosion

typically causes severe, chronic back pain; extreme cases can present with spinal instability and neurologic deficits from spinal cord compression. Although mycotic aneurysms have a peculiar propensity to destroy vertebral bodies, spinal erosion also occurs with degenerative aneurysms. Descending thoracic aortic aneurysms may cause varying degrees of airway obstruction, manifested as cough, wheezing, stridor, or pneumonitis. Pulmonary or airway erosion presents as hemoptysis. Compression or erosion of the esophagus creates dysphagia and hematemesis, respectively. Thoracoabdominal aortic aneurysms can cause duodenal obstruction, or upon bowel wall erosion, gastrointestinal bleeding. Jaundice due to compression of the liver or porta hepatis is uncommon. Erosion into the inferior vena cava or iliac vein will present with an abdominal bruit, widened pulse pressure, edema, and heart failure. (See Schwartz 8th ed., p 694.)

6. The most useful imaging study for thoracic aneurysms is
   A. Echocardiography
   B. Computed tomography scan
   C. Magnetic resonance angiography
   D. Aortography

**Answer: B**
Computed tomographic (CT) scanning is widely available and provides visualization of the entire thoracic and abdominal aorta. Consequently, it is the most common—and arguably the most useful—imaging modality for evaluating thoracic aortic aneurysms. Systems capable of constructing multiplanar images and three-dimensional aortic reconstructions are becoming increasingly available. In addition to establishing the diagnosis, CT provides information regarding location, extent, anatomic anomalies, and relationship to major branch vessels. Contrast-enhanced CT provides information regarding the aortic lumen, and can detect mural thrombus, aortic dissection, inflammatory periaortic fibrosis, and mediastinal or retroperitoneal hematoma due to contained aortic rupture. It is particularly useful in determining the absolute diameter of the aorta, especially in the presence of laminated clot. (See Schwartz 8th ed., p 695.)

7. A patient with Marfan's syndrome who has undergone "aortic surgery" most likely had
   A. Aortic valve annuloplasty (annular plication)
   B. Aortic root replacement (valve and ascending aorta)
   C. Total arch replacement with reattachment of the brachiocephalic branches
   D. Elephant trunk repair of thoracic aneurysm

**Answer: B**
Many patients undergoing proximal aortic operations have aortic valve pathology that requires concomitant surgical correction. When aortic valvular disease is present and the sinus segment is normal, separate repair or replacement of the aortic valve and graft replacement of the tubular segment of the ascending aorta are carried out. Mild to moderate valve insufficiency with annular dilatation in this setting can be addressed by plicating the annulus with mattress sutures placed below each commissure. Valve replacement with a stented biologic or mechanical prosthesis is performed in patients with more severe valvular insufficiency or with valvular stenosis. Separate replacement of the aortic valve and ascending aorta are not performed in patients with Marfan syndrome, because progressive dilatation of the remaining sinus segment eventually leads to complications requiring reoperation. Therefore, patients with Marfan syndrome or annuloaortic ectasia require some form of aortic root replacement. (See Schwartz 8th ed., p 697.)

8. The proximal extent of a Crawford type III thoracoab-dominal aneurysm is
   A. Aortic annulus
   B. Mid arch
   C. Left subclavian artery
   D. Mid descending thoracic aorta

**Answer: D**

By definition, descending thoracic aortic aneurysms involve the aorta in between the left subclavian artery and the diaphragm. Thoracoabdominal aneurysms can involve the entire thoracoabdominal aorta, from the origin of the left subclavian artery to the aortic bifurcation, and are categorized based on the Crawford classification (Fig. 21-7). Extent I thoracoabdominal aortic aneurysms involve most of the descending thoracic aorta, usually beginning near the left subclavian artery, and extend down to encompass the aorta at the origins of the celiac axis and superior mesenteric arteries; the renal arteries may also be involved. Extent II aneurysms also arise near the left subclavian artery, but extend distally into the infrarenal abdominal aorta and often reach the aortic bifurcation. Extent III aneurysms originate in the lower descending thoracic aorta (below the sixth rib) and extend into the abdomen. Extent IV aneurysms begin within the diaphragmatic hiatus and often involve the entire abdominal aorta. (See Schwartz 8th ed., p 699.)

9. Which of the following reduces the risk of paraplegia after repair of a thoracoabdominal aneurysm?
   A. Intraoperative drainage of cerebrospinal fluid
   B. Heparinization
   C. Retrograde perfusion of visceral arteries
   D. Reimplantation of segemental arteries above T8

**Answer: A**

**Table 21-2.**
**Current Strategy for Spinal Cord, Visceral, and Renal Protection during Repair of Distal Thoracic Aortic Aneurysms**

All extents
- Permissive mild hypothermia (32–34°C, nasopharyngeal)
- Moderate heparinization (1 mg/kg)
- Aggressive reattachment of segmental arteries, especially between T8 and L1
- Sequential aortic clamping when possible
- Perfusion of renal arteries with 4°C crystalloid solution when possible

Crawford extent I and II thoracoabdominal repairs
- Cerebrospinal fluid drainage
- Left heart bypass during proximal anastomosis
- Selective perfusion of celiac axis and superior mesenteric artery during intercostal and visceral/renal anastomoses

See Schwartz 8th ed., p 700.

10. Which of the following is the most typical presenting symptom in a patient with an aortic dissection?
    A. "Tearing" pain
    B. Paraplegia
    C. Abdominal pain
    D. Cold left arm

**Answer: A**

The onset of dissection is often associated with severe chest or back pain—classically described as "tearing"—that migrates distally as the dissection progresses along the length of the aorta. The location of the pain often indicates which aortic segments are involved. Pain in the anterior chest suggests involvement of the proximal aorta, whereas pain in the back and abdomen generally indicates involvement of the distal segment. Additional clinical sequelae of acute aortic dissection are best considered in terms of the potential anatomic manifestations at each level of the aorta. (See Schwartz 8th ed., p 704.)

**Table 21-3.**
**Anatomic Complications of Aortic Dissection and Their Associated Symptoms and Signs**

| Anatomic Manifestation | Symptoms and Signs |
| --- | --- |
| Aortic valve insufficiency | Dyspnea |
| | Murmur |
| | Pulmonary rales |
| | Shock |
| Coronary malperfusion | Chest pain with characteristics of angina |
| | Nausea/vomiting |
| | Shock |
| | Ischemic changes on electrocardiogram |
| | Elevated cardiac enzymes |
| Pericardial tamponade | Dyspnea |
| | Jugular venous distention |
| | Pulsus paradoxus |
| | Muffled cardiac tones |
| | Shock |
| | Low-voltage electrocardiogram |
| Subclavian or iliofemoral artery malperfusion | Cold, painful extremity |
| | Extremity sensory and motor deficits |
| | Peripheral pulse deficit |
| Carotid artery malperfusion | Syncope |
| | Focal neurologic deficit (transient or persistent) |
| | Carotic pulse deficit |
| | Coma |
| Spinal malperfusion | Paraplegia |
| | Incontinence |
| Visceral malperfusion | Nausea/vomiting |
| | Abdominal pain |
| Renal malperfusion | Oliguria or anuria |
| | Hematuria |

See Schwartz 8th ed., p 705.

11. Formation of an aortic aneurysm results from all of the following EXCEPT
    A. Thickening of the adventitia
    B. Change in structure of collagen and elastin within the vessel wall
    C. Increased collagenase activity
    D. Loss of elastin from the media

**Answer: A**

Aneurysm formation is not simply secondary to tension related to passive dilatation. It is a complex process that involves remodeling in the structure of collagen and elastin within the vessel wall. This is associated with activation of inflammatory mediators, especially in patients with atherosclerotic infections or autoimmune disorders. Initially, a proteolytic process develops, with loss of elastin in the media. Adventitial thickening compensates for weakness of the media until increased collagenase activity leads to degradation of the adventitial layer. (See Schwartz 7th ed.)

12. A patient with a moderate-sized aneurysm of the descending thoracic aorta is likely to have
    A. Back pain
    B. Diaphragmatic paralysis
    C. Tracheal compression
    D. No symptoms

**Answer: D**

Most patients with moderate-sized aneurysms of the descending thoracic aorta are asymptomatic until the aneurysm begins to enlarge. When this happens, back pain, recurrent nerve palsy, or tracheal compression may occur depending on the location of the aneurysm. The phrenic nerve is not frequently disturbed by the aneurysm. Diaphragmatic paralysis is not a common symptom. (See Schwartz 7th ed.)

13. Mortality rates for operative repair of an aortic arch aneurysm have been significantly reduced intraoperatively by
    A. Deep hypothermia to allow circulatory arrest
    B. Innominate and left carotid artery cannulation to permit oxygenation of the brain
    C. Right heart to left subclavian artery bypass to continue brain perfusion
    D. Use of an intraaortic balloon pump to maintain distal circulation

**Answer: A**
It has been found that the brain will tolerate up to 45 min of circulatory arrest if the cerebral temperature is 15° to 17°C. During this time, the aneurysm is opened and a synthetic graft sutured in place inside the shell of the aneurysm. The graft is protected by closing the aneurysm over it. Attempting to maintain cerebral circulation by cannulation of the innominate and left carotid arteries or by right heart to left subclavian artery bypass lengthens an already complex operation. An aortic balloon pump would not protect the cerebral circulation in this situation, and heparinization of the patient would be inappropriate. (See Schwartz 7th ed.)

14. The first step in the management of a descending aneurysm arising distal to the left subclavian artery is
    A. Establishment of controlled hypothermia
    B. Vigorous antihypertensive therapy
    C. Fenestration of the dissection back into the aortic lumen
    D. Placement of an intraaortic stent to exclude the tear site from the circulation

**Answer: B**
Lowering the blood pressure in dissecting aneurysms that arise distal to the left subclavian artery may stop the dissection and prevent exsanguination by rupture through the adventitia. β-adrenergic blockade and afterload reduction are effective therapy. Early operative management is restricted to controlling problems that arise when the dissection occludes a renal or mesenteric artery. Continuing pain, threatened ruptures, and compromise of the lower extremities are other causes for operative intervention. Fenestration, at one time a popular operative choice, has been disappointing. (See Schwartz 7th ed.)

15. When a dissecting aortic aneurysm is suspected, the initial diagnostic procedure of choice is
    A. Arch aortography
    B. Cardiac catheterization
    C. Computed tomography of the chest with contrast
    D. Transesophageal echocardiography

**Answer: D**
Transesophageal echocardiography is sensitive and specific, with a 99% accuracy. The procedure can be performed in the emergency department without delay. Computed tomography with contrast and magnetic resonance angiography are effective but time consuming and require moving a critically ill patient to the scanner. Arch aortography is highly accurate, but it is seldom necessary. Cardiac catheterization may be useful with problems in the right heart and pulmonary circulation, but it would not be an effective method of evaluating the descending aorta. (See Schwartz 7th ed.)

16. On the second day after repair of coarctation of the aorta, a patient develops abdominal pain with some tenderness. Correct management for the patient's problem is most likely to include
    A. Antibiotic agents
    B. Antacids
    C. Steroids
    D. Antihypertensive drugs

**Answer: D**
Hypertension may rebound paradoxically in the postoperative period after repair of coarctation of the aorta, with diastolic pressures exceeding 110 mm Hg. Apparently, the hypertension is related to sudden perfusion of visceral arteries that previously were functioning with a lower perfusion pressure. If untreated, the hypertension can produce significant abdominal pain or even intestinal necrosis, which is probably attributable to a mesenteric arteritis. The condition will almost always resolve with the use of antihypertensive medication, usually reserpine, and if the condition is treated promptly, serious complications virtually are unknown. (See Schwartz 7th ed.)

17. Paraplegia after operative repair of coarctation of the aorta is usually caused by
    A. Aortic cross clamping
    B. Hypotension during anesthetic induction
    C. Intraoperative hypovolemia
    D. Ligation of intercostal arteries

**Answer: A**

Paraplegia is an infrequent but disastrous complication of the operation. It is usually caused by aortic cross clamping and is associated with a fall in distal aortic pressure. When a long cross-clamping period (longer than 20–30 min) or a drop in distal aortic pressure below 50–60 mm Hg is anticipated, the use of an intraoperative shunt may prevent this problem. (See Schwartz 7th ed.)

18. The most common complication in a patient with an aneurysm of the ascending thoracic aorta is
    A. Aortic valve insufficiency
    B. Cardiac tamponade
    C. Distal dissection
    D. Rupture into the right pleural cavity

**Answer: A**

Aneurysms in the ascending thoracic aorta, once common in patients with syphilis, are unusual events. These aneurysms may develop in patients with Marfan syndrome. Isolated arteriosclerotic aneurysms in this location are unusual. As the aneurysm enlarges, the aortic root is enlarged, and aortic insufficiency is more frequent than rupture or compression of adjacent structures. (See Schwartz 7th ed.)

1. Abdominal aortic aneurysms should be repaired if their diameter is larger than
   A. 3 cm
   B. 4 cm
   C. 5 cm
   D. 6 cm

**Answer: C**
Abdominal aortic aneurysms grow on average 0.4 cm/y. Risk of rupture is exponentially related to aneurysm diameter. Aneurysms 5.0 cm in diameter have an average yearly rupture rate of 3 to 5% (Fig. 22-16). However, a 7-cm aneurysm carries a rupture rate of 19% per year. Szilagyi and colleagues demonstrated that repair of aneurysms greater than 6 cm prolonged patient survival, despite the fact that at that time a 14% operative mortality rate existed. Currently, with perioperative mortality rates of 3 to 5%, intervention is recommended for all aneurysms greater than 5 cm. (See Schwartz 8th ed., p 733.)

2. In the United States, the most common organism responsible for mycotic aneurysms of the abdominal aorta is
   A. *Streptococcus*
   B. *Staphylococcus*
   C. *Salmonella*
   D. *Treponema*

**Answer: B**
Although mycotic aneurysms can occur in any artery, they are most frequently found in the aorta. The most common organisms cultured are staphylococci, followed by *Salmonella*. (See Schwartz 8th ed., p 742.)

3. The most common peripheral artery aneurysm is
   A. Brachial
   B. Radial
   C. Popliteal
   D. Tibial

**Answer: C**
Popliteal arterial aneurysms are the most common peripheral arterial aneurysms, accounting for 70%, and are commonly bilateral in 50 to 75%. Finding one popliteal aneurysm mandates evaluation of the contralateral popliteal artery, usually with ultrasound. They are more common in males. These aneurysms present by a process of chronic distal embolization or sudden-onset acute occlusion of the popliteal artery. Consequently the clinical presentation is by development of claudication; chronic foot ischemia; or sudden-onset, limb-threatening, acute ischemia below the knee. Rupture is rare. Frequently a pattern of acute or chronic ischemia occurs, and the presence of chronic embolization of the infrapopliteal vessels can markedly complicate revascularization. (See Schwartz 8th ed., p 750.)

4. The compartment most commonly affected in a lower leg compartment syndrome is the
   A. Anterior compartment
   B. Lateral compartment
   C. Deep posterior compartment
   D. Superficial posterior compartment

**Answer: A**
The most commonly affected compartment is the anterior compartment in the leg (Fig. 22-64). Numbness in the web space between the first and second toes is diagnostic due to compression of the deep peroneal nerve. When skin changes occur over the compartment, this indicates advanced ischemia. Compartment pressure is measured by inserting an arterial line into the compartment and recording the pres-

sure. Although controversial, pressures greater than 30 mm Hg or below 30 mm Hg diastolic are frequently cited. Treatment is by fasciotomy. In the leg, medial and lateral incisions are utilized via the medial incision. Long openings are then made in the fascia of the superficial and deep posterior compartments. Through the lateral incision, the anterior and peroneal compartments are opened. Both skin and fascial incisions should be of adequate length to ensure full compartment decompression. (See Schwartz 8th ed., p 763.)

5. The preferred procedure for treatment of typical occlusive disease of the aorta and both iliac arteries is
   A. Endovascular stenting
   B. Extra-anatomic bypass
   C. Aortoiliac endarterectomy
   D. Aortobifemoral bypass

**Answer: D**

In most cases aortobifemoral bypass grafting is the procedure of choice of these authors. Bilateral bypass is virtually always performed since patients usually have disease in both iliac systems. Although one side may be more severely affected than the other, progression may occur, and bilateral bypass adds little to the procedure. Aortobifemoral bypass grafting is a satisfactory operation, it reliably relieves symptoms, has an excellent long-term patency of 60 to 75% at 10 years, and can be completed with a tolerable mortality of 2 to 3%. (See Schwartz 8th ed., p 765.)

6. The treatment of acute embolic mesenteric ischemia is
   A. Observation
   B. Anticoagulation
   C. Thrombolysis
   D. Operative embolectomy

**Answer: D**

The primary goal of surgical treatment in embolic mesenteric ischemia is to restore arterial perfusion with removal of the embolus from the vessel. The abdomen is explored through a midline incision, which often reveals variable intestinal ischemia from the midjejunum to the ascending or transverse colon. The transverse colon is lifted superiorly, and the small intestine is reflected toward the right upper quadrant. The superior mesenteric artery (SMA) is approached at the root of the small bowel mesentery (Fig. 22-76), usually as it emerges from beneath the pancreas to cross over the junction of the third and fourth portions of the duodenum. Alternatively, the SMA can be approached by incising the retroperitoneum lateral to the fourth portion of the duodenum, which is rotated medially to expose the SMA. Once the proximal SMA is identified and controlled with vascular clamps, a transverse arteriotomy is made to extract the embolus, using standard balloon embolectomy catheters (Fig. 22-77). (See Schwartz 8th ed., p 773.)

7. The treatment of nonocclusive mesenteric ischemia is
   A. Observation
   B. Catheter infusion of papaverine
   C. Stenting to prevent further spasm
   D. Operative bypass of the superior mesenteric artery

**Answer: B**

The treatment of nonocclusive mesenteric ischemia is primarily pharmacologic, with selective mesenteric arterial catheterization followed by infusion of vasodilatory agents such as tolazoline or papaverine. Once the diagnosis is made via mesenteric arteriography, intra-arterial papaverine is given at a dose of 30 to 60 mg/h. This must be coupled with the cessation of other vasoconstricting agents. (See Schwartz 8th ed., p 774.)

8. The most accurate diagnostic test with the lowest morbidity in the diagnosis of renal artery stenosis is
   A. Angiography
   B. Computed tomography scan
   C. Magnetic resonance angiography
   D. Renal systemic renin index

**Answer: C**

Magnetic resonance angiography (MRA), particularly with gadolinium contrast enhancement, has become a useful diagnostic tool for renal artery occlusive disease, because of its ability to provide high-resolution images (Fig. 22-83). The minimally invasive nature of MRA plus the low risk of nephrotoxicity of gadolinium contrast makes it an appealing diagnostic modality. With continuous refinement in imaging software, it will likely become a widely accepted imaging modality in patients suspected of renovascular hypertension. (See Schwartz 8th ed., p 778.)

9. The bypass graft of choice in children with renovascular hypertension is
   A. Saphenous vein
   B. Hypogastric artery
   C. Prosthetic
   D. Dacron

**Answer: B**

Use of the saphenous vein should be avoided in children, because it is prone to the development of aneurysmal change. The hypogastric artery is the best choice for aortorenal grafting in the pediatric patient. (See Schwartz 8th ed., p 779.)

10. Which of the following is the most prevalent inherited risk factor for peripheral vascular disease?
    A. Elevated high-density lipoprotein (HDL)
    B. Elevated low-density lipoprotein (LDL)
    C. Elevated very low-density lipoprotein (VLDL)
    D. Elevated lipoprotein a [Lp(a)]

**Answer: D**

Elevated plasma lipids have been reported in one third to one half of patients with peripheral vascular disease (PVD). Low levels of HDL cholesterol are associated with PVD. There are several apoprotein levels and apoprotein ratios which are predictive of PVD: A-I and A-II levels, and A-I:B and A-I:C-III ratios.

Lp(a), a cholesterol ester, is a low-density lipoprotein-like particle associated with an increased risk of cardiovascular disease. Elevated Lp(a) may represent the most prevalent inherited risk factor for atherosclerosis. Lp(a) levels are insensitive to dietary and drug manipulations. (See Schwartz 8th ed., p 720.)

11. Which of the following statements concerning carotid body tumors is true?
    A. Occur more commonly in patients who live at high altitudes
    B. Require resection of the underlying carotid artery with reconstruction for cure
    C. Are associated with catecholamine release
    D. Are usually malignant

**Answer: A**

Carotid body tumors originate from the chemoreceptor cells located at the carotid bifurcation (Fig. 22-93). Because the cells of the carotid body typically detect changes in partial oxygen pressure ($Po_2$), partial pressure of carbon dioxide ($Pco_2$), and pH levels, carotid body tumors have been reported to be more prevalent in individuals who live at high altitudes, suggesting that chronic hypoxia may be a causative factor in carotid body cell hyperplasia. A carotid body tumor typically presents as a palpable and painless mass over the carotid bifurcation region in the neck. Cranial nerve palsy may occur in up to 25% of patients, particularly involving the vagus and hypoglossal nerves. The differential diagnosis includes cervical lymphadenopathy, carotid artery aneurysm, brachial cleft cyst, laryngeal carcinoma, and metastatic tumor. (See Schwartz 8th ed., p 784.)

12. Rest pain seen with occlusive peripheral vascular disease in the lower extremity most commonly occurs in
    A. The buttock
    B. The quadriceps
    C. The calf muscles
    D. The metatarsophalangeal joint

**Answer: D**

Symptoms are elicited based on the presenting complaint (Table 22-2). The patient with lower extremity pain on ambulation has intermittent claudication that occurs in certain muscle groups; for example, calf pain upon exercise usually reflects superficial femoral artery disease, while pain in the buttocks reflects iliac disease. In most cases, the pain manifests in one muscle group below the level of the affected artery, occurs only with exercise, and is relieved with rest only to recur at the same location, hence the term "window-gazers disease." Rest pain (a manifestation of severe underlying occlusive disease) is constant and occurs in the foot (not the muscle groups), typically at the metatarsophalangeal junction, and is relieved by dependency. Often the patient is prompted to sleep with their foot hanging off one side of the bed to increase the hydrostatic pressure. (See Schwartz 8th ed., p 722.)

13. A patient with a creatinine of 1.8 who is scheduled for angiography should
    A. Not proceed with angiography
    B. Be given oral acetylcysteine the day before and day of the study
    C. Be given Lasix and a fluid bolus after the study
    D. Have a dialysis catheter inserted at the time of the study

**Answer: B**
The preangiography checklist includes serum creatinine; medications such as anticoagulants and oral hypoglycemics, specifically metformin (which can cause lactic acidosis when combined with contrast agents); history of dye allergy; and hydration status. Contrast angiography should be avoided if possible in all patients with a serum creatinine level greater than 3.0. It should be performed only if it is truly necessary, and other imaging modalities cannot provide equivalent information in patients with a serum creatinine level greater than 2.0. All patients with a serum creatinine level greater than 1.7 mg/dL are premedicated with acetylcysteine 600 mg by mouth twice daily on the day before and the day of angiography. (See Schwartz 8th ed., p 726.)

14. Which of the following can be used in the treatment of hyperhomocysteinemia?
    A. Statin drugs
    B. Aspirin
    C. Niacin
    D. Folic acid

**Answer: D**
The incidence of hyperhomocysteinemia is as high as 60% in patients with vascular disease, compared with 1% in the general population. It has been reported that hyperhomocysteinemia was detected in 28 to 30% of patients with premature peripheral arterial disease (PAD). Hyperhomocysteinemia has been established as an independent risk factor for atherosclerosis by several studies. It may be a stronger risk factor for PAD than for coronary artery disease (CAD). A meta-analysis of studies concluded that the odds ratios for CAD were 1.6 and 1.8 in men and women, respectively, compared with 6.8 for patients with PAD. Elevated homocysteine levels can be treated with folic acid supplementation of 0.5 to 1.0 mg/d. (See Schwartz 8th ed., p 729.)

15. The best initial treatment for a groin pseudoaneurysm after angiography is
    A. Surgical repair
    B. Ultrasound-guided compression
    C. Ultrasound-guided injection of thrombin
    D. Observation

**Answer: C**
Postcatheterization groin pseudoaneurysms present with local tenderness, swelling, and the presence of a tender pulsatile mass. The diagnosis is confirmed with ultrasound scanning. Treatment depends on the size of the pseudoaneurysm and whether the patient is anticoagulated. Spontaneous resolution is less likely if the patient is anticoagulated. Treatment has evolved from surgical repair of all pseudoaneurysms, through ultrasound-guided compression to the current standard therapy, which is ultrasound-guided thrombin injection. Surgical repair is reserved for those who fail injection or have a contraindication to thrombin injection such as wide neck, inability to compress the neck, or presence of an arteriovenous fistula. (See Schwartz 8th ed., p 727.)

16. Which of the following statements concerning cilostazol is true?
    A. Is more effective than pentoxifylline in the treatment of claudication
    B. Works by inhibiting platelets and lowering low-density lipoprotein cholesterol
    C. Works within 2 weeks of starting the drug
    D. Should not be used in patients with acute coronary syndromes

**Answer: A**
Cilostazol inhibits platelet aggregation, increases vasodilation, inhibits smooth muscle proliferation (via inhibition of phosphodiesterase type 3), and lowers high density lipoprotein cholesterol and triglyceride levels. This drug has been more effective than pentoxifylline in the treatment of claudication at doses of 100 mg twice daily (Fig. 22-14). Cilostazol has been shown to significantly increase walking distance in patients with claudication in several randomized trials and to result in improvement in physical functioning and quality of life. Improvement has ranged from 35 to 100%. A trial of the drug is indicated in symptomatic patients. It should be continued for at least 3 months before a decision is made about efficacy. The most common adverse effects are headache, transient diarrhea, palpitations, and dizziness. It is contraindicated in patients with congestive heart failure because of its effects on phosphodiesterase. (See Schwartz 8th ed., p 730.)

17. The most common nonatherosclerotic disease of the internal carotid artery is
    A. Thrombosis from protein C deficiency
    B. Trauma
    C. Takayasu's arteritis
    D. Fibromuscular dysplasia

**Answer: D**
Fibromuscular dysplasia (FMD) is the most common non-atherosclerotic disease affecting the internal carotid artery (Fig. 22-90). Approximately one quarter of patients with carotid FMD have associated intracranial aneurysms, and up to two-thirds of these patients will have bilateral carotid FMD. (See Schwartz 8th ed., p 782.)

18. The earliest detectable lesion of atherosclerosis is
    A. Fatty streak
    B. Fibrous plaques
    C. Subendothelial monocytes
    D. Platelet deposition

**Answer: A**
The fatty streak is the earliest identifiable lesion of atherosclerosis. It has been detected in children as young as 10 years of age and consists of lipid-laden macrophages overlying lipid-laden smooth muscle cells. They occur at the same anatomic sites as subsequent fibrous plaques. McGill demonstrated that increased surface involvement of fatty streaks precedes development of fibrous plaques, further supporting a precursor role for the fatty streak. (See Schwartz 8th ed., p 719.)

19. Carotid artery dissection is best treated by
    A. Surgical resection and reconstruction with graft
    B. Surgical resection and reconstruction with vein
    C. Endoluminal stenting
    D. Anticoagulation

**Answer: D**
Acute carotid dissection can complicate atherosclerosis, fibromuscular dysplasia, cystic medial necrosis, and blunt trauma. Angiographic studies suggest that the most likely mechanism of acute carotid dissection is an intimal tear followed by an acute intimal dissection, which produces luminal occlusion due to secondary thrombosis. This appears as a flame-shaped occlusion 2 to 3 cm beyond the bifurcation. Autopsy studies typically reveal a sharply demarcated transition between the normal carotid artery and the dissected carotid segment. The internal carotid artery is commonly affected, with the dissection plane typically occurring in the outer medial layer. Treatment is with anticoagulation, and in most cases this results in complete resolution within 1 to 2 months. Recently there has been increasing use of stenting in severely symptomatic patients. (See Schwartz 8th ed., p 783.)

20. A patient who develops dizziness, drop attacks, and diplopia with exercise most likely has
    A. Carotid stenosis
    B. Subclavian steal syndrome
    C. Coronary subclavian steal syndrome
    D. Coronary artery disease

**Answer: B**

The most common location for atherosclerosis affecting the upper limb is at the origin of the subclavian artery, most commonly the left subclavian artery. Frequently there are no symptoms, due to rich collaterals and reversed flow in the ipsilateral vertebral artery. Symptoms when they do occur manifest as arm pain, described as aching and weakness in the extremity, made worse with exercise of the arm and relieved by rest. Subclavian steal syndrome occurs when posterior circulation symptoms (dizziness, drop attacks, and diplopia) occur during arm exercise in patients with proximal subclavian artery occlusion. This syndrome is relatively rare. Another unusual manifestation of subclavian artery occlusion is coronary-subclavian steal syndrome. This occurs in the setting of proximal (usually left) subclavian artery occlusion in a patient with a prior left internal mammary artery (LIMA) to left anterior descending artery graft. Arm exercise may lead to reversed flow in the LIMA and lead to development of chest pain from myocardial ischemia. Because of the collaterals, the limb is threatened only rarely; however, distal embolization can occur from atherosclerotic stenoses or from an axillosubclavian aneurysm, both of which can complicate thoracic outlet syndrome. Embolization usually manifests as small areas of digital gangrene. (See Schwartz 8th ed., p 796.)

21. A patient who is taking metformin has an increased risk of which of these complications after angiography?
    A. Renal failure
    B. Coagulopathy
    C. Lactic acidosis
    D. Hyperkalemia

**Answer: C**

The preangiography checklist includes serum creatinine; medications such as anticoagulants and oral hypoglycemics, specifically metformin (which can cause lactic acidosis when combined with contrast agents); history of dye allergy; and hydration status. Contrast angiography should be avoided if possible in all patients with a serum creatinine level greater than 3.0. It should be performed only if it is truly necessary, and other imaging modalities cannot provide equivalent information in patients with a serum creatinine level greater than 2.0. All patients with a serum creatinine level greater than 1.7 mg/dL are premedicated with acetylcysteine 600 mg by mouth twice daily on the day before and the day of angiography. (See Schwartz 8th ed., p 726.)

22. Which of the following is a risk factor specific for peripheral vascular disease?
    A. Family history
    B. Hyperhomocysteinemia
    C. Elevated high-density lipoprotein (HDL)
    D. Elevated low-density lipoprotein (LDL)

**Answer: B**

Risk factors for peripheral arterial disease (PAD) are similar to those for coronary and cerebrovascular disease, but some factors appear to be even stronger for peripheral disease. Risk factors strongly linked to peripheral vascular disease include smoking, diabetes, elevated triglycerides, hyperhomocysteinemia, and low HDL cholesterol. Although a positive family history has been definitely linked with coronary heart disease and stroke, it has not been confirmed as a significant risk factor for PAD. (See Schwartz 8th ed., p 728.)

23. Cholesterol-lowering drugs (statin therapy) should be recommended in patients with peripheral vascular disease who have
    A. High-density lipoprotein (HDL) <40 mg/dL
    B. Triglycerides >150 mg/dL
    C. Low-density lipoprotein cholesterol (LDL-C) >130 mg/dL
    D. Cholesterol >185 mg/dL

**Answer: C**

Therefore lipid-lowering therapy has benefits in patients with peripheral arterial disease (PAD), who often have co-existing coronary and cerebral arterial disease. In the recent recommendation, patients with PAD are to be treated in a similar manner as patients with coronary artery disease. Drug therapy should be initiated in patients with LDL-C greater than or equal to 130 mg/dL, with a target LDL-C of less than 100 mg/dL. Specific targets of therapy for HDL-C and triglycerides are not provided, but the definition of a low HDL-C is now less than or equal to 40 mg/dL, and optimal triglyceride levels are less than or equal to 150 mg/dL. (See Schwartz 8th ed., p 721.)

24. The osmolality of most contrast agents used for angiography is
    A. 100–300 mOsm
    B. 300–600 mOsm
    C. 600–900 mOsm
    D. 900–1200 mOsm

**Answer: C**

Modern contrast agents are low in osmolality (600 to 900 mOsm), compared with up to 2000 mOsm in the agents used in the past. The low-osmolar agents are associated with less pain during injection and may be associated with a reduced incidence of minor allergic reactions. (See Schwartz 8th ed., p 727.)

25. All patients with peripheral vascular disease should have medical treatment aimed to achieve which of the following goals?
    A. Statin therapy to lower C-reactive protein (CRP) to <1.0
    B. Treatment of blood pressure to attain 130/85 mm Hg
    C. Management of diabetes to obtain glycohemoglobin level <12%
    D. Niacin to achieve normal homocysteine levels

**Answer: B**

Because of the systemic nature of atherosclerosis, all patients with peripheral arterial disease, whether they have a history of coronary disease or not, should benefit from medical prevention strategies. These include aggressive management of smoking, statin therapy with a goal of lowering low-density lipoprotein (LDL) cholesterol to at least 100 mg/dL, treatment of blood pressure to attain 130/85 mm Hg, and management of diabetes mellitus to a glycohemoglobin level of 7%. Drugs shown to have particular benefit in these patients include the statins for LDL reduction, angiotensin converting enzyme (ACE) inhibitors to treat blood pressure, and beta blockers for their cardioprotective effects. In addition, all patients should be given a trial of cilostazol, clopidogrel, or aspirin. Patients should also be investigated for other dyslipidemias and hyperhomocysteinemia and treated accordingly. (See Schwartz 8th ed., p 730.)

26. An ankle-brachial index of 0.7
    A. Is normal
    B. Indicates an increased risk of cardiovascular events
    C. Is indicative of moderate ischemia with rest pain
    D. Is indicative of severe ischemia with a risk for gangrene

**Answer: B**

There is increasing interest in the use of the ankle-brachial index (ABI) to evaluate patients at risk for cardiovascular events. An ABI less than 0.9 correlates with increased risk of myocardial infarction and indicates significant, although perhaps asymptomatic, underlying peripheral vascular disease. The ankle-brachial index is determined in the following ways. Blood pressure (BP) is measured in both upper extremities using the highest systolic BP as the denominator for the ABI. The ankle pressure is determined by placing a BP cuff above the ankle and measuring the return to flow of the posterior tibial and dorsalis pedis arteries using a pencil Doppler over each artery. The ratio of the systolic pressure in each vessel divided by the highest arm systolic pressure can be used to express the ABI in both the posterior tibial and dorsalis pedis arteries. Normal is more than 1. Claudicants are in the 0.6 to 0.9 range, with rest pain and gangrene occurring at less than 0.3. The test is less reliable in patients with heavily calcified vessels due to noncompressibility (i.e., diabetes and end-stage renal disease). (See Schwartz 8th ed., p 724.)

27. The primary event in the occlusion of a coronary artery is
    A. Arterial narrowing at a bifurcation site
    B. Development of an atrial arrhythmia
    C. Episodes of hypotension
    D. Episodes of plaque disruption

**Answer: D**
An occluded coronary artery appears to result from recurrent episodes of plaque disruption that were serially covered with layered thrombus in a repetitive process. These events characteristically occur at bifurcation sites. (See Schwartz 7th ed.)

28. The most common presenting symptom of acute arterial occlusion is
    A. Pain
    B. Pallor
    C. Paresthesia
    D. Pulselessness

**Answer: A**
Pain is usually the first symptom or sign in a cascade that includes all of the other listed items in addition to poikilothermia (coolness). Pain may be absent because of diabetic neuropathy or the rapid progression to advanced ischemia with immediate anesthesia. (See Schwartz 7th ed.)

29. Platelets are derived from
    A. Eosinophils
    B. Lymphocytes
    C. Megakaryocytes
    D. Monocytes

**Answer: C**
Platelets are membrane-bound cytoplasmic remnants of bone marrow megakaryocytes. They act essentially to plug defects in vascular endothelium. (See Schwartz 7th ed.)

30. Chronic occlusion of the popliteal artery may produce
    A. Brawny discoloration of the skin over the ankle
    B. Dilated collateral vessels in calf and foot
    C. Pain in the calf that is relieved by dependency
    D. Ulceration over the medial malleolus

**Answer: C**
The excessive pain associated with arterial occlusion is frequently relieved by holding the foot quiet in a dependent position, taking advantage of gravity to increase blood flow. Collateral vessels around the knee are usually insufficient to maintain circulation after popliteal artery occlusion. The other listed symptoms and signs are characteristic of chronic venous disease. (See Schwartz 7th ed.)

31. The most common type of aneurysm is
    A. Degenerative
    B. Dissecting
    C. Poststenotic
    D. Traumatic

**Answer: A**
The common aortic aneurysm below the renal arteries is frequently called an *atherosclerotic aneurysm*. Because the role of atherosclerosis in aneurysmal disease is unclear, the term "degeneration" is more appropriate. A dissecting aneurysm is a longitudinal splitting of the arterial wall, not a true aneurysm. Mycotic aneurysms, aneurysms that are infected, can occur anywhere in the body. At one time, luetic aneurysms in the proximal aorta were the freest type of aneurysm, but they are now rare in the Western world. At present, the most common organisms in infected aneurysms are *Salmonella* and *Staphylococcus*. Poststenotic aneurysms can develop at any site because of the turbulent flow found just beyond an arterial stenosis. The most frequent traumatic aneurysms today follow arterial catheterization or penetrating violence. (See Schwartz 7th ed.)

32. Each of the following is characteristic of causalgia of an extremity EXCEPT
    A. Anhydrosis
    B. Burning pain
    C. Coolness
    D. Skin hypersensitivity

**Answer: A**

Causalgia occurs after partial nerve transection. The burning pain is severe, and the skin hypersensitivity may make contact with clothing intolerable. Coolness, cyanosis, hyperhydrosis, and edema are also characteristic of the syndrome. (See Schwartz 7th ed.)

33. The first change encountered in acute mesenteric ischemia is
    A. Severe periumbilical pain
    B. Elevation of creatine phosphokinase levels
    C. Hyperkalemia
    D. Metabolic acidosis

**Answer: A**

Severe periumbilical pain out of proportion to the physical findings, especially in an older patient, must be considered evidence of mesenteric ischemia until proved otherwise. All the other findings listed occur later in the course of the disease. (See Schwartz 7th ed.)

34. A 55-year-old woman presents 6 days after experiencing an acute arterial occlusion in her left leg. After she undergoes an arterial reconstruction, pulses return to her foot, but 6 h postoperatively, her urine becomes reddish brown and is found by dipstick to be positive for hemoglobin. Which of the following treatments would be absolutely contraindicated for this patient?
    A. Administration of mannitol
    B. Administration of glucose and insulin
    C. Administration of sodium bicarbonate
    D. Administration of ammonium chloride

**Answer: D**

The revascularization of an extremity may initiate rhabdomyolysis and lead to the release of myoglobin and potassium. Treatment in this situation consists of the administration of fluids to increase intravascular volume, mannitol to promote diuresis, sodium bicarbonate to alkalinize the urine and prevent myoglobin precipitation in the renal tubules, and glucose and insulin if hyperkalemia is a problem. If the myoglobin is severely damaging the kidneys, then amputation sometimes may be necessary. Ammonium chloride would never be indicated in the presence of rhabdomyolysis because it would acidify the urine and cause myoglobin to precipitate in the renal tubules. (See Schwartz 7th ed.)

35. Which of the following statements concerning patients who have an asymptomatic bruit located at the carotid bifurcation is true?
    A. Approximately 50% of these bruits originate in the external carotid artery
    B. The loudest bruits are heard when the stenosis is tightest
    C. If these patients develop symptoms, transient ischemic attacks usually precede frank strokes
    D. Almost 50% of these patients will develop neurologic symptoms within 5 years

**Answer: D**

Roughly 90% of asymptomatic carotid bruits are due to disease at the bifurcation of the common carotid and internal carotid artery, and only 1% reflect disease in the external carotid artery. The bruits may disappear completely when stenosis approaches the 85–90% range. Thompson's study of 138 nonoperated patients who had asymptomatic carotid bruits showed that over a mean follow-up period of 4–5 years, 77 patients remained asymptomatic (56%), whereas 37 patients had transient ischemic attacks, 21 patients had nonfatal strokes, and 3 patients had fatal strokes. The 61 patients (44%) of the last three groups developed neurologic symptoms. Frank strokes in the study population were not preceded by transient ischemic attacks and often were related to total occlusion of the internal carotid artery. In the past, prophylactic carotid endarterectomy was recommended for patients who had asymptomatic lesions and who were about to undergo a major abdominal or thoracic operation with the risk of hypotension. However, recent reports question the validity of this approach and instead recommend noninvasive studies, which, if positive, should be followed by angiography before aortocoronary bypass or major arterial reconstructions. (See Schwartz 7th ed.)

36. Which of the following treatments is contraindicated in the management of frostbite of an extremity?
    A. Rapid warming in warm water
    B. Antibiotics and tetanus antiserum
    C. Elevation of the extremity
    D. Early amputation of demarcated areas

**Answer: D**

The most important aspects of treating frostbite is the rapid immersion of the affected part in a warm water bath with a temperature in the range of 40°–44°C (104°–112°F). Hot water should never be used. Antibiotics and tetanus antiserum to prevent infection and elevation to reduce edema are also important. Sympathectomy, performed between 36 and 72 h after injury, should be done for injuries that may result in loss of tissue to minimize the extent of necrosis and to prevent the usual late vasomotor sequelae. Amputation should be delayed despite demarcation because ultimate loss of tissue cannot be determined early, and although the skin may be gangrenous, the underlying tissue may be viable. Although theoretically plausible, consistent benefit has not been demonstrated from the routine use of either heparin or dextran. The use of intra-arterial reserpine and other fast-acting vasodilators may, however, be appropriate. (See Schwartz 7th ed.)

37. A major difference between congenital and acquired arteriovenous fistulas is
    A. The locations affected
    B. The hemodynamic stresses involved
    C. The character of the bruits
    D. The rates of surgical cure

**Answer: D**

A major difference between acquired and congenital arteriovenous fistulas is the rate of surgical cure. In the acquired form, a single communication usually exists that can be cured by division and reconstruction of the involved artery and, preferably, of the injured vein. A single communication is rare, however, in the congenital form, and a complete cure thus is almost impossible unless the lesion is localized sufficiently to permit excision of adjacent soft tissues. Additionally, there is an almost uniform recurrence of fistulas in patients who have the congenital type, which suggests the presence of a basic defect in these patients' peripheral vascular trees. The locations affected, the hemodynamic stresses involved, the character of the bruits, and the physical characteristics of the typical pulsatile masses are generally similar in the two conditions, although a bruit can be obliterated completely by digital compression with traumatic fistulas but not with congenital ones. (See Schwartz 7th ed.)

38. All of the following statements concerning popliteal artery aneurysms are true EXCEPT
    A. Approximately 50% are associated with aneurysms at other sites
    B. Rupture into the popliteal space is a frequent complication
    C. Associated thrombosis carries a high risk of amputation
    D. Associated distal embolization may result in tissue loss

**Answer: B**

Popliteal aneurysms usually are associated with either distal embolization or thrombosis, both of which can cause limb-threatening ischemia and gangrene. Although rupture is a serious threat with abdominal or thoracic aneurysms, with popliteal aneurysms, it occurs in only 5–10% of reported series. Approximately 50% of popliteal aneurysms are associated with aneurysms elsewhere in the body, particularly in the abdominal aorta or the contralateral popliteal artery. Because these lesions typically are small, excision usually is not necessary, and bypass is acceptable when combined with ligation of the aneurysms. (See Schwartz 7th ed.)

# CHAPTER 23

# Venous and Lymphatic Disease

1. Which of the following veins has valves?
   A. Portal vein
   B. Superior vena cava
   C. Inferior vena cava
   D. Iliac veins

**Answer: B**
The inferior vena cava, the common iliac veins, the portal venous system, and the cranial sinuses are valveless. (See Schwartz 8th ed., p 809.)

2. What is the risk of developing venous stasis changes in the 20 years after a single episode of deep venous thrombosis (DVT)?
   A. 4%
   B. 14%
   C. 27%
   D. 48%

**Answer: C**
Not only does DVT pose an immediate threat to life with pulmonary embolism, it can also cause long-term impairment due to resultant venous insufficiency. The 20-year cumulative incidence rate is 26.8% and 3.7% for the development of venous stasis changes and venous ulcers, respectively, after an episode of DVT. (See Schwartz 8th ed., p 812.)

3. Which of the following is NOT seen in phlegmasia cerulean dolens?
   A. Pain
   B. Edema
   C. Blanching
   D. Cyanosis

**Answer: C**
Clinical symptoms may worsen as deep venous thrombosis (DVT) propagates and involves the major proximal deep veins. Massive DVT that obliterates the major deep venous channel of the extremity with relative sparing of collateral veins causes a condition called phlegmasia alba dolens (Fig. 23-4). This condition is characterized by pain, pitting edema, and blanching. There is no associated cyanosis. When the thrombosis extends to the collateral veins, massive fluid sequestration and more significant edema ensues, resulting in a condition known as phlegmasia cerulea dolens. Phlegmasia cerulea dolens is preceded by phlegmasia alba dolens in 50 to 60% of patients. The affected extremity in phlegmasia cerulea dolens is extremely painful, edematous, and cyanotic, and may be associated with arterial insufficiency or compartment syndrome. If untreated, venous gangrene can ensue, leading to amputation. (See Schwartz 8th ed., p 813.)

4. What percentage of patients undergoing laparotomy for malignancy will develop deep venous thrombosis (DVT)?
   A. 5%
   B. 15%
   C. 25%
   D. 35%

**Answer: C**
Without prophylaxis, patients undergoing surgery for intra-abdominal malignancy have a 25% incidence of DVT, while orthopedic patients undergoing hip fracture surgery have a 40 to 50% incidence of DVT in the postoperative period. Patients at highest risk are elderly patients undergoing major surgery or those with previous venous thromboembolism, malignancy, or paralysis. (See Schwartz 8th ed., p 815.)

5. The initial dose of unfractionated heparin (UFH) to fully heparinize a patient is
   A.  20 IU/kg IV
   B.  40 IU/kg IV
   C.  60 IU/kg IV
   D.  80 IU/kg IV

**Answer: D**

Weight-based UFH dosages have been shown to be more effective than standard fixed boluses in rapidly achieving therapeutic levels. Weight-based dosing of UFH is initiated with a bolus of 80 IU/kg IV, and a maintenance continuous infusion is started at 18 IU/kg per hour IV. (See Schwartz 8th ed., p 817.)

6. The half-life of unfractionated heparin (UFH) is
   A.  ½ h
   B.  1½ h
   C.  3 h
   D.  5 h

**Answer: B**

The half-life of UFH is approximately 90 minutes. The level of anticoagulation should be monitored every 6 hours with activated partial thromboplastin time (aPTT) determinations until aPTT levels reach a steady state. Thereafter, aPTT can be obtained daily. aPTT levels must be kept at or above 1.5 times the control level for venous thromboembolism (VTE) treatment. (See Schwartz 8th ed., p 817.)

7. Which of the following treatments for deep vein thrombosis is contraindicated in pregnancy?
   A.  Unfractionated heparin
   B.  Low molecular weight heparin
   C.  Warfarin
   D.  Inferior vena cava filter

**Answer: C**

Warfarin is not recommended for use in pregnant patients. In animal studies, it has been associated with spontaneous abortion and birth defects. Pregnant patients with venous thromboembolism (VTE) should be treated with heparin and monitored for the development of osteopenia. Heparin is discontinued 24 to 36 hours prior to labor induction. (See Schwartz 8th ed., p 818.)

8. Which of the following statements concerning hirudin is true?
   A.  It works by tightly binding to thrombin.
   B.  It binds to platelet factor 4.
   C.  It cross reacts with heparin antibodies and cannot be used in patients with heparin-induced thrombocytopenia (HIT).
   D.  It is given orally.

**Answer: A**

Hirudin is a class of direct thrombin inhibitors that was first derived from the leech, *Hirudo medicinalis*. The commercially available hirudin, lepirudin, is manufactured by recombinant DNA technology. Hirudins form a tight complex with thrombin. They inhibit thrombin conversion of fibrinogen to fibrin as well as thrombin-induced platelet aggregation. These actions are independent of antithrombin. Unlike the larger heparin-antithrombin complex, the smaller hirudins can inhibit thrombin and fibrin deposition in the interstices of a developing thrombus. Hirudins do not bind to platelet factor 4. They can be used in patients who develop HIT as a complication of heparin therapy. Hirudin is administered intravenously with a loading dose of 0.4 mg/kg followed by a continuous infusion of 0.15 mg/kg per hour. The activated partial thromboplastin time (aPTT) is used to monitor the effects of hirudins. The dose of hirudin must be adjusted in patients with renal failure because it is metabolized in the kidneys. There is no reversal agent currently available for hirudin. When necessary, plasma exchange may be useful to reverse the anticoagulant effect of hirudin. (See Schwartz 8th ed., p 819.)

9. Initial therapy of a patient with mesenteric venous thrombosis (MVT) without peritonitis is
   A.  Bowel rest and observation
   B.  IV dobutamine
   C.  Anticoagulation
   D.  Laparotomy

**Answer: C**

Patients with MVT should have adequate fluid resuscitation and be anticoagulated with heparin. Urgent laparotomy is undertaken in patients presenting with peritoneal findings. Perioperative broad-spectrum antibiotics are administered. Findings at laparotomy consist of edema and cyanotic discoloration of the mesentery and bowel wall with thrombus involving the distal mesenteric veins. Complete thrombosis of the superior mesenteric vein is rare, occurring in only 12% of patients undergoing laparotomy for suspected MVT. The arterial supply to the involved bowel is usually intact. Nonviable bowel is resected, and primary anastomoses can be performed. If the viability of the remaining bowel is in question, a second-look operation is performed within 24 to 48 hours.

In patients without peritoneal findings, anticoagulation with intravenous unfractionated heparin (UFH) is promptly initiated. Patients are maintained on bowel rest and are fluid resuscitated. Close clinical observation is warranted with serial abdominal examinations. Once the patient's clinical status improves, oral intake can be carefully started. The patient is transitioned to oral anticoagulation over 3 to 4 days and is usually maintained on lifelong oral anticoagulation. (See Schwartz 8th ed., p 823.)

10. The most common form of primary lymphedema is
    A. Congenital lymphedema
    B. Lymphedema praecox
    C. Lymphedema intermedius
    D. Lymphedema tarda

**Answer: B**

The original classification system, described by Allen, is based on the etiology of the lymphedema. Primary lymphedema is further subdivided into congenital, praecox, and tarda. *Congenital lymphedema* can involve a single lower extremity, multiple limbs, the genitalia, or the face. The edema is typically present at birth. *Lymphedema praecox* is the most common form of primary lymphedema, accounting for 94% of cases. *Lymphedema praecox* is far more common in women, with the gender ratio favoring women 10:1. The onset of swelling is during the childhood or teenage years and involves the foot and calf. *Lymphedema tarda* is uncommon, accounting for less than 10% of cases of primary lymphedema. The onset of edema is later in life than in *lymphedema praecox*. (See Schwartz 8th ed., p 828.)

11. The primary treatment for lymphedema is
    A. Excision of lymphedematous tissue with reconstruction
    B. Microvascular lymphovenous anastomosis
    C. Microvascular lympholymphatic anastomosis
    D. Compression garments

**Answer: D**

Graded compression stockings are widely used in the treatment of lymphedema. The stockings reduce the amount of swelling in the involved extremity by preventing the accumulation of edema while the extremity is dependent. When worn daily, compression stockings have been associated with long-term maintenance of reduced limb circumference. They may also protect the tissues against chronically elevated intrinsic pressures, which lead to thickening of the skin and subcutaneous tissue. Compression stockings also offer a degree of protection against external trauma. (See Schwartz 8th ed., p 829.)

12. Risk factors for the development of thrombocytopenia during heparin therapy include
    A. Female patient
    B. Heparin given for more than 10 days
    C. Use of unfractionated heparin
    D. None of the above

**Answer: D**

The development of heparin-induced thrombocytopenia (HIT) is not predictable, and there are no known risk factors. In the mild form of the disease, the platelet count remains >100,000/mm$^3$, and the process reverses even if heparin is continued. In contrast, type II HIT, which occurs in approximately 20% of affected patients, is associated with a platelet count <100,000/mm$^3$. These patients have an antibody that binds to the platelet-heparin complex, and they are prone to develop arterial and venous thromboses, with a high mortality rate. Heparin must be stopped immediately when type II HIT is diagnosed. (See Schwartz 7th ed.)

13. In a patient after a moderate-risk general surgical operation, such as a low anterior resection of the colon, the most effective step in the prevention of postoperative pulmonary embolization is
   A. Early ambulation
   B. Leg elevation
   C. Use of elastic stockings
   D. Use of intermittent pneumatic leg compression

**Answer: D**

Superficial femoral vein ligation was suggested at one time as a prophylactic measure, but results did not substantiate its use. Each of the other methods is currently used. Intermittent pneumatic leg compression is the most effective measure. Application of the boots in the operating room and their postoperative management is not complicated. (See Schwartz 7th ed.)

14. The most common symptom after major pulmonary embolism is
   A. Cough
   B. Dyspnea
   C. Hemoptysis
   D. Pleural pain

**Answer: B**

Pulmonary embolism may be responsible for each of the listed symptoms. Data from a national urokinase pulmonary embolism trial found that dyspnea, present in 80% of patients, was the most frequent symptom. Although many physicians associate hemoptysis with pulmonary embolism, it occurred in only 27% of the patients in the same study. (See Schwartz 7th ed.)

15. The first-choice diagnostic study for suspected deep venous thrombosis of the lower extremity is
   A. Contrast sonography
   B. Impedance plethysmography
   C. Radioactive-labeled fibrinogen uptake
   D. Real-time Doppler imaging

**Answer: D**

All these methods have been advocated for detecting deep venous thrombosis. Real-time B-mode Doppler imaging is the method of choice because it is noninvasive and has sensitivity, specificity, and accuracy in the 90–95% range. (See Schwartz 7th ed.)

16. The best initial therapy for deep venous thrombosis of the common femoral vein is
   A. Heparin
   B. Placement of a vena caval filter
   C. Streptokinase
   D. Venous thrombectomy

**Answer: A**

Primary management of deep venous thrombosis involves heparin followed by a 3- to 6-month course of warfarin. Streptokinase and urokinase have no advantage over heparin, and they have a relatively high incidence of hemorrhagic complications. Venous thrombectomy carries a disappointing recurrence rate. A vena caval filter should be used if primary anticoagulant therapy is ineffective in preventing pulmonary embolization. (See Schwartz 7th ed.)

# CHAPTER 24

# Esophagus and Diaphragmatic Hernia

1. Grade II esophagitis on endoscopy is defined by
   A. Erythema extending circumferentially in the mucosa
   B. Any ulceration
   C. Linear ulcerations with friable granulation tissue
   D. Circumferential loss of epithelium

**Answer: C**

Grade I esophagitis is defined as small, circular, nonconfluent erosions. Grade II esophagitis is defined by the presence of linear erosions lined with granulation tissue that bleeds easily when touched. Grade III esophagitis represents a more advanced stage, in which the linear or circular erosions coalesce into circumferential loss of the epithelium, or the appearance of islands of epithelium which on endoscopy appears as a "cobblestone" esophagus. Grade IV esophagitis is the presence of a stricture. Its severity can be assessed by the ease of passing a 36F endoscope. When a stricture is observed, the severity of the esophagitis above it should be recorded. The absence of esophagitis above a stricture suggests a chemical-induced injury or a neoplasm as a cause. The latter should always be considered and is ruled out only by evaluation of a tissue biopsy of adequate size. (See Schwartz 8th ed., p 845.)

2. A healthy person may experience gastroesophageal reflux (pH <4 in the distal esophagus) for what percent of the day?
   A. 0.5%
   B. 2%
   C. 4.5%
   D. 6%

**Answer: C**

**Table 24-1.**
**Normal Values for Esophageal Exposure to pH <4 (n = 50)**

| Component | Mean | SD | 95% |
|---|---|---|---|
| Total time | 1.51 | 1.36 | 4.45 |
| Upright time | 2.34 | 2.34 | 8.42 |
| Supine time | 0.63 | 1.0 | 3.45 |
| No. of episodes | 19.00 | 12.76 | 46.90 |
| No. >5 min | 0.84 | 1.18 | 3.45 |
| Longest episode | 6.74 | 7.85 | 19.80 |

SD = standard deviation.
Source: Reproduced with permission from DeMeester TR, Stein HJ: Gastroesophageal reflux disease, in Moody FG, Carey LC, et al (eds): *Surgical Treatment of Digestive Disease*. Chicago: Year Book Medical, 1990, p 68.
See Schwartz 8th ed., p 853.

3. The incidence of metaplastic Barrett's epithelium progressing to adenocarcinoma is
   A. 1% per year
   B. 3% per year
   C. 5% per year
   D. 10% per year

**Answer: A**

Endoscopically, Barrett's esophagus can be quiescent or associated with complications of esophagitis, stricture, Barrett's ulceration, and dysplasia. The complications associated with Barrett's esophagus may be due to the continuous irritation from refluxed duodenogastric juice. This continued injury is pH dependent and may be modified by medical therapy. The incidence of metaplastic Barrett's epithelium becoming dysplastic and progressing to adenocarcinoma is approximately 1% per year. (See Schwartz 8th ed., p 861.)

4. Which of the following patients should be offered anti-reflux surgery as the first treatment option in the treatment of gastroesophageal reflux disease?
   A. Hiatal hernia
   B. Symptoms of >5-year duration
   C. Barrett's esophagitis on endoscopy
   D. pH <4 for >20% of the day

**Answer: C**

Patients presenting for the first time with symptoms suggestive of gastroesophageal reflux may be given initial therapy with $H_2$ blockers. In view of the availability of these as over-the-counter medications, many patients will have already self-medicated their symptoms. Failure of $H_2$ blockers to control the symptoms, or immediate return of symptoms after stopping treatment, suggests either that the diagnosis is incorrect or that the patient has relatively severe disease. Endoscopic examination at this stage of the patient's evaluation provides the opportunity for assessing the severity of mucosal damage and the presence of Barrett's esophagus. Both of these findings on initial endoscopy are associated with a high probability that medical treatment will fail. A measurement of the degree and pattern of esophageal exposure to gastric and duodenal juice, via 24-hour pH and bilirubin monitoring, should be obtained at this point. The status of the lower esophageal sphincter (LES) and the function of the esophageal body should also be measured. These studies identify features such as the following, which are predictive of a poor response to medical therapy, frequent relapses, and the development of complications: supine reflux, poor esophageal contractility, erosive esophagitis (or a columnar-lined esophagus at initial presentation), bile in the refluxate, and a structurally defective sphincter. Patients who have these risk factors should be given the option of surgery as a primary therapy, with the expectation of long-term control of symptoms and complications. (See Schwartz 8th ed., p 863.)

5. Which of the following is an indication for a partial fundoplication?
   A. Minimal reflux (pH <4 for <10% of the measured time)
   B. Absence of a hiatal hernia
   C. Amplitude of esophageal contraction <20 mm Hg in the lower esophagus
   D. Barrett's esophagus

**Answer: C**

Before proceeding with an antireflux operation, several factors should be evaluated. First, the propulsive force of the body of the esophagus should be evaluated by esophageal manometry to determine if it has sufficient power to propel a bolus of food through a newly reconstructed valve. Patients with normal peristaltic contractions do well with a 360 degree Nissen fundoplication. When peristalsis is absent or severely disordered, or the amplitude of the contraction is below 20 mm Hg throughout the lower esophagus, a two-thirds partial fundoplication may be the procedure of choice. (See Schwartz 8th ed., p 863.)

6. Which of the following is an indication for a gastroplasty?
   A. Presence of a sliding hiatal hernia that does not reduce in the standing position
   B. Large paraesophageal hernia
   C. Redundant fundus
   D. Gastric outlet obstruction

**Answer: A**

Anatomic shortening of the esophagus can compromise the ability to do an adequate repair without tension, and lead to an increased incidence of breakdown or thoracic displacement of the repair. Esophageal shortening is identified on a barium swallow roentgenogram by a sliding hiatal hernia that will not reduce in the upright position, or that measures larger than 5 cm between the diaphragmatic crura and gastroesophageal junction on endoscopy. When esophageal shortening is present, the motility of the esophageal body must be carefully evaluated, and if inadequate, a gastroplasty should be performed. In patients who have a global absence of contractility, more than 50% interrupted or dropped contractions, or a history of several failed previous antireflux procedures, esophageal resection should be considered as an alternative. (See Schwartz 8th ed., p 863.)

7. Which of the following is a relative indication for a transthoracic approach for a Nissen fundoplication?
   A. Previous hiatal hernia repair
   B. Large hiatal hernia
   C. Paraesophageal hernia
   D. Previous splenectomy

**Answer: A**

The indications for performing an antireflux procedure by a transthoracic approach are as follows:

1. A patient who has had a previous hiatal hernia repair. In this situation, a peripheral circumferential incision in the diaphragm is made to provide simultaneous exposure of the upper abdomen. This allows safe dissection of the previous repair from both the abdominal and thoracic sides of the diaphragm.
2. A patient who requires a concomitant esophageal myotomy for achalasia or diffuse spasm.
3. A patient who has a short esophagus. This is usually associated with a stricture or Barrett's esophagus. In this situation, the thoracic approach is preferred to allow maximum mobilization of the esophagus, and to perform a Collis gastroplasty in order to place the repair without tension below the diaphragm.
4. A patient with a sliding hiatal hernia that does not reduce below the diaphragm during a roentgenographic barium study in the upright position. This can indicate esophageal shortening, and again, a thoracic approach is preferred for maximum mobilization of the esophagus, and if necessary, the performance of a Collis gastroplasty.
5. A patient who has associated pulmonary pathology. In this situation, the nature of the pulmonary pathology can be evaluated and the proper pulmonary surgery, in addition to the antireflux repair, can be performed.
6. An obese patient. In this situation, the abdominal repair is difficult because of poor exposure, particularly in men, in whom the intra-abdominal fat is more abundant.

(See Schwartz 8th ed., p 866.)

8. Which incision is used for a transthoracic Nissen fundoplication?
   A. Left posterolateral thoracotomy in the 6th intercostal space
   B. Left posterolateral thoracotomy in the 4th intercostal space
   C. Right posterolateral thoracotomy in the 6th intercostal space
   D. Right posterolateral thoracotomy in the 4th intercostal space

**Answer: A**

In the thoracic approach the hiatus is exposed through a left posterior lateral thoracotomy incision in the sixth intercostal space (i.e., over the upper border of the seventh rib). When necessary, the diaphragm is incised circumferentially 2 to 3 cm from the lateral chest wall for a distance of approximately 10 to 15 cm. The esophagus is mobilized from the level of the diaphragm to underneath the aortic arch. Mobilization up to the aortic arch is usually necessary to place the repair in a patient with a shortened esophagus into the abdomen without undue tension. Failure to do this is one of the major causes for subsequent breakdown of a repair and return of symptoms. The cardia is then freed from the diaphragm. When all the attachments between the cardia and diaphragmatic hiatus are divided, the fundus and part of the body of the stomach are drawn up through the hiatus into the chest. The vascular fat pad that lies at the gastroesophageal junction is excised. Crural sutures are then placed to close the hiatus, and the fundoplication is constructed by enveloping the fundus around the distal esophagus in a manner similar to that described for the abdominal approach. When complete, the fundoplication is placed into the abdomen by compressing the fundic ball with the hand and manually maneuvering it through the hiatus. (See Schwartz 8th ed., p 865.)

9. Primary treatment of a Zenker's diverticulum is
   A. Reassurance and dietary changes
   B. Open resection of the diverticulum
   C. Cervical myotomy with resection of large diverticulum
   D. Esophagectomy

**Answer: C**
The low morbidity and mortality associated with cricopharyngeal and upper esophageal myotomy have encouraged a liberal approach toward its use for almost any problem in the oropharyngeal phase of swallowing. (See Schwartz 8th ed., p 876.)

10. The most common primary esophageal motility disorder is
    A. Achalasia
    B. Segmental esophageal spasm
    C. Diffuse esophageal spasm
    D. "Nutcracker" esophagus

**Answer: D**
The disorder, termed "nutcracker" or "supersqueezer" esophagus, was recognized in the late 1970s. Other terms used to describe this entity are "hypertensive peristalsis" or "high-amplitude peristaltic contractions." It is the most common of the primary esophageal motility disorders. By definition the so-called nutcracker esophagus is a manometric abnormality in patients with chest pain characterized by peristaltic esophageal contractions with peak amplitudes greater than two standard deviations above the normal values in individual laboratories. Contraction amplitudes in these patients can easily be above 400 mm Hg. Ambulatory 24-hour monitoring of esophageal motor function in patients diagnosed as having nutcracker esophagus has identified a subgroup of patients with a motor pattern characteristic of diffuse esophageal spasm. These patients usually complain of dysphagia in addition to chest pain, and probably are misclassified on the basis of standard manometric findings. The identification of these patients is important, since esophageal myotomy is a therapeutic option for patients with dysphagia and diffuse esophageal spasm, but is of questionable value in patients with chest pain secondary to nutcracker esophagus. (See Schwartz 8th ed., p 879.)

11. Which of the following is the most effective treatment for achalasia?
    A. Repeated balloon dilatation
    B. Laparoscopic Heller myotomy
    C. Thoracoscopic Heller myotomy
    D. Dietary changes and observation

**Answer: B**
In a randomized long-term follow-up by Csendes and colleagues of 81 patients treated for achalasia, either by forceful dilation or by surgical myotomy, myotomy was associated with a significant increase in the diameter at the gastroesophageal junction and a decrease in the diameter at the middle third of the esophagus on follow-up radiographic studies. There was a greater reduction in sphincter pressure and improvement in the amplitude of esophageal contractions after myotomy. Thirteen percent of patients regained some peristalsis after dilation, compared with 28% after surgery. These findings were shown to persist over a 5-year follow-up period, at which time 95% of those treated with surgical myotomy were doing well. Of those

who were treated with dilation, only 54% were doing well, while 16% required redilation and 22% eventually required surgical myotomy to obtain relief. (See Schwartz 8th ed., p 887.)

12. The overall success rate of cervical myotomy for patients with a pharyngoesophageal swallowing dysfunction is
    A. 20%
    B. 35%
    C. 65%
    D. 90%

**Answer: C**
The more liberal application of myotomy to problems of the oropharyngeal phase of swallowing has resulted in an overall success rate in the relief of symptoms of only 64%. When patients are selected using radiographic or motility markers of disease as outlined above, it is unusual for patients not to see benefit. (See Schwartz 8th ed., p 874.)

13. Patients with hiatal hernias on barium swallow
    A. Are usually symptomatic (gastrointestinal reflux disease)
    B. Should be treated initially with proton pump inhibitors
    C. Require surgical therapy only if the hernia is large
    D. Should be further evaluated by endoscopy

**Answer: C**
A small hiatal hernia is usually not associated with significant symptoms or illness, and its presence is an irrelevant finding unless the hiatal hernia is large (Fig. 24-17), the hiatal opening is narrow and interrupts the flow of barium into the stomach (Fig. 24-18), or the hernia is of the paraesophageal variety. (See Schwartz 8th ed., p 845.)

14. Alginic acid
    A. Neutralizes gastric acid
    B. Neutralizes bile reflux in the stomach
    C. Promotes gastric emptying
    D. Creates a barrier for gastric and esophageal epithelium

**Answer: D**
Used in combination with simple antacids, alginic acid may augment the relief of symptoms by creating a physical barrier to reflux, as well as by acid reduction. Alginic acid reacts with sodium bicarbonate in the presence of saliva to form a highly viscous solution that floats like a raft on the surface of the gastric contents. When reflux occurs, this protective layer is refluxed into the esophagus, and acts as a protective barrier against the noxious gastric contents. Medications to promote gastric emptying such as metoclopramide, domperidone, or cisapride are beneficial in early disease, but of little value in more severe disease. (See Schwartz 8th ed., p 863.)

15. What percentage of patients on long-term follow up, will have persistent, pathologic esophageal acid exposure after a Nissen fundoplication?
    A. <1%
    B. 5%
    C. 15%
    D. 25%

**Answer: D**
Long-term outcome studies suggest that as many as 25% of post-Nissen patients will have persistent pathologic esophageal acid exposure confirmed by positive 24-hour pH studies. (See Schwartz 8th ed., p 862.)

16. Which of the following is one of the five principles of anti-reflux surgery?
    A. A 360-degree fundoplication should be used.
    B. The posterior wall of the fundoplication should be sutured to the crura to maintain the inferior fixation of the esophagus.
    C. A fundoplication should restore the lower esophageal sphincter pressure to twice that of the resting gastric pressure.
    D. At least 5 cm of intra-abdominal esophagus should be created.

**Answer: C**
The five principles:

1. Restore the pressure of the distal esophageal sphincter to twice the resting gastric pressure and it's length to at least 3 cm
2. Place an adequate length of the distal esophageal sphincter in the abdomen (positive pressure)
3. The reconstructed cardia should be able to relax with swallowing
4. Do not exceed the peristaltic ability of the distal esophagus
5. The fundoplication should be maintained in the abdomen without undue tension

(See Schwartz 8th ed., p 864.)

17. Pharyngoesophageal dysfunction is often caused by
    A. Acquired disease of the nervous system
    B. Cleft palate
    C. Thyromegaly
    D. Cervical spine injury

**Answer: A**

Pharyngoesophageal swallowing disorders are usually congenital or due to acquired disease involving the central and peripheral nervous system. This includes cerebrovascular accidents, brain stem tumors, poliomyelitis, multiple sclerosis, Parkinson's disease, pseudobulbar palsy, peripheral neuropathy, and operative damage to the cranial nerves involved in swallowing. Muscular diseases such as radiation-induced myopathy, dermatomyositis, myotonic dystrophy, and myasthenia gravis are less common causes. Rarely, extrinsic compression by thyromegaly, cervical lymphadenopathy, or hyperostosis of the cervical spine can cause pharyngoesophageal dysphagia. (See Schwartz 8th ed., p 873.)

18. Valves involved in the act of swallowing include all of the following EXCEPT
    A. Cricopharyngeus
    B. Epiglottis
    C. Lower esophageal sphincter
    D. Tongue

**Answer: D**

Relaxation of the cricopharyngeus allows food to enter the esophagus. The epiglottis tilts backward to cover the larynx and prevent aspiration. The soft palate is elevated, closing the passage between the nasopharynx and the oropharynx. The lower esophageal sphincter provides a pressure barrier between the esophagus and the stomach. The tongue acts as a piston, moving the bolus of food into the posterior oropharynx and hypopharynx. (See Schwartz 7th ed.)

19. The most significant risk factor for the development of adenocarcinoma of the esophagus is
    A. Alcohol abuse
    B. Barrett's esophagus
    C. Long-standing achalasia
    D. Smoking

**Answer: B**

In Barrett's esophagus, there is a metaplastic change in the esophageal mucous membrane. The resulting columnar epithelium is susceptible to the development of adenocarcinoma. If 100 patients with Barrett's esophagus are followed prospectively for 1 year, one adenocarcinoma can be expected in the group. Alcohol abuse, achalasia, lye stricture, and smoking are all risk factors for the development of squamous carcinoma in the esophagus. (See Schwartz 7th ed.)

20. A 65-year-old patient has a carcinoma of the esophagus at the level of the sternal notch. There are no palpable lymph nodes in the neck. The appropriate management of this patient is
    A. Chemotherapy
    B. Combination chemotherapy and radiation therapy
    C. Preoperative radiation therapy and surgical resection
    D. Surgical resection

**Answer: D**

Lesions at this level have a poor prognosis. Local recurrence, however, is more common after radiation therapy or chemotherapy than after surgical resection, and the recurrent lesion usually is difficult to treat. Preoperative radiation therapy should be considered if the lesion is fixed to the spine or if cervical lymph node metastases are present. (See Schwartz 7th ed.)

21. All of the following statements concerning Schatzki's ring are true EXCEPT
    A. Drug ingestion is involved in the development of the ring in many patients.
    B. Esophageal dilatation is the treatment of choice unless the patient has gastric reflux.
    C. Patients with Schatzki's ring have an increased incidence of carcinoma at the gastroesophageal junction.
    D. Short-duration dysphagia is the most frequent presenting symptom.

**Answer: C**

Schatzki's ring is a submucosal ring in the lower esophagus, and drug ingestion is present in many people with the ring. Dysphagia after rapid ingestion of solid food is the most common symptom. Unless the patient has significant reflux symptoms, dilatation is appropriate therapy. An increased incidence of gastroesophageal cancer occurs with Barrett's esophagus rather than Schatzki's ring. (See Schwartz 7th ed.)

22. Spontaneous perforation of the esophagus most frequently occurs in the
    A. Left pleural cavity
    B. Pericardium
    C. Posterior mediastinum
    D. Retropharyngeal region

**Answer: A**
Spontaneous perforation usually occurs in a patient with gastroesophageal reflux disease. Perforation usually occurs either in the left pleural cavity or just above the gastroesophageal junction. (See Schwartz 7th ed.)

23. Diagnosis of esophageal perforation is best established by
    A. Contrast esophagograms
    B. Esophagoscopy with a flexible esophagoscope
    C. Esophagoscopy with a rigid esophagoscope
    D. Upright X-rays of the chest, including lateral and oblique films

**Answer: A**
X-rays of the chest may demonstrate mediastinal air, but this finding may not be present for several hours. Esophagoscopy is an appropriate early diagnostic study after caustic ingestion. Transesophageal ultrasound study affords good visualization of cardiac valve function and ventricular activity. Esophagograms demonstrate extravasation in 90% of patients with esophageal perforation. A water-soluble contrast medium should be used, and the patient should be positioned in the right lateral decubitus position so that the entire esophagus can be visualized. (See Schwartz 7th ed.)

24. All of the following statements about achalasia are true EXCEPT
    A. In most affected persons, ganglion cells in the body of the esophagus either are absent or have degenerated.
    B. Pressure in the body of the esophagus is lower than normal.
    C. Affected persons usually experience more difficulty swallowing cold foods than warm foods.
    D. Esophageal cancer is seven times as common in affected persons as in the general population.

**Answer: B**
Achalasia, a disorder of the esophagus, is associated with loss or degeneration of ganglion cells in the body of the esophagus. The cause of the nerve changes in Auerbach's plexus in the esophagus is unknown. Pain is not a common complaint of affected persons, and, if it occurs, it is likely to mark an early stage of the disease. Regurgitation, however, is a common symptom, and dysphagia is more pronounced for cold than for warm foods. Esophageal motility is uncoordinated, and pressure in the body of the esophagus usually is higher than normal. Achalasia most commonly affects people between the ages of 30 and 50 years. Because of the risk of carcinoma, careful follow-up of these patients is important. (See Schwartz 7th ed.)

25. After a patient has ingested lye, esophagoscopy should be performed
    A. Shortly after the event to establish the degree of injury
    B. After several weeks have passed to prevent early perforation
    C. Only if evidence of dysphagia occurs
    D. After several days of antibiotic therapy

**Answer: A**
Early esophagoscopy to, but not beyond, the level of injury is safe, and it is the best method of evaluating the degree of injury. The physician should attempt to prevent rather than to treat dysphagia. As soon as the patient is able to swallow saliva, a string should be passed to facilitate later dilatation. Although antibiotic therapy is appropriate, it need not delay esophagoscopy. Steroid therapy is controversial and may mask serious problems. (See Schwartz 7th ed.)

26. All of the following statements about paraesophageal hernia are true EXCEPT
    A. Heartburn is the usual chief complaint of affected persons.
    B. Symptoms can stem from obstruction and hemorrhage.
    C. The herniated portion of the stomach may become gangrenous and perforate.
    D. Surgical repair generally is indicated.

**Answer: A**
Obstruction and hemorrhage are the chief complications of paraesophageal hernia, in which a part of the stomach has herniated into the thorax. The herniated portion of the stomach can become gangrenous and perforate. Unlike sliding hiatal hernia, for which surgical repair is indicated only if symptoms warrant, paraesophageal hernia requires prompt surgical repair because of the potentially life-threatening complications of the underlying anatomic defect. The repair of paraesophageal hernias is by an abdominal approach; reflux control procedures usually are not indicated. True paraesophageal hernia is not associated with reflux. (See Schwartz 7th ed.)

27. The treatment of choice for perforation of the cervical esophagus is
    A. Bed rest and use of antibiotics
    B. Nasogastric intubation and use of antibiotics
    C. Cervical exploration, drainage of superior mediastinum, and use of antibiotics
    D. Resection and colonic interposition

**Answer: C**
Surgical exploration of the neck combined with drainage of the retrovisceral space is the preferred treatment of persons who have a cervical esophageal perforation. Drainage can be performed under local anesthesia, and improvement is prompt. Suture closure may be required for major lacerations. All persons who have an esophageal injury should receive parenterally administered antibiotics and appropriate fluid and electrolyte solutions; however, relying on these measures alone—without surgery—is dangerous and may be fatal. (See Schwartz 7th ed.)

28. The most effective treatment of achalasia is
    A. Antispasmodic medication
    B. Dilation of the lower esophageal sphincter
    C. Esophagomyotomy
    D. Resection of the cardioesophageal junction

**Answer: C**
Esophagomyotomy is currently the treatment of choice for patients who have achalasia. In one series, 94% of patients who underwent esophagomyotomy experienced some improvement after the procedure, and 83% of patients experienced good to excellent results. By contrast, in the same study, only 65% of patients treated with hydrostatic dilation had good to excellent results. The late results of esophagomyotomy are far superior to those of forceful dilation, and the latter treatment should be reserved for those for whom surgery is contraindicated. Although resection of the region of the lower esophageal sphincter has been associated with severe reflux, only a 3% incidence of esophageal incompetence after esophagomyotomy has been reported. (See Schwartz 7th ed.)

# CHAPTER 25

# Stomach

1. The consistently largest artery to the stomach is the
   A. Right gastroepiploic
   B. Left gastroepiploic
   C. Right gastric
   D. Left gastric

**Answer: D**

The consistently largest artery to the stomach is the left gastric artery, which usually arises directly from the celiac trunk and divides into an ascending and descending branch along the lesser gastric curvature. Approximately 15% of the time, the left gastric artery supplies an aberrant vessel which travels in the gastrohepatic ligament (lesser omentum) to the left side of the liver. Rarely, this is the only arterial blood supply to this part of the liver, and inadvertent ligation may lead to clinically significant hepatic ischemia. (See Schwartz 8th ed., p 935.)

2. The left gastroepiploic artery arises from
   A. The left gastric artery
   B. The splenic artery
   C. The right hepatic artery
   D. The gastroduodenal artery

**Answer: B**

The second largest artery to the stomach is usually the right gastroepiploic artery, which arises fairly consistently from the gastroduodenal artery behind the first portion of the duodenum. The left gastroepiploic artery arises from the splenic artery, and together with the right gastroepiploic artery, forms the rich gastroepiploic arcade along the greater curvature. (See Schwartz 8th ed., p 935.)

3. Which of the following is secreted by gastric chief cells?
   A. Somatostatin
   B. Gastrin
   C. Pepsinogen
   D. Histamine
   E. Glucagon

**Answer: C**

See Table 25-1 on p 182.

| Cell Type | Substance(s) Secreted |
|---|---|
| Chief cells | Lipase, pepsinogen |
| Oxyntic (parietal) cells | Acid, intrinsic factor |
| D cells | Somatostatin |
| G cells | Gastrin |
| Superficial epithelial cells | Bicarbonate, mucous |
| Enterochromaffin-like cells | Histamine |

**Table 25-1.**
**Epithelial Cells of the Stomach**

| Cell Type | Distinctive Ultrastructural Features | Major Functions |
|---|---|---|
| Surface-foveolar mucous cells | Apical stippled granules up to 1 μm in diameter | Production of neutral glycoprotein and bicarbonate to form a gel on the gastric luminal surface, neutralization of hydrochloric acid[a] |
| Mucous neck cell | Heterogeneous granules 1–2 μm in diameter dispersed throughout the cytoplasm | Progenitor cell for all other gastric epithelial cells, glycoprotein production, production of pepsinogens I and II |
| Oxyntic (parietal) cell | Surface membrane invaginations (canaliculi), tubulovesicle structures, numerous mitochondria | Production of hydrochloric acid production of intrinsic factor production of bicarbonate |
| Chief cell | Moderately dense apical granules up to 2 μm in diameter, prominent supranuclear Golgi apparatus, extensive basolateral granular endoplasmic reticulum | Production of pepsinogens I and II, and of lipase |
| Cardiopyloric mucous cell | Mixture of granules like those in mucous neck and chief cells, extensive basolateral granular endoplasmic reticulum | Production of glycoprotein, production of pepsinogen II |
| Endocrine cells | See Fig. 25-14 | |

[a]Bicarbonate is probably produced by other gastric epithelial cells in addition to surface-foveolar mucous cells.
Source: Reproduced with permission from Antonioli DA, Madara JL, in Ming SC, Goldman H (eds): *Pathology of the Gastrointestinal Tract*. Baltimore: Williams & Wilkins, 1998, p 13.
See Schwartz 8th ed., pp 939–941.

4. The effect of erythromycin on gastric emptying is through its function as a
   A. Dopamine antagonist
   B. Cholinergic agonist
   C. Motilin agonist
   D. Cholinergic antagonist

**Answer: C**

**Table 25-2.**
**Promotility Agents That Accelerate Gastric Emptying**

| Drug | Mechanism |
|---|---|
| Metoclopramide | Dopamine antagonist |
| Domperidone | Dopamine antagonist |
| Erythromycin | Motilin agonist |
| Bethanechol | Cholinergic agonist |
| Neostigmine | Cholinergic agonist |

See Schwartz 8th ed., p 950.

5. Which of the following is the best test to use to confirm eradication of *Helicobacter pylori* infection after treatment?
   A. Serologic test
   B. Urea breath test
   C. Histology
   D. Rapid urease test

6. What percentage of patients with a bleeding peptic ulcer will stop bleeding if made n.p.o. and given acid suppression?
   A. 10%
   B. 25%
   C. 50%
   D. 75%

**Answer: B**

A positive serologic test is presumptive evidence of active infection if the patient has never been treated for *H. pylori*. Histologic examination of an antral mucosal biopsy using special stains is the gold standard test. Other sensitive tests include commercially available rapid urease tests, which assay for the presence of urease in mucosal biopsies (strong presumptive evidence of infection). Urease is an omnipresent enzyme in *H. pylori* strains that colonize the gastric mucosa. The labeled carbon urea breath test has recently become available (Fig. 25-29). This has become the standard test to confirm eradication of *H. pylori* following appropriate treatment. In this test the patient ingests urea labeled with radioactive $^{14}C$ or nonradioactive $^{13}C$. The labeled urea is acted upon by the urease present in the *H. pylori* and converted into ammonia and carbon dioxide. The radiolabeled carbon dioxide is excreted from the lungs and can be detected in the expired air. It also can be detected in a blood sample. The fecal antigen test also is quite sensitive and specific for active *H. pylori* infection and may prove useful in confirming a cure. (See Schwartz 8th ed., p 953.)

**Answer: D**

Three quarters of the patients who come to the hospital with bleeding peptic ulcer will stop bleeding if given acid suppression and kept n.p.o. (non per os, meaning nothing by mouth). However, one fourth will continue to bleed or will rebleed after an initial quiescent period, and virtually all the mortalities (and all the operations for bleeding) occur in this group. This group can be fairly well delineated based on clinical factors related to the magnitude of the hemorrhage and endoscopic findings (Table 25-10). Shock, hematemesis, transfusion requirement exceeding four units in 24 hour, and high-risk endoscopic stigmata (active bleeding or visible vessel) define this high-risk group. These patients benefit from endoscopic therapy to stop the bleeding. The most common endoscopic hemostatic modalities used are injection with epinephrine, and electrocautery. Persistent bleeding or rebleeding after endoscopic therapy is an indication for operation, although repeat endoscopic treatment has been successful in treating rebleeding. Elderly and high-risk patients do not tolerate repeated episodes of hemodynamically significant hemorrhage, and may benefit from early elective operation after initially successful endoscopic treatment, especially if they have one or more of the risk factors mentioned above or a high-risk ulcer. Planned surgery under controlled circumstances often yields better outcomes than emergent surgery performed in the middle of the night. Deep bleeding ulcers on the posterior duodenal bulb or lesser gastric curvature are high-risk lesions, because they often erode large arteries not amenable to nonoperative treatment, and early operation should be considered. (See Schwartz 8th ed., p 959.)

7. The most accurate diagnostic test for Zollinger-Ellison syndrome (ZES) is
   A. Fasting serum gastrin
   B. Computed tomography scan
   C. Endoscopy
   D. Secretin stimulation test

**Answer: D**

Hypergastrinemia in the presence of elevated basal acid output (BAO) suggests gastrinoma. Despite this relatively simple guideline, most patients with ZES have been symptomatic for several years prior to diagnosis. In patients on antisecretory therapy, medication should be stopped for several days prior to checking the serum gastrin level, since acid suppression may falsely elevate gastrin levels. Causes of hypergastrinemia can be divided into those associated with hyperacidity and those associated with hypoacidity (Table 25-15). The diagnosis of ZES is confirmed by the secretin stimulation test. An intravenous bolus of secretin (2 U/kg) is given and gastrin levels are checked before and after injection. An increase in serum gastrin of 200 pg/mL or greater suggests the presence of gastrinoma. Other provocative tests such as calcium stimulation or standard meal are usually unnecessary. Patients with gastrinoma should have serum calcium and parathyroid hormone levels determined to rule out multiple endocrine neoplasia type I (MEN-I). (See Schwartz 8th ed., p 970.)

8. Which blood group is associated with an increased risk of gastric cancer?
   A. A
   B. B
   C. AB
   D. O

**Answer: A**

Gastric cancer is more common in patients with pernicious anemia, blood group A, or a family history of gastric cancer. When patients migrate from a high incidence region to a low incidence region, the risk of gastric cancer decreases in the subsequent generations born in the new region. This strongly suggests an environmental influence on the development of gastric cancer. Environmental factors appear to be more related etiologically to the intestinal form of gastric cancer than the more aggressive diffuse form. The commonly accepted risk factors for gastric cancer are listed in Table 25-3. (See Schwartz 8th ed., p 972.)

**Table 25-3.**
**Factors Increasing and Decreasing the Risk for Gastric Cancer**

*Increase risk*
   Family history
   Diet (high in nitrates, salt, fat)
   Familial polyposis
   Gastric adenomas
   Hereditary nonpolyposis colorectal cancer
   *Helicobacter pylori* infection
      Atrophic gastritis, intestinal metaplasia, dysplasia
   Previous gastrectomy or gastrojejunostomy (>10 years ago)
   Tobacco use
   Ménétrier's disease
*Decrease risk*
   Aspirin
   Diet (high fresh fruit and vegetable intake)
   Vitamin C

See Schwartz 8th ed., p 973.

9. The standard surgical treatment of a gastrointestinal stromal tumor (GIST) of the stomach is
   A. Endoscopic ablation
   B. Wedge resection with clear margins
   C. Subtotal gastrectomy
   D. Total gastrectomy

**Answer: B**

GISTs are submucosal tumors that are slow growing. Smaller lesions are usually found incidentally, though they occasionally may ulcerate and cause impressive bleeding. Larger lesions generally produce symptoms of weight loss, abdominal pain, fullness, early satiety, and bleeding. An abdominal mass may be palpable. Spread is by the hematogenous route, often to liver and/or lung, though positive lymph nodes are occasionally seen in resected specimens. Diagnosis is by endoscopy and biopsy, though the interpretation of the latter may be problematic. Endoscopic ultrasound may be helpful, but symptomatic tumors and tumors over 2 cm in size should be removed. Metastatic workup entails computed tomography (CT) of the chest, abdomen, and pelvis (chest X-ray may suffice in lieu of CT of the chest). Most gastric GISTs occur in the body of the stomach, but they also can occur in the fundus or antrum. They are almost always solitary. Wedge resection with clear margins is adequate treatment, and prognosis depends on tumor size and mitotic count. True invasion of adjacent structures is evidence of malignancy. If safe, en bloc resection of involved surrounding organs is appropriate to remove all tumor when the primary is large and invasive. Most patients with low-grade lesions are cured (80% 5-year survival), but most patients with high-grade lesions are not (30% 5-year survival). (See Schwartz 8th ed., p 981.)

10. Watermelon stomach is best treated by
    A. Acid-reducing agents
    B. Motility agents
    C. Antrectomy
    D. Total gastrectomy

**Answer: C**

The parallel red stripes atop the mucosal folds of the distal stomach give the rare entity of "watermelon stomach" (gastric antral vascular ectasia) its name. Histologically, gastric antral vascular ectasia is characterized by dilated mucosal blood vessels that often contain thrombi, in the lamina propria. Mucosal fibromuscular hyperplasia and hyalinization often are present (Fig. 25-66). The histologic appearance can resemble portal gastropathy, but the latter usually affects the proximal stomach, whereas watermelon stomach predominantly affects the distal stomach. Patients with gastric antral vascular ectasia are usually elderly women with chronic gastrointestinal (GI) blood loss requiring transfusion. Most have an associated autoimmune connective tissue disorder, and at least 25% have chronic liver disease. Antrectomy may be required to control blood loss, but in patients with portal hypertension, transvenous intrahepatic portosystemic shunt should be considered first. (See Schwartz 8th ed., p 983.)

11. Dieulafoy's lesion most commonly results in
    A. Progression to gastric cancer
    B. Gastroparesis
    C. Gastric outlet obstruction
    D. Upper gastrointestinal bleed

**Answer: D**

Dieulafoy's lesion is a congenital arteriovenous malformation characterized by an unusually large tortuous submucosal artery. If this artery is eroded, impressive bleeding may occur. To the operating surgeon, this appears as a stream of arterial blood emanating from what appears grossly to be a normal gastric mucosa. The lesion typically occurs in middle-aged or elderly men. Patients typically present with upper gastrointestinal (GI) bleeding, which may be intermittent, and endoscopy can miss the lesion if it is not actively bleeding. Treatment options include endoscopic hemostatic therapy (usually injection), angiographic embolization, or operation. At surgery, the lesion may be oversewn or resected. (See Schwartz 8th ed., p 984.)

12. Initial treatment for severe early dumping after gastrectomy is
    A. Expectant management
    B. Oral glucose for symptoms
    C. Octreotide
    D. Surgical conversion to a Roux-en-Y drainage

**Answer: C**
The medical therapy for the dumping syndrome consists of dietary management and somatostatin analogue (octreotide). Often symptoms improve if the patient avoids liquids during meals. Hyperosmolar liquids (e.g., milk shakes) may be particularly troublesome. There is some evidence that adding dietary fiber compounds at mealtime may improve the syndrome. If dietary manipulation fails, the patient is started on octreotide, 100 µg subcutaneously twice daily. This can be increased up to 500 µg twice daily if necessary. Octreotide ameliorates the abnormal hormonal pattern seen in patients with dumping symptoms. It also promotes restoration of a fasting motility pattern in the small intestine (i.e., restoration of the migrating motor complex). The alpha-glucosidase inhibitor acarbose may be particularly helpful in ameliorating the symptoms of late dumping. (See Schwartz 8th ed., p 987.)

13. A 55-year-old executive who is seen because of severe epigastric pain is found by gastroduodenal endoscopy to have a large ulcer in the duodenal bulb. He is placed on a diet and $H_2$ blocker, but his symptoms persist. At this time, it would be most appropriate to suggest a
    A. Course of metronidazole, tetracycline, and bismuth
    B. Highly selective vagotomy
    C. Truncal vagotomy and antrectomy
    D. Truncal vagotomy and pyloroplasty

**Answer: A**
Surgery is no longer commonly offered to patients with severe ulcer pain. Careful medical management with acid reduction and control of *Helicobacter pylori* infection is effective for most patients, and the need for operation is unusual. If an operation is done, highly selective vagotomy is the treatment of choice, because this operation preserves the normal functional anatomy of the stomach and pylorus. (See Schwartz 7th ed.)

14. All of the following occur after highly selective vagotomy EXCEPT
    A. Basal acid secretion is reduced.
    B. Basal gastrin production is decreased.
    C. Liquids pass more rapidly into the duodenum.
    D. Solids pass into the duodenum at a normal rate.

**Answer: B**
After highly selective vagotomy, basal gastrin production is increased, but the gastrin response to a meal is reduced. Basal and stimulated acid secretion are reduced by more than 75 and 50%, respectively. Liquids pass into the duodenum more rapidly than normal, but solids are handled in the usual manner. (See Schwartz 7th ed.)

15. A 65-year-old woman with a known duodenal ulcer is being treated with diet and $H_2$ blocker therapy. She is admitted with a major upper gastrointestinal hemorrhage. After blood replacement is begun, the next step in her management should be
    A. Beginning bismuth, tetracycline, and metronidazole
    B. Beginning omeprazole
    C. Endoscopy and coagulation of the bleeding vessel
    D. Pyloroduodenotomy and oversewing of the bleeding vessel

**Answer: C**
In the presence of an acute hemorrhage, none of the listed drug regimens provides immediate control. Endoscopy with coagulation of the bleeding vessel should be attempted. If the procedure is unsuccessful or if bleeding recurs within a few hours, direct surgical intervention with ligation of the bleeding vessel can be life-saving. (See Schwartz 7th ed.)

16. The normal stomach secretes all of the following EXCEPT
    A. Bicarbonate
    B. Intrinsic factor
    C. Lipase
    D. Pepsinogen
    E. Glucagon

**Answer: E**

In response to acetylcholine, the chief cells secrete pepsinogen and lipase, and in the acid gastric content, this compound is broken down to release pepsin. Intrinsic factor is secreted to facilitate the absorption of vitamin $B_{12}$ in the terminal ileum. The surface epithelial cells of the stomach secrete a combination of mucus and bicarbonate, probably to protect the stomach from all acid digestion. (See Schwartz 7th ed.)

17. Patients at increased risk for gastric carcinoma include all of the following EXCEPT
    A. Those who have undergone gastric resection for duodenal ulcer
    B. Those with pernicious anemia
    C. Those who have undergone gastric bypass for morbid obesity
    D. Those with blood group A

**Answer: C**

The incidence of gastric carcinoma in the United States has declined significantly since 1930, and the reasons for the decline are not clear. In Japan, Chile, and Iceland the disease remains common, and it is believed that smoked fish in the diet contributes to this situation. Patients with pernicious anemia who have atrophic gastritis are at increased risk. Patients with blood group A are also at risk, although this observation has never been explained. Carcinoma may develop in the gastric remnant many years after gastric resection for duodenal ulcer, probably on the basis of bile-induced gastritis. Gastric cancer is not recognized as a complication of gastric bypass procedures. (See Schwartz 7th ed.)

18. A patient with the Zollinger-Ellison syndrome is found to have the multiple endocrine neoplasia type I (MEN-I) syndrome. Appropriate management for the ulcer symptoms should be
    A. Cimetidine
    B. Omeprazole
    C. Pancreatic resection
    D. Streptozocin

**Answer: B**

Patients with MEN-I syndrome have multiple small pancreatic tumors not amenable to resection. Omeprazole, a protein pump blocker, has been more effective than cimetidine in managing the ulcer diathesis in these patients. Streptozocin and fluorouracil may provide palliation. Total gastrectomy is appropriate for MEN-I patients refractory to medical therapy. In contrast, the initial approach to sporadic gastrinoma without metastasis should be exploratory celiotomy with resection of the pancreatic neoplasm if it is localized. (See Schwartz 7th ed.)

19. Fat absorption occurs primarily in the
    A. Stomach
    B. Third portion of the duodenum
    C. Jejunum
    D. Ileum

**Answer: C**

Fat digestion and absorption occur in the jejunum where triglycerides are partially hydrolyzed by pancreatic lipase. (See Schwartz 7th ed.)

20. The treatment of choice for a 40-year-old man who is found on endoscopy and biopsy to have a gastric lymphoma would be
    A. Subtotal gastrectomy
    B. Radiotherapy
    C. Chemotherapy
    D. Wide local excision

**Answer: B**

Lymphoma accounts for about 2% of all gastric malignancies. The treatment of choice once a histologic diagnosis has been confirmed is radiation therapy. This lesion is quite radiosensitive, and morbidity from radiation is low. An 85% 5-year survival has been reported when the tumor is confined to the stomach. Operative resection is reserved for bulky lesions with gastric outlet obstruction. (See Schwartz 7th ed.)

# CHAPTER 26

# The Surgical Management of Obesity

1. The body mass index (BMI) of a patient who weighs 220 lb (100 k) and is 68 in. tall (172 cm) is
   A. 27.5
   B. 32.4
   C. 33.9
   D. 38.1

**Answer: C**

Obesity is a serious disease that carries substantial morbidity and mortality and has mixed genetic and environmental etiologies. Obesity is defined as the accumulation of excess body fat that leads to pathology. Severity is based on the degree of excess body fat, which is commonly assessed using the body mass index [BMI = weight (kg)/height (m)$^2$], which correlates body weight with height. Patients are classified as overweight, obese, or severely obese (sometimes referred to as morbidly obese) (Table 26-1). Obesity may also be defined as body weight that exceeds ideal body weight by 20%, with ideal body weight determined by population studies. Morbidly obese individuals generally exceed ideal body weight by 100 lb or more, or are 100% over ideal body weight. In 1991, the National Institutes of Health defined morbid obesity as a BMI of 35 kg/m$^2$ or greater with severe obesity-related comorbidity, or BMI of 40 kg/m$^2$ or greater without comorbidity. Superobesity is a term sometimes used to define individuals who have a body weight exceeding ideal body weight by 225% or more, or a BMI of 50 kg/m$^2$ or greater. (See Schwartz 8th ed., p 997.)

2. The mortality of laparoscopic Roux-en-Y gastric bypass is approximately
   A. 1:10,000 patients
   B. 1:1,000 patients
   C. 1:500 patients
   D. 1:100 patients

**Answer: D**

Postoperative complications include pulmonary embolism (0 to 1.5%), anastomotic leak (1.5 to 5.8%), bleeding (0 to 3.3%), and pulmonary complications (0 to 5.8%). Stenosis of the gastrojejunostomy is observed in 1.6 to 6.3%. Other complications include internal hernia (2.5%), gallstones (1.4%), marginal ulcer (1.4%), and staple-line failure (1%). Conversion to an open procedure occurs in 3 to 9%. The mortality rate is 0 to 1.5%. (See Schwartz 8th ed., p 1007.)

3. Obesity is defined as a body mass index (BMI) greater than or equal to
   A. 25
   B. 30
   C. 35
   D. 40

**Answer: B**

**Table 26-1.**
**Assessing Disease Risk Using Body Mass Index and Waist Size**

| Category | BMI | Men (<40 in.), Women (<35 in.) | Men (>40 in.), Women (>35 in.) |
|---|---|---|---|
| Underweight | <18.5 | – | – |
| Normal | 18.5–24.9 | – | – |
| Overweight | 25.0–29.9 | + | + |
| Obesity | 30 | | |
| Class I | 30.0–34.9 | + | ++ |
| Class II | 35.0–39.9 | ++ | ++ |
| Class III (extreme obesity) | 40 | +++ | |

See Schwartz 8th ed., p 998.

4. Which of the following patients is a candidate for bariatric surgery?
   A. Body mass index (BMI) >25, major comorbidities
   B. BMI >30, minor comorbidities
   C. BMI >35, with or without comorbidities
   D. BMI >40, with or without comorbidities

**Answer: D**

Patients that have a BMI of 35 kg/m$^2$ or more with comorbidity, or those with a BMI of 40 kg/m$^2$ or greater regardless of comorbidity, are eligible for bariatric surgery. Candidates must have attempted weight loss in the past by medically supervised diet regimens, exercise, or medications. Furthermore, they must be motivated to comply with postoperative dietary and exercise regimens and follow-up. Traditionally, surgeons have offered bariatric surgery to patients aged 18 to 60 years. However, bariatric surgery is now offered to some older adults at some institutions with no reported increase in morbidity or mortality. Adolescent patients with morbid obesity may be considered for bariatric surgery under select circumstances. (See Schwartz 8th ed., p 1000.)

5. The most common early (<30 day) complication of a Roux-en-Y gastric bypass is
   A. Wound dehiscence
   B. Pulmonary embolism
   C. Anastomotic stricture
   D. Small bowel obstruction due to internal hernia

**Answer: C**

Major complications after Roux-en-Y gastric bypass occur early (<30 days), and include pulmonary embolus (1 to 2%), gastrointestinal leak (1 to 5%), and anastomotic stricture (3 to 10%). Common late complications include hernia (5 to 24%), marginal ulcers (3 to 10%), and bowel obstructions (1 to 5%). Vitamin $B_{12}$ deficiency and iron deficiency anemia are the most common nutritional sequelae after gastric bypass arising in approximately 15 and 30%, respectively. Both can be prevented with supplementation in most patients. Unlike malabsorptive procedures, significant protein-calorie malnutrition is rare in the absence of infection, obstruction, or other medical disorders. (See Schwartz 8th ed., p 1003.)

6. Which of the following is NOT a component of syndrome X?
   A. Glucose intolerance
   B. Hypercholesterolemia
   C. Sleep apnea
   D. Hypertension

**Answer: C**

The combination of central obesity, glucose intolerance, dyslipidemia, and hypertension is known as syndrome X. Those with syndrome X have an elevated risk of developing coronary artery disease and diabetes mellitus. Once diagnosed with syndrome X, an individual should initiate dietary changes, exercise, and weight loss; medical intervention may be necessary as well. (See Schwartz 8th ed., p 998.)

7. To lose 1 lb of weight, what calorie deficit (i.e., calories burned over calories ingested) is required?
   A. 250 kcal
   B. 750 kcal
   C. 1250 kcal
   D. 3500 kcal

8. Which of the following is an advantage of the laparoscopic band when compared to a Roux-en-Y gastric bypass (RYGB)?
   A. Frequent visits for adjustment of port
   B. Better weight loss
   C. Better control of gastroesophageal reflux
   D. Lower leak rate

9. The most common complication after a biliopancreatic diversion (BPD) is
   A. Ulceration
   B. Hypocalcemia
   C. Anemia
   D. Osteoporosis

**Answer: D**
As a rule of thumb, a deficit of 500 kcal per day, resulting in a weekly deficit of 3500 kcal, translates to the loss of one pound of fat a week. (See Schwartz 8th ed., p 999.)

**Answer: D**
**Advantages.** Laparoscopic adjustable gastric banding is a relatively simple procedure that takes less operative time than the more complex procedures such as laparoscopic RYGB or laparoscopic biliopancreatic diversion. The mortality rate is low (0.06%), as are conversion rates (0 to 4%). No staple lines or anastomoses are required. Recovery is rapid and hospital stay is short. The adjustable nature of the laparoscopic band allows the degree of restriction to be optimized for the patient's weight loss. Increasing band diameter may relieve postoperative vomiting.

    **Disadvantages.** With this procedure, there is a potential for port site complications and the need for frequent postoperative visits for band adjustment. Some patients (5 to 10%) experience band slipping or gastric prolapse, which usually requires reoperation. Other potential problems include band erosion, port-related complications, gastroesophageal reflux, alterations in esophageal motility, and esophageal dilatation. Should inadequate weight loss occur, revision to Roux-en-Y gastric bypass is feasible, but may be technically difficult because of adhesions in the area surrounding the band. (See Schwartz 8th ed., p 1005.)

**Answer: C**
The incidence of postoperative complications is quite high following BPD. The most common morbidities include anemia (30%), protein-calorie malnutrition (20%), dumping syndrome, and marginal ulceration (10%). The duodenal switch modification is associated with a lower ulceration rate (1%) and a lower incidence of dumping syndrome. Other complications include vitamin $B_{12}$ deficiency, hypocalcemia, fat-soluble vitamin deficiencies, osteoporosis, night blindness, and prolongation of prothrombin time. The postoperative mortality rate ranges from 0.4 to 0.8%. (See Schwartz 8th ed., p 1008.)

1. The sensitivity of plain radiographs in the diagnosis of small bowel obstruction is
   A. 30–40%
   B. 50–60%
   C. 70–80%
   D. 90–100%

**Answer: C**

The diagnosis of small-bowel obstruction is usually confirmed with radiographic examination. The abdominal series consists of a radiograph of the abdomen with the patient in a supine position, a radiograph of the abdomen with the patient in an upright position, and a radiograph of the chest with the patient in an upright position. The finding most specific for small-bowel obstruction is the triad of dilated small-bowel loops (>3 cm in diameter), air–fluid levels seen on upright films, and a paucity of air in the colon. The sensitivity of abdominal radiographs in the detection of small-bowel obstruction ranges from 70 to 80%. Specificity is low, because ileus and colonic obstruction can be associated with findings that mimic those observed with small-bowel obstruction. False-negative findings on radiographs can result when the site of obstruction is located in the proximal small bowel and when the bowel lumen is filled with fluid but no gas, thereby preventing visualization of air–fluid levels or bowel distention. The latter situation is associated with closed-loop obstruction. Despite these limitations, abdominal radiographs remain an important study in patients with suspected small-bowel obstruction because of their widespread availability and low cost. (See Schwartz 8th ed., p 1029.)

2. The best examination for the diagnosis of partial small bowel obstruction is
   A. Plain radiographs
   B. Upper gastrointestinal (UGI) with small bowel follow-through
   C. Computed tomography (CT) scan with contrast
   D. Magnetic resonance imaging (MRI)

**Answer: C**

A limitation of CT scanning is its low sensitivity (<50%) in the detection of low-grade or partial small-bowel obstruction. A subtle transition zone may be difficult to identify in the axial images obtained during CT scanning. In such cases, contrast examinations of the small bowel, either small-bowel series (small-bowel follow-through) or enteroclysis, can be helpful. For standard small-bowel series, contrast is swallowed or instilled into the stomach through a nasogastric tube. Abdominal radiographs are then taken serially as the contrast travels distally in the intestine. Although barium can be used, water-soluble contrast agents, such as Gastrografin, should be used if the possibility of intestinal perforation exists. These examinations are more labor intensive and less-rapidly performed than CT scanning, but may offer greater sensitivity in the detection of luminal and mural etiologies of obstruction, such as primary intestinal tumors. For enteroclysis, 200 to

250 mL of barium followed by 1 to 2 L of a solution of methylcellulose in water is instilled into the proximal jejunum via a long nasoenteric catheter. Enteroclysis is rarely performed in the acute setting, but offers greater sensitivity than small-bowel series in the detection of lesions that may be causing partial small-bowel obstruction. The double-contrast technique used in enteroclysis permits assessment of mucosal surface detail and detection of relatively small lesions, even through overlapping small-bowel loops. (See Schwartz 8th ed., p 1029.)

3. Which of the following has been shown to decrease the duration of postoperative ileus after laparotomy?
   A. Nasogastric decompression
   B. Early ambulation
   C. Early post-operative feeding
   D. Use of ketorolac

**Answer: D**
Given the frequency of postoperative ileus, a large number of investigations have been conducted to define strategies to reduce its duration. Although often used, the use of early ambulation, early postoperative feeding protocols, and routine nasogastric intubation have not been demonstrated to be associated with earlier resolution of postoperative ileus. The administration of nonsteroidal anti-inflammatory drugs such as ketorolac and concomitant reductions in opioid dosing have been shown to reduce the duration of ileus in most studies. Similarly, the use of perioperative thoracic epidural anesthesia/analgesia with regimens containing local anesthetics combined with limitation or elimination of systemically administered opioids has been shown to reduce duration of postoperative ileus. (See Schwartz 8th ed., p 1032.)

4. The most common tumor of the small bowel is
   A. Carcinoma
   B. Adenoma
   C. Fibroma
   D. Hemangioma

**Answer: B**
Adenomas are the most common benign neoplasm of the small intestine. Other benign tumors include fibromas, lipomas, hemangiomas, lymphangiomas, and neurofibromas. These lesions are most frequently encountered in the duodenum as incidental findings during esophagogastroduodenoscopy (EGD) examinations (Fig. 27-23). Their reported prevalence rates, as detected during EGD performed for other reasons, range from 0.3 to 4.6%. (See Schwartz 8th ed., p 1038.)

5. The most common small bowel cancer is
   A. GIST (gastrointestinal stromal tumor)
   B. Carcinoid tumors
   C. Adenocarcinoma
   D. Lymphoma

**Answer: C**
Primary small-bowel cancers are rare, with an estimated incidence of 5300 cases per year in the United States (Table 27-7). Among small-bowel cancers, adenocarcinomas comprise 35 to 50% of all cases, carcinoid tumors comprise 20 to 40%, and lymphomas comprise approximately 10 to 15%. GISTs are the most common mesenchymal tumors arising in the small intestine and comprise up to 15% of small-bowel malignancies. GISTs comprise the vast majority of tumors that were formerly classified as leiomyomas, leiomyosarcomas, and smooth muscle tumors of the intestine. The small intestine is frequently affected by metastases from or local invasion by cancers originating at other sites. Melanoma, in particular, is associated with a propensity for metastasis to the small intestine. (See Schwartz 8th ed., p 1038.)

6. The appropriate treatment of localized small bowel lymphoma is
   A. Segmental resection only
   B. Adjuvant chemotherapy followed by segmental resection
   C. Segmental resection followed by chemotherapy
   D. Resection, chemotherapy, and X-ray therapy

**Answer: C**
Localized small-intestinal lymphoma should be treated with segmental resection of the involved intestine and adjacent mesentery. If the small intestine is diffusely affected by lymphoma, chemotherapy, rather than surgical resection, should be the primary therapy. The value to adjuvant chemotherapy after resection of localized lymphoma is controversial. (See Schwartz 8th ed., p 1042.)

7. Appropriate therapy for a bleeding Meckel's diverticulum is
   A. H$_2$ blockade followed by diverticulectomy
   B. Diverticulectomy alone
   C. Diverticulectomy and oversewing of the bleeding point
   D. Segmental small bowel resection to include the Meckel's diverticulum

**Answer: D**
The surgical treatment of symptomatic Meckel's diverticula should consist of diverticulectomy with removal of associated bands connecting the diverticulum to the abdominal wall or intestinal mesentery. If the indication for diverticulectomy is bleeding, segmental resection of ileum that includes both the diverticulum and the adjacent ileal peptic ulcer should be performed. Segmental ileal resection may also be necessary if the diverticulum contains a tumor, or if the base of the diverticulum is inflamed or perforated. (See Schwartz 8th ed., p 1045.)

8. The treatment of choice for an asymptomatic acquired duodenal diverticulum is
   A. Observation
   B. Endoscopic resection
   C. Surgical resection
   D. Surgical bypass

**Answer: A**
Asymptomatic acquired diverticula should be left alone. Bacterial overgrowth associated with acquired diverticula is treated with antibiotics. Other complications, such as bleeding and diverticulitis, are treated with segmental intestinal resection for diverticula located in the jejunum or ileum. Bleeding and obstruction related to lateral duodenal diverticula are generally treated with diverticulectomy alone. (See Schwartz 8th ed., p 1047.)

9. Which of the following DOES NOT contribute to small bowel epithelial defenses?
   A. Tight junctions
   B. Immunoglobulin A
   C. Immunoglobulin G
   D. Mucins

**Answer: C**
Factors contributing to epithelial defense include immunoglobulin A (IgA), mucins, and the relative impermeability of the brush border membrane and tight junctions to macromolecules and bacteria. Recently described factors likely to play important roles in intestinal mucosal defense include antimicrobial peptides such as the defensins. (See Schwartz 8th ed., p 1024.)

10. What percentage of the body's immune cells are located in the intestine?
    A. 10%
    B. 30%
    C. 50%
    D. 70%

**Answer: D**
Although the intestinal epithelium allows for efficient absorption of dietary nutrients, it must discriminate between pathogens and harmless antigens, such as food proteins and commensal bacteria, and it must resist invasion by pathogens. Factors contributing to epithelial defense include immunoglobulin A (IgA), mucins, and the relative impermeability of the brush border membrane and tight junctions to macromolecules and bacteria. Recently described factors likely to play important roles in intestinal mucosal defense include antimicrobial peptides such as the defensins. The intestinal component of the immune system, known as the gut-associated lymphoid tissue (GALT), contains more than 70% of the body's immune cells. (See Schwartz 8th ed., p 1024.)

11. Which of the following is NOT a common etiology of ileus?
    A. Pneumonia
    B. Hypernatremia
    C. Calcium channel blockers
    D. Hypothyroidism

**Answer: B**

**Table 27-1.**
**Ileus: Common Etiologies**

| | |
|---|---|
| Abdominal surgery | Anticholinergics |
| Infection | Opiates |
| Sepsis | Phenothiazines |
| Intra-abdominal abscess | Calcium channel blockers |
| Peritonitis | Tricyclic antidepressants |
| Pneumonia | Hypothyroidism |
| Electrolyte abnormalities | Ureteral colic |
| Hypokalemia | Retroperitoneal hemorrhage |
| Hypomagnesemia | Spinal cord injury |
| Hypermagnesemia | Myocardial infarction |
| Hyponatremia | Mesenteric ischemia |
| Medications | |

See Schwartz 8th ed., p 1031.

12. Which of the following is NOT an extraintestinal manifestation of Crohn's disease?
    A. Pyoderma gangrenosum
    B. Erythema nodosum
    C. Ankylosing spondylitis
    D. Nodular arthritis

**Answer: D**

**Table 27-2.**
**Extraintestinal Manifestations of Crohn's Disease**

| | |
|---|---|
| Dermatologic | Primary sclerosing cholangitis |
| Erythema nodosum | Pericholangitis |
| Pyoderma gangrenosum | Urologic |
| Rheumatologic | Nephrolithiasis |
| Peripheral arthritis | Ureteral obstruction |
| Ankylosing spondylitis | Miscellaneous |
| Sacroiliitis | Thromboembolic disease |
| Ocular | Vasculitis |
| Conjunctivitis | Osteoporosis |
| Uveitis/iritis | Endocarditis, myocarditis, |
| Episcleritis | pleuropericarditis |
| Hepatobiliary | Interstitial lung disease |
| Hepatic steatosis | Amyloidosis |
| Cholelithiasis | Pancreatitis |

See Schwartz 8th ed., p 1034.

13. Chronic radiation enteritis usually presents how long after the exposure to radiation?
    A. 7–10 days
    B. 6–12 months
    C. 2–4 years
    D. 8–10 years

**Answer: B**

The clinical manifestations of chronic radiation enteritis usually become evident within 2 years of radiation administration, although they can begin as early as several months or as late as decades afterwards. The most common clinical presentation is one of partial small-bowel obstruction with nausea, vomiting, intermittent abdominal distention, crampy abdominal pain, and weight loss being the most common symptoms. The terminal ileum is the most frequently affected segment. Other manifestations of chronic radiation enteritis include complete bowel obstruction, acute or chronic intestinal hemorrhage, and abscess or fistula formation. (See Schwartz 8th ed., p 1031.)

14. The surgical treatment of radiation enteritis is indicated for
    A. Persistent low-grade stenosis
    B. Persistent crampy pain
    C. Prevention of malignant degeneration
    D. Enteroenteric fistula

**Answer: D**

In contrast, the treatment of chronic radiation enteritis represents a formidable challenge. Surgery for this condition is difficult, is associated with high morbidity rates, and should be avoided in the absence of specific indications such as high-grade obstruction, perforation, hemorrhage, intra-abdominal abscesses, and fistulas. The goal of surgery is limited resection of diseased intestine with primary anastomosis between healthy bowel segments. However, the characteristically diffuse nature of fibrosis and dense adhesions among bowel segments can make limited resection difficult to achieve. Furthermore, it is difficult to distinguish between normal and irradiated intestine intraoperatively by either gross inspection or frozen-section analysis. This distinction is important because anastomoses between irradiated segments of intestine are associated with leak rates as high as 50%. If limited resection is not achievable, an intestinal bypass procedure may be an option, except in cases for which hemorrhage is the surgical indication. There remain cases in which resections extensive enough to cause short-bowel syndrome are unavoidable. (See Schwartz 8th ed., p 1042.)

15. Secretin has all of the following actions EXCEPT
    A. Inhibition of the flow of bile
    B. Inhibition of gastrin release
    C. Stimulation of release of bicarbonate from pancreatic ductal cells
    D. Stimulation of release of water from pancreatic ductal cells

**Answer: A**

Secretin stimulates bicarbonate and water release from pancreatic ductal cells. It also stimulates the flow of bile and inhibits gastrointestinal mobility. Although secretin releases gastrin from gastrinomas, it inhibits gastrin release from the normal stomach. (See Schwartz 7th ed.)

16. Cholecystokinin has all of the following actions EXCEPT
    A. It inhibits bowel motility.
    B. It produces relaxation of the sphincter of Oddi.
    C. It stimulates gallbladder contractility.
    D. It stimulates release of insulin.

**Answer: A**

Cholecystokinin stimulates release of bile by producing gallbladder contractions and relaxing the sphincter of Oddi. It also stimulates release of insulin, stimulates secretion of enzymes by pancreatic acinar cells, and increases bowel motility. (See Schwartz 7th ed.)

17. Vasoactive intestinal peptide (VIP) has all of the following actions EXCEPT
    A. It leads to the watery diarrhea syndrome.
    B. It produces potent vasodilatation.
    C. It stimulates gastric acid secretion.
    D. It stimulates intestinal secretion.

**Answer: C**

VIP is a potent vasodilator, which is the chief agent responsible for the watery diarrhea syndrome. It also stimulates intestinal and pancreatic secretion but inhibits gastric acid secretion. (See Schwartz 7th ed.)

18. The most common small bowel malignancy in children under 10 years of age is
    A. Carcinoid
    B. Carcinoma
    C. Leiomyosarcoma
    D. Lymphoma

**Answer: D**

Lymphomas, especially in the ileum, are the most common small bowel malignancy in children. Many of these lesions are cured after small bowel resection. (See Schwartz 7th ed.)

19. The most common sarcoma in the small intestine in adults is
    A. Angiosarcoma
    B. Fibrosarcoma
    C. Kaposi's sarcoma
    D. Leiomyosarcoma

**Answer: D**
Leiomyosarcomas are evenly distributed throughout the small intestine. They spread by direct invasion of adjacent structures by transperitoneal seeding or by hematogenous dissemination. (See Schwartz 7th ed.)

20. After massive small bowel resection the body compensates by
    A. Increased number of villi
    B. Lengthened individual villi
    C. Increased life span for absorptive cells
    D. Increased synthesis of digestive enzymes by absorptive cells

**Answer: B**
When a massive small bowel resection is necessary, the body attempts to adapt by increasing digestion and absorption of nutrients. This is accomplished by lengthening the individual villi and the number of active cells on the villous surface, which effectively increases the absorptive area available. However, the number of villi is not increased. The individual epithelial cell does not have a greater life span, and the cell does not increase its synthesis of digestive enzymes or its absorptive capacity. (See Schwartz 7th ed.)

21. A 55-year-old nonsmoking, postmenopausal woman has had intermittent flushing of her face, upper body, and hands for the last 8 months. Approximately 3 months ago she began to develop cramping abdominal pain followed by the sudden onset of watery, nonbloody diarrhea stools. Physical examination now reveals the following vital signs: temperature, normal; pulse, 110 beats per minute; blood pressure, 130/80 mm Hg; and respiratory rate, 18 breaths per minute. Telangiectasis is noted on the cheeks, nose, and forehead. Rectal examination yields guaiac-positive stool. Extremities show mild peripheral edema. Which of the following tests would be most helpful in reaching a diagnosis in this case?
    A. Endoscopy
    B. Tagged red cell nuclear medicine study
    C. Quantitative determination of urinary vanillylmandelic acid excretion
    D. Quantitative determination of urinary 5-hydroxyindoleacetic acid excretion

**Answer: D**
Patients who have the malignant carcinoid syndrome present with symptoms related at least in part to excessive circulating levels of serotonin. Episodic attacks of cutaneous flushing, hyperperistalsis, and diarrhea are usual manifestations, and mild tachycardia and occasionally symptoms of asthma also can accompany this condition. Permanent changes associated with carcinoid syndrome include peripheral edema, valvular heart lesions, and cutaneous manifestations of pellagra. The most useful test in diagnosing carcinoid syndrome is the urinary concentration of 5-hydroxyindoleacetic acid (5-HIAA), the breakdown product of serotonin. (See Schwartz 7th ed.)

22. In response to antigen stimulation the secretory immune system in the gut is a major source of
    A. Immunoglobulin A (IgA)
    B. Immunoglobulin G (IgG)
    C. Interleukin-4
    D. Interleukin-5

**Answer: A**
The gut serves a major immune function in dealing with the bacteria, viruses, and enterotoxins present in the bowel lumen. Antigens entering the gut wall stimulate the production of IgA by plasma cells within the lamina propria. IgG is the antibody that mediates general humoral immunity. T cells secrete the various interleukins that induce the differentiation and proliferation of B cells. The B cells mature into plasma cells that produce the necessary IgA. (See Schwartz 7th ed.)

23. A 25-year-old man presents to the emergency room having swallowed two open safety pins 6 h ago. X-rays show the pins to be located in the small intestine. The most appropriate management at this point would be
    A. Administration of a broad-spectrum antibiotic intravenously
    B. Administration of 250 mL of magnesium citrate to induce catharsis and increase the rapidity of passage
    C. Follow-up with serial X-rays and abdominal examinations
    D. Immediate surgery

**Answer: C**
Most swallowed foreign bodies pass through the alimentary tract without causing intestinal perforation. However, persons who have swallowed objects capable of piercing the intestinal wall should be carefully observed by way of repeated abdominal examinations and plain X-rays of the abdomen. Catharsis is contraindicated in the treatment of affected patients. There is no indication for antibiotic therapy unless bowel perforation occurs. (See Schwartz 7th ed.)

24. All of the following conditions are associated with resection of the terminal ileum EXCEPT
    A. Megaloblastic anemia
    B. Choleretic diarrhea
    C. Low levels of serum iron
    D. Vitamin $B_{12}$ deficiency

**Answer: C**
Resection of the terminal ileum can have several complications. The terminal ileum is the sole site of absorption of vitamin $B_{12}$ and a primary site of absorption for bile salts. Therefore, 3 to 6 months after resection of the terminal ileum, megaloblastic anemia is likely to develop as a result of low serum levels of vitamin $B_{12}$; parenteral supplementation of this vitamin after resection is thus essential. The loss of absorptive capability for bile salts can result in a relative bile-salt deficiency, as the salts fail to recirculate but are infused instead into the colon. Unabsorbed fatty acids and soaps then irritate the colonic mucosa and, together with the increased amount of bile salts in the colon that interferes with water and electrolyte absorption, produce choleretic diarrhea. The terminal ileum is not the site of absorption for iron. (See Schwartz 7th ed.)

# CHAPTER 28

# Colon, Rectum, and Anus

1. Diversion colitis after ileostomy is caused by
   A. Change in bacterial flora
   B. Change in the sodium transported across the colonic mucosa
   C. Insufficient short chain fatty acids to fuel the colonic mucosa
   D. Insufficient long chain fatty acids to fuel the colonic mucosa

**Answer: C**

Short-chain fatty acids (acetate, butyrate, and propionate) are produced by bacterial fermentation of dietary carbohydrates. Short-chain fatty acids are an important source of energy for the colonic mucosa, and metabolism by colonocytes provides energy for processes such as active transport of sodium. Lack of a dietary source for production of short-chain fatty acids, or diversion of the fecal stream by an ileostomy or colostomy, may result in mucosal atrophy and "diversion colitis." (See Schwartz 8th ed., p 1061.)

2. Which of the following extraintestinal manifestations of ulcerative colitis improves with colectomy?
   A. Sclerosing cholangitis
   B. Arthritis
   C. Erythema nodosum
   D. Uveitis

**Answer: B**

Arthritis is also a common extracolonic manifestation of inflammatory bowel disease, and the incidence is 20 times greater than in the general population. Arthritis usually improves with treatment of the colonic disease. Sacroiliitis and ankylosing spondylitis are associated with inflammatory bowel disease, although the relationship is poorly understood. Medical and surgical treatment of the colonic disease does not impact symptoms. (See Schwartz 8th ed., p 1077.)

3. Which of the following is a first-line agent in the treatment of mild to moderate colitis from inflammatory bowel disease?
   A. Salicylates
   B. Steroids
   C. 6-Mercaptopurine
   D. Methotrexate

**Answer: A**

Sulfasalazine (Azulfidine), 5-aminosalicylic acid (5-ASA), and related compounds are first-line agents in the medical treatment of mild to moderate inflammatory bowel disease. These compounds decrease inflammation by inhibition of cyclooxygenase and 5-lipooxygenase in the gut mucosa. They require direct contact with affected mucosa for efficacy. Multiple preparations are available for administration to different sites in the small intestine and colon (sulfasalazine, mesalamine [Pentasa], Asacol, Rowasa). (See Schwartz 8th ed., p 1078.)

4. Infliximab (Remicade)
   A. Is a monoclonal antibody against interleukin-6 (IL-6)
   B. Is effective in approximately 50% of patients with moderate to severe Crohn's disease
   C. Is never effective in perianal Crohn's disease
   D. Is given orally

**Answer: B**

Infliximab (Remicade) is a monoclonal antibody against tumor necrosis factor alpha (TNF-α). Intravenous infusion of this agent decreases inflammation systemically. More than 50% of patients with moderate to severe Crohn's disease will improve with infliximab therapy. This agent also has been useful in treating patients with perianal Crohn's disease. Recurrence is common, however, and many patients require infusions on a bimonthly basis. Infliximab has not been used as extensively for treatment of ulcerative colitis; however, there are reports of efficacy in this setting. (See Schwartz 8th ed., p 1078.)

5. The risk of developing adenocarcinoma after 10 years of ulcerative colitis is
   A. <10%
   B. 10–20%
   C. 20–30%
   D. >50%

**Answer: A**

Indications for elective surgery in ulcerative colitis include intractability despite maximal medical therapy and high-risk development of major complications of medical therapy such as aseptic necrosis of joints secondary to chronic steroid use. Elective surgery is also indicated in patients at significant risk of developing colorectal carcinoma. Risk of malignancy increases with pancolonic disease and the duration of symptoms is approximately 2% after 10 years, 8% after 20 years, and 18% after 30 years. (See Schwartz 8th ed., p 1097.)

6. Which of the following is associated with increased risk of colorectal cancer?
   A. Inactivation of the adenomatous polyposis coli gene
   B. Inactivation of the K-ras gene
   C. Activation of the DCC (deleted in colorectal cancer) gene
   D. Activation of the *p*53 gene

**Answer: A**

Approximately 80% of colorectal cancers occur sporadically, while 20% arise in patients with a known family history of colorectal cancer. Advances in the understanding of these familial disorders have led to interest in early diagnosis using genetic testing. Assays currently exist to detect the most common defects in the adenomatous polyposis coli (APC) gene and in mismatch repair genes. Because of the medical, legal, and ethical considerations that are involved in this type of testing, all patients should be offered genetic counseling if a familial syndrome is suspected. (See Schwartz 8th ed., p 1084.)

7. The initial diagnostic examination in a 50-year-old patient who is febrile and tender in the left lower quadrant of the abdomen should be
   A. Flexible sigmoidoscopy
   B. Water soluble contrast enema
   C. Ultrasound
   D. Computed tomography scan

**Answer: D**

Diverticulitis refers to inflammation and infection associated with a diverticulum and is estimated to occur in 10 to 25% of people with diverticulosis. Peridiverticular and pericolic infection results from a perforation (either macroscopic or microscopic) of a diverticulum, which leads to contamination, inflammation, and infection. The spectrum of disease ranges from mild, uncomplicated diverticulitis that can be treated in the outpatient setting, to free perforation and diffuse peritonitis that requires emergency laparotomy. Most patients present with left-sided abdominal pain, with or without fever, and leukocytosis. A mass may be present. Plain radiographs are useful for detecting free intra-abdominal air. Computed tomography (CT) scan is extremely useful for defining pericolic inflammation, phlegmon, or abscess. Contrast enemas and/or endoscopy are relatively contraindicated because of the risk of perforation. The differential diagnosis includes malignancy, ischemic colitis, infectious colitis, and inflammatory bowel disease. (See Schwartz 8th ed., p 1082.)

8. What percentage of patients with diverticulitis have a second (recurrent) episode?
   A. <20%
   B. 20–30%
   C. 30–40%
   D. >50%

**Answer: C**

Most patients with uncomplicated diverticulitis will recover without surgery and 50 to 70% will have no further episodes. However, the risk of complications increases with recurrent disease. For this reason, elective sigmoid colectomy is often recommended after the second episode of diverticulitis, especially if the patient has required hospitalization. Resection may be indicated after the first episode in very young patients and in immunosuppressed patients, and is often recommended after the first episode of complicated diverticulitis. Medical comorbidity should be considered when evaluating a patient for elective resection, and the risks of recurrent disease weighed against the risks of the operation. Because colon carcinoma may have an identical clinical presentation to diverticulitis (either complicated or uncomplicated), all patients must be evaluated for malignancy after resolution of the acute episode. Sigmoidoscopy or colonoscopy is recommended 4 to 6 weeks after recovery. Inability to exclude malignancy is another indication for resection. (See Schwartz 8th ed., p 1083.)

9. Which of the following is most likely to harbor a colorectal cancer?
   A. Hamartomatous polyp
   B. Tubular adenomatous polyp
   C. Tubulovillous adenomatous polyp
   D. Villous adenomatous polyp

**Answer: D**
Adenomatous polyps are common, occurring in up to 25% of the population older than 50 years of age in the United States. By definition, these lesions are dysplastic. The risk of malignant degeneration is related to both the size and type of polyp. Tubular adenomas are associated with malignancy in only 5% of cases, whereas villous adenomas may harbor cancer in up to 40%. Tubulovillous adenomas are at intermediate risk (22%). Invasive carcinomas are rare in polyps smaller than 1 cm; the incidence increases with size. The risk of carcinoma in a polyp larger than 2 cm is 35 to 50%. Although most neoplastic polyps do not evolve to cancer, most colorectal cancers originate as a polyp. It is this fact that forms the basis for secondary prevention strategies to eliminate colorectal cancer by targeting the neoplastic polyp for removal before malignancy develops. (See Schwartz 8th ed., p 1086.)

10. The treatment of a patient who has undergone appropriate surgery to resect a colon cancer which is T3, N0, M0 is
    A. Chemotherapy and radiation for all patients
    B. Chemotherapy alone for all patients
    C. Chemotherapy alone for patients with high-risk histology
    D. Surgery alone

**Answer: C**
Stages I and II: Localized Colon Carcinoma (T1-3, N0, M0). The majority of patients with stages I and II colon cancer will be cured with surgical resection. Few patients with completely resected stage I disease will develop either local or distant recurrence, and adjuvant chemotherapy does not improve survival in these patients. However, up to 46% of patients with completely resected stage II disease will ultimately die from colon cancer. For this reason, adjuvant chemotherapy has been suggested for selected patients with stage II disease (young patients, tumors with "high-risk" histologic findings). Data is controversial as to whether chemotherapy improves survival rates in these patients. Improved staging to detect micrometastases and/or more sensitive prognostic tumor markers may improve patient selection for adjuvant therapy. (See Schwartz 8th ed., p 1092.)

11. The treatment of cecal volvulus is
    A. Observation alone
    B. Colonoscopic detorsion, bowel prep, and elective resection
    C. Operative detorsion and cecopexy
    D. Operative detorsion, right hemicolectomy with ileocolostomy

**Answer: D**
Cecal volvulus results from nonfixation of the right colon. Rotation occurs around the ileocolic blood vessels and vascular impairment occurs early. Plain X-rays of the abdomen show a characteristic kidney-shaped, air-filled structure in the left upper quadrant (opposite the site of obstruction), and a Gastrografin enema confirms obstruction at the level of the volvulus. Unlike sigmoid volvulus, cecal volvulus can almost never be detorsed endoscopically. Moreover, because vascular compromise occurs early in the course of cecal volvulus,

surgical exploration is necessary when the diagnosis is made. Right hemicolectomy with a primary ileocolic anastomosis can usually be performed safely and prevents recurrence. Simple detorsion or detorsion and cecopexy are associated with a high rate of recurrence. (See Schwartz 8th ed., p 1099.)

12. The most common cause of emergency laparotomy in patients with acquired immunodeficiency syndrome is
    A. Cytomegalovirus (CMV) enterocolitis
    B. *Clostridium difficile* enterocolitis
    C. Gastrointestinal (GI) perforation from Kaposi's sarcoma
    D. GI perforation from lymphoma

**Answer: A**
Patients infected with human immunodeficiency virus (HIV) may present with a myriad of gastrointestinal symptoms. Diarrhea, in particular, is extremely common. The severity of gastrointestinal disease depends in part upon the degree of immunosuppression; however, both ordinary and opportunistic pathogens may affect patients at any stage of the disease. Opportunistic infections with bacteria (*Salmonella*, *Shigella*, *Campylobacter*, *Chlamydia*, and *Mycobacterium* species), fungi (*Histoplasmosis*, *Coccidiosis*, *Cryptococcus*), protozoa (*Toxoplasmosis*, *Cryptosporidiosis*, *Isosporiasis*), and viruses (Cytomegalovirus, herpes simplex virus) can cause diarrhea, abdominal pain, and weight loss. CMV in particular may cause severe enterocolitis and is the most common infectious cause of emergency laparotomy in acquired immunodeficiency syndrome (AIDS) patients. (See Schwartz 8th ed., p 1114.)

13. The origin of the parasympathetic innervation of the left colon is
    A. T6-T12
    B. L1-L3
    C. Vagus nerve
    D. S2-S4

**Answer: D**
The colon is innervated by both sympathetic (inhibitory) and parasympathetic (stimulatory) nerves, which parallel the course of the arteries. Sympathetic nerves arise from T6-T12 and L1-L3. The parasympathetic innervation to the right and transverse colon is from the vagus nerve; the parasympathetic nerves to the left colon arise from sacral nerves S2-S4 to form the nervi erigentes. (See Schwartz 8th ed., p 1057.)

14. Which of the following statements concerning hepatobiliary manifestations of ulcerative colitis (UC) is true?
    A. 70–80% of patients with UC have fatty infiltration of the liver.
    B. Liver failure is the leading cause of death in patients with UC.
    C. Bile duct carcinoma is a rare but possible complication of UC.
    D. Common bile duct occlusion from stones is the most common hepatobiliary complication of UC.

**Answer: C**
The liver is a common site of extracolonic disease in inflammatory bowel disease. Fatty infiltration of the liver is present in 40 to 50% of patients and cirrhosis is found in 2 to 5%. Fatty infiltration may be reversed by medical or surgical treatment of colonic disease, but cirrhosis is irreversible. Primary sclerosing cholangitis is a progressive disease characterized by intra- and extrahepatic bile duct strictures. Forty to 60% of patients with primary sclerosing cholangitis have ulcerative colitis. Colectomy will not reverse this disease and the only effective therapy is liver transplantation. Pericholangitis is also associated with inflammatory bowel disease and may be diagnosed with a liver biopsy. Bile duct carcinoma is a rare complication of long-standing inflammatory bowel disease. Patients who develop bile duct carcinoma in the presence of inflammatory bowel disease are, on average, 20 years younger than other patients with bile duct carcinoma. (See Schwartz 8th ed., p 1077.)

15. Which of the following increases the risk of developing a colon cancer?
    A. A diet high in saturated fat
    B. A diet high in oleic acid
    C. A diet high in selenium
    D. A diet high in calcium

**Answer: A**
The observation that colorectal carcinoma occurs more commonly in populations that consume diets high in animal fat and low in fiber has lead to the hypothesis that dietary factors contribute to carcinogenesis. A diet high in saturated or polyunsaturated fats increases risk of colorectal cancer, while a diet high in oleic acid (olive oil, coconut oil, fish oil) does not increase risk. (See Schwartz 8th ed., p 1084.)

16. The adenomatous polyposis coli (APC) gene
    A. Is an oncogene
    B. Leads to development of polyps with mutation in a single allele
    C. Can be used (by determining the specific mutation) to predict clinical severity of disease in patients with familial polyposis
    D. Was discovered in patients with familial juvenile polyposis

**Answer: C**
The APC gene is a *tumor-suppressor gene*. Mutations in both alleles are necessary to initiate polyp formation. The majority of mutations are premature stop codons, which result in a truncated APC protein. In familial adenomatous polyposis (FAP), the site of mutation correlates with the clinical severity of the disease. For example, mutations in either the 3 or 5 end of the gene result in attenuated forms of FAP, while mutations in the center of the gene result in more virulent disease. Thus, knowledge of the specific mutation in a family may help guide clinical decision making. (See Schwartz 8th ed., p 1085.)

17. Which of the following is associated with Cronkite-Canada syndrome?
    A. Alopecia and atrophy of the fingernails and toenails
    B. Melanin spots on the mucosa of the lips
    C. Adenomatous polyps, particularly in the small bowel
    D. Breast cancer

**Answer: A**
Cronkite-Canada syndrome is a disorder in which patients develop gastrointestinal polyposis in association with alopecia, cutaneous pigmentation, and atrophy of the fingernails and toenails. Diarrhea is a prominent symptom, and vomiting, malabsorption, and protein-losing enteropathy may occur. Most patients die of this disease despite maximal medical therapy, and surgery is reserved for complications of polyposis such as obstruction. (See Schwartz 8th ed., p 1086.)

18. Contraindications to primary repair of traumatic left colon injuries include
    A. Injury to one other organ
    B. Mesenteric vascular injury
    C. Any fecal soilage with formed stool
    D. 4-h delay between injury and laparotomy

**Answer: B**
Management of colonic injury depends upon the mechanism of injury, the delay between the injury and surgery, the overall condition and stability of the patient, the degree of peritoneal contamination, and the condition of the injured colon. A primary repair may be considered in hemodynamically stable patients with few additional injuries and minimal contamination if the colon appears otherwise healthy. Contraindications to primary repair include shock, injury to more than two other organs, mesenteric vascular damage, and extensive fecal contamination. A delay of greater than 6 hours between the injury and the operation is also associated with increased morbidity and mortality and is a relative contraindication to primary repair. Injuries caused by high-velocity gunshot wounds or blast injuries are often associated with multiple intra-abdominal injuries and tissue loss and therefore are usually treated by fecal diversion after débridement of all nonviable tissue. Patient factors, such as medical comorbidities, advanced age, and the presence of tumor or radiation injury, must also be considered (Table 28-5). (See Schwartz 8th ed., p 1112.)

19. Right-sided colonic diverticula
    A. Occur in elderly patients
    B. Are more common in patients of Asian ancestry
    C. Can usually be treated by simple diverticulectomy
    D. Most commonly present with lower gastrointestinal bleeding

**Answer: B**

The cecum and ascending colon infrequently are involved in diverticulosis coli. Even more uncommon is a true solitary diverticulum, which contains all layers of the bowel wall and is thought to be congenital in origin. Right-sided diverticula occur more often in younger patients than do left-sided diverticula, and are more common in people of Asian descent than in other populations. Most patients with right-sided diverticula are asymptomatic. However, diverticulitis does occur occasionally. Because patients are young and present with right lower quadrant pain, they are often thought to suffer from acute appendicitis, and the diagnosis of right-sided diverticulitis is subsequently made in the operating room. If there is a single large diverticulum and minimal inflammation, a diverticulectomy may be performed, but an ileocecal resection is usually the preferred operation in this setting. Hemorrhage rarely occurs and should be treated in the same fashion as hemorrhage from a left-sided diverticulum. (See Schwartz 8th ed., p 1084.)

20. The marginal artery of Drummond is present and complete in what percentage of people?
    A. 3–5%
    B. 15–20%
    C. 50–65%
    D. 85–95%

**Answer: B**

The arterial supply to the colon is highly variable (Fig. 28-1). In general, the superior mesenteric artery branches into the ileocolic artery (absent in up to 20% of people), which supplies blood flow to the terminal ileum and proximal ascending colon, the right colic artery, which supplies the ascending colon, and the middle colic artery, which supplies the transverse colon. The inferior mesenteric artery branches into the left colic artery, which supplies the descending colon, several sigmoidal branches, which supply the sigmoid colon, and the superior rectal artery, which supplies the proximal rectum. The terminal branches of each artery form anastomoses with the terminal branches of the adjacent artery and communicate via the marginal artery of Drummond. This arcade is complete in only 15 to 20% of people. (See Schwartz 8th ed., p 1057.)

21. Anatomic characteristics of the anoderm include
    A. Hair follicles
    B. Sebaceous glands
    C. Sensory nerves
    D. Sweat glands

**Answer: C**

The anal canal below the dentate line is covered with a squamous epithelium that contains numerous sensory nerve fibers, but is devoid of the secondary skin appendages. Above the dentate line there is a transitional zone with first, cuboidal and then, columnar epithelium. (See Schwartz 7th ed.)

22. Anal incontinence will result from division of
    A. The first sacral nerve roots bilaterally
    B. The second sacral nerve roots bilaterally
    C. The third sacral nerve roots bilaterally
    D. The fourth sacral nerve roots bilaterally

**Answer: C**

Division of both third sacral nerve roots leads to incontinence. (See Schwartz 7th ed.)

23. Which of the following is absorbed from the colon?
    A. Dextrose
    B. Fatty acid
    C. Fiber
    D. Lactulose

**Answer: B**

Active absorption of nutrients from the colon is minimal. However, short-chain fatty acids produced by intraluminal bacterial fermentation of unabsorbed carbohydrates can be possibly absorbed. This absorption can account for up to 540 kcal/day. (See Schwartz 7th ed.)

24. The most common bacterial organism present in the colon is
    A. *Bacteroides*
    B. *Clostridium difficile*
    C. *Escherichia coli*
    D. *Salmonella*

**Answer: A**

The human colon is sterile at birth but the intestine is colonized within hours after birth. *Bacteroides* is the dominant bacterial organism in the colon. (See Schwartz 7th ed.)

25. Colorectal pseudo-obstruction has been associated with all of the following EXCEPT
    A. Excess parasympathetic tone
    B. Malignant infiltration of the celiac plexus
    C. Neuroleptic medications
    D. Opiate usage

**Answer: A**

Ogilvie first described a profound colonic ileus in the absence of bowel pathology. His patients suffered from malignant infiltration of the celiac plexus. Neuroleptic medications, opiate usage, and severe metabolic disease have produced a similar clinical picture. Although the exact cause for colonic ileus has not been defined, excess sympathetic tone has been advanced as a probable mechanism. (See Schwartz 7th ed.)

26. The most common site of volvulus is
    A. Cecum
    B. Proximal jejunum
    C. Sigmoid colon
    D. Stomach

**Answer: C**

Although volvulus can occur at any point in the gastrointestinal tract, sigmoid volvulus accounts for about 90% of the volvulus concentrated in the United States. It is most commonly encountered in older or institutionalized patients. (See Schwartz 7th ed.)

27. An 80-year-old woman is seen with abdominal pain and obstipation. On examination, she is afebrile with slight tachycardia. Her abdomen is distended and tympanitic, but there are no peritoneal signs. Abdominal X-rays suggest the presence of sigmoid volvulus. The first step in her management should be
    A. Administration of laxatives and cleansing enemas
    B. Barium enema
    C. Rigid sigmoidoscopy
    D. Sigmoid resection

**Answer: C**

Advancing a sigmoidoscope past the point of obstruction allows immediate decompression of the dilated and gas-filled bowel segment. The disease process is likely to recur, and elective sigmoid resection should be done once her condition is stabilized. Laxatives, cleansing enemas, and barium enema are dangerous and should not be done. Transverse colostomy is not effective since it does not relieve the marked sigmoid distention. (See Schwartz 7th ed.)

28. Normally the colon secretes
    A. Ammonia
    B. Chloride
    C. Sodium
    D. Potassium

**Answer: D**

The colonic mucosa absorbs sodium, chloride, and water. Sodium is absorbed against a concentration and electrical gradient using energy provided by the metabolism of short-chain fatty acids. As sodium is absorbed, potassium diffuses into the colonic lumen. Ammonia that results from degradation of protein and urea by colonic bacteria diffuses across the colonic mucosa and is carried to the liver via the portal vein. Ammonium ions are metabolized by the normal liver, but the diseased liver may be unable to carry this out effectively, and ammonia intoxication results. (See Schwartz 7th ed.)

29. A 24-year-old woman who has ulcerative colitis is admitted to the hospital because of fever, bloody diarrhea, and abdominal tenderness. Medical treatment, including the use of parenteral steroids, is started. During the next several days, the woman becomes increasingly ill; an abdominal X-ray now shows a transverse-colon diameter of 12 cm but no free intraperitoneal air. The treatment of choice would be
    A. Cecostomy
    B. Transverse colostomy
    C. Transverse colectomy
    D. Total proctocolectomy

**Answer: D**
Toxic megacolon is a complication of fulminant ulcerative colitis and affects 2 to 5% of persons with the disorder. Although toxic megacolon can be a reversible process, operative intervention is indicated if clinical deterioration and marked colon dilation have not been controlled by a trial of medical therapy, including administration of steroids. The operation of choice, in the absence of perforation, is total proctocolectomy and ileostomy. (See Schwartz 7th ed.)

1. Which of the following are usual locations for the tip of the appendix?
   A. Retrocecal, pelvic, subcecal
   B. Preileal, right pericolic, subovarian
   C. Retrocecal, subcecal, supracecal
   D. Right pericolic, subovarian, pelvic

**Answer: A**
The relationship of the base of the appendix to the cecum remains constant, whereas the tip can be found in a retrocecal, pelvic, subcecal, preileal, or right pericolic position (Fig. 29-1). (See Schwartz 8th ed., p 1119.)

2. Which of the following best describes the immunologic function of the appendix?
   A. Essential function of the gut-associated lymphoid tissue system
   B. Not associated with the gut-associated lymphoid tissue system
   C. Secretes immunoglobulin G immunoglobins
   D. Secretes immunoglobulin A immunoglobins

**Answer: D**
For many years, the appendix was erroneously viewed as a vestigial organ with no known function. It is now well recognized that the appendix is an immunologic organ that actively participates in the secretion of immunoglobulins, particularly immunoglobulin A (IgA). Although the appendix is an integral component of the gut-associated lymphoid tissue (GALT) system, its function is not essential and appendectomy is not associated with any predisposition to sepsis or any other manifestation of immune compromise. Lymphoid tissue first appears in the appendix approximately 2 weeks after birth. The amount of lymphoid tissue increases throughout puberty, remains steady for the next decade, and then begins a steady decrease with age. After the age of 60 years, virtually no lymphoid tissue remains within the appendix, and complete obliteration of the appendiceal lumen is common. (See Schwartz 8th ed., p 1119.)

3. The rate of negative appendectomy is highest in which of the following groups?
   A. Younger females
   B. Younger males
   C. Older females
   D. Older males

**Answer: C**
Despite an increased use of ultrasonography, computed tomography (CT) scanning, and laparoscopy between 1987 and 1997, the rate of misdiagnosis of appendicitis has remained constant (15.3%), as has the rate of appendiceal rupture. The percentage of misdiagnosis of appendicitis is significantly higher among women than men (22.2 vs. 9.3%). The negative appendectomy rate for women of reproductive age is 23.2%, with the highest rates identified in women age 40 to 49 years. The highest negative appendectomy rate is reported for women older than 80 years of age. (See Schwartz 8th ed., p 1120.)

4. The optimal duration for postoperative antibiotics after appendectomy is
   A. 1–2 days for perforated appendicitis
   B. 7–10 days for nonperforated appendicitis
   C. 7–10 days for perforated appendicitis
   D. Intravenous antibiotics until the patient is afebrile and has a normal white blood cell count

**Answer: D**
Antibiotic coverage is limited to 24 to 48 hours in cases of nonperforated appendicitis. For perforated appendicitis, 7 to 10 days is recommended. Intravenous antibiotics are usually given until the white blood cell count is normal and the patient is afebrile for 24 hours. (See Schwartz 8th ed., p 1121.)

5. Which of the following is most commonly confused with appendicitis in children?
   A. Meckel's diverticulitis
   B. Mesenteric adenitis
   C. Pelvic inflammatory disease
   D. Acute gastroenteritis

**Answer: B**
Acute mesenteric adenitis is the disease most often confused with acute appendicitis in children. Almost invariably, an upper respiratory infection is present or has recently subsided. The pain is usually diffuse, and tenderness is not as sharply localized as in appendicitis. Voluntary guarding is sometimes present, but true rigidity is rare. Generalized lymphadenopathy may be noted. Laboratory procedures are of little help in arriving at the correct diagnosis, although a relative lymphocytosis, when present, suggests mesenteric adenitis. Observation for several hours is in order if the diagnosis of mesenteric adenitis seems likely, because mesenteric adenitis is a self-limited disease. However, if the differentiation remains in doubt, immediate exploration is the safest course of action. (See Schwartz 8th ed., p 1127.)

6. Which of the following statements concerning appendicitis during pregnancy is true?
   A. Surgery should be performed with an open technique.
   B. The risk of premature labor is the same as with any abdominal procedure.
   C. Surgery should be performed only if the diagnosis is sure.
   D. Appendicitis is most common in the third trimester.

**Answer: B**
Appendicitis is the most frequently encountered extrauterine disease requiring surgical treatment during pregnancy. The incidence is approximately 1 in 2000 pregnancies. Acute appendicitis can occur at any time during pregnancy, but is more frequent during the first two trimesters. As fetal gestation progresses, the diagnosis of appendicitis becomes more difficult as the appendix is displaced laterally and superiorly. Nausea and vomiting after the first trimester or new-onset nausea and vomiting should raise the consideration of appendicitis. Abdominal pain and tenderness will be present, although rebound and guarding are less frequent because of laxity of the abdominal wall. Elevation of the white blood cell count above the normal pregnancy levels of 15,000 to 20,000/$\mu$L, with a predominance of polymorphonuclear cells, is usually present. When the diagnosis is in doubt, abdominal ultrasound may be beneficial. Laparoscopy may be indicated in equivocal cases, especially early in pregnancy. The performance of any operation during pregnancy carries a risk of premature labor of 10 to 15%, and the risk is similar for both negative laparotomy and appendectomy for simple appendicitis. The most significant factor associated with both fetal and maternal death is appendiceal perforation. Fetal mortality increases from 3 to 5% in early appendicitis to 20% with perforation. The suspicion of appendicitis during pregnancy should prompt rapid diagnosis and surgical intervention. (See Schwartz 8th ed., p 1129.)

7. Open appendectomy differs from laparoscopic appendectomy in that
   A. The laparoscopic approach decreases hospital stay.
   B. The laparoscopic approach decreases pain.
   C. The open approach decreases wound infection rate.
   D. The open approach is most appropriate for obese patients.

**Answer: B**
A principal proposed benefit of laparoscopic appendectomy has been decreased postoperative pain. Patient-reported pain on the first postoperative day is significantly less after laparoscopic appendectomy. However, the difference has been calculated to be only 8 on a 100-point visual analogue scale. This difference is under the level of pain that an average patient is able to perceive. Hospital length of stay also is statistically significantly less after laparoscopic appendectomy. However, in most studies this difference is less than 1 day. It appears that the more important determinant of length of

stay after appendectomy is the pathology at operation, specifically whether a patient has perforated or nonperforated appendicitis. In nearly all studies, laparoscopic appendectomy is associated with a shorter period prior to return to normal activity, return to work, and return to sports. However, treatment and subject bias may have a significant impact on the data. Although the majority of studies have been performed in adults, similar data has been obtained in children. (See Schwartz 8th ed., p 1131.)

8. Which of the following statements concerning appendiceal adenocarcinoma is true?
   A. These tumors are most commonly found incidentally.
   B. Treatment is by appendectomy with adjuvant chemotherapy.
   C. Perforation does not change prognosis.
   D. Synchronous tumors are rare.

**Answer: C**
Primary adenocarcinoma of the appendix is a rare neoplasm of three major histologic subtypes: mucinous adenocarcinoma, colonic adenocarcinoma, and adenocarcinoid. The most common mode of presentation for appendiceal carcinoma is that of acute appendicitis. Patients may also present with ascites or a palpable mass, or the neoplasm may be discovered during an operative procedure for an unrelated cause. The recommended treatment for all patients with adenocarcinoma of the appendix is a formal right hemicolectomy. Appendiceal adenocarcinomas have a propensity for early perforation, although they are not clearly associated with a worsened prognosis. Overall 5-year survival is 55% and varies with stage and grade. Patients with appendiceal adenocarcinoma are at significant risk for both synchronous and metachronous neoplasms, approximately half of which will originate from the gastrointestinal tract. (See Schwartz 8th ed., p 1134.)

9. Which of the following is appropriate surgical treatment for an appendiceal carcinoid without mesenteric extension?
   A. Right hemicolectomy for a tumor 0.8 cm in diameter
   B. Right hemicolectomy for a tumor 1.6 cm in diameter
   C. Extended right hemicolectomy for a tumor 2.5 cm in diameter
   D. Appendectomy for a tumor 1.1 cm in diameter

**Answer: B**
The majority of carcinoids are located in the tip of the appendix. Malignant potential is related to size, with tumors less than 1 cm rarely resulting in extension outside of the appendix or adjacent to the mass. In one report, 78% of appendiceal carcinoids were less than 1 cm, 17% were 1 to 2 cm, and only 5% were greater than 2 cm. Treatment rarely requires more than simple appendectomy. For tumors smaller than 1 cm with extension into the mesoappendix, and for all tumors larger than 1.5 cm, a right hemicolectomy should be performed. (See Schwartz 8th ed., p 1134.)

10. The treatment of choice for pseudomyxoma peritonei is
    A. Observation
    B. Chemotherapy
    C. Chemotherapy and radiation therapy
    D. Surgical debulking

**Answer: D**
Thorough surgical debulking is the mainstay of treatment. All gross disease should be removed. Appendectomy is routinely performed. Hysterectomy with bilateral salpingo-oophorectomy is performed in women. Ultra-radical surgery has not been shown to be of significant benefit. Additionally, adjuvant intraperitoneal chemotherapy (with or without hyperthermia) or systemic postoperative chemotherapy have not been shown to be of benefit. Pseudomyxoma is a disease that progresses slowly and in which recurrences may take years to develop or become symptomatic. In a series from the Mayo Clinic, 76% of patients developed recurrences within the abdomen. Lymph node metastasis and distant

metastasis are uncommon. Any recurrence should be investigated completely. Recurrences are usually treated by additional surgery. It is important to note that surgery for recurrent disease is usually difficult and associated with an increased incidence of unintentional enterotomies, anastomotic leaks, and fistulas. With adequate primary surgery and debulking of recurrences, the median survival of pseudomyxoma is 5.9 years, with 53% of patients surviving 5 years. (See Schwartz 8th ed., p 1135.)

11.  In which decade of life would a patient be most likely to get appendicitis?
    A.  First
    B.  Second
    C.  Sixth
    D.  Seventh

**Answer: B**
The lifetime rate of appendectomy is 12% for men and 25% for women, with approximately 7% of all people undergoing appendectomy for acute appendicitis. Over a 10-year period from 1987 to 1997, the overall appendectomy rate decreased parallel to a decrease in incidental appendectomy. However, the rate of appendectomy for appendicitis has remained constant at 10 per 10,000 patients per year. Appendicitis is most frequently seen in patients in their second through fourth decades of life, with a mean age of 31.3 years and a median age of 22 years. There is a slight male to female predominance (M:F 1.2 to 1.3:1). (See Schwartz 8th ed., p 1120.)

12.  At operation for presumed appendicitis, a 26-year-old patient was found to have a firm, yellow, bulbar mass at the tip of the appendix. You estimate its size to be 0.5 cm. You should
    A.  Perform a right hemicolectomy
    B.  Perform an appendectomy
    C.  Leave the appendix in place and look for a Meckel's diverticulum
    D.  Inspect the entire bowel for a synchronous lesion

**Answer: B**
The finding of a firm, yellow, bulbar mass in the appendix should raise the suspicion of an appendiceal carcinoid. The appendix is the most common site of gastrointestinal carcinoid, followed by the small bowel and then rectum. Carcinoid syndrome is rarely associated with appendiceal carcinoid unless widespread metastases are present, which occur in 2.9% of cases. Symptoms attributable directly to the carcinoid are rare, although the tumor can occasionally obstruct the appendiceal lumen much like a fecalith and result in acute appendicitis. The majority of carcinoids are located in the tip of the appendix. Malignant potential is related to size, with tumors less than 1 cm rarely resulting in extension outside of the appendix or adjacent to the mass. In one report, 78% of appendiceal carcinoids were less than 1 cm, 17% were 1 to 2 cm, and only 5% were greater than 2 cm. Treatment rarely requires more than simple appendectomy. For tumors smaller than 1 cm with extension into the mesoappendix, and for all tumors larger than 1.5 cm, a right hemicolectomy should be performed. (See Schwartz 8th ed., p 1134.)

13.  Peritoneal fluid from a patient with a ruptured appendix is likely to grow
    A.  *Bacteroides fragilis* alone
    B.  *Bacteroides fragilis*, *Escherichia coli*, and a variety of other organisms
    C.  *Campylobacter jejuni*
    D.  *Escherichia coli* alone

**Answer: B**
Ruptured appendicitis is associated with peritonitis, and it is almost always a multiorganism infection. *Bacteroides fragilis* and *Escherichia coli* are almost always present with an average of eight additional organisms. (See Schwartz 7th ed.)

14. The predominant organism cultured from the peritoneal fluid of a patient with acute unruptured appendicitis is
    A. *Bacteroides fragilis*
    B. *Campylobacter jejuni*
    C. *Escherichia coli*
    D. No organism would be cultured

**Answer: D**
The peritoneal fluid found in association with acute unruptured appendicitis is sterile. This situation changes dramatically after perforation, emphasizing the need for prompt diagnosis and therapy. (See Schwartz 7th ed.)

15. All of the following symptoms and signs are suggestive of acute unruptured appendicitis EXCEPT
    A. Anorexia
    B. Paraumbilical shifting to the right lower quadrant
    C. Patient writhing in discomfort
    D. Vomiting

**Answer: C**
A patient with acute appendicitis remains quiet because any motion exacerbates discomfort. Writhing in search of a more comfortable position is characteristic of biliary or renal colic. The other listed signs and symptoms are typical of acute appendicitis. (See Schwartz 7th ed.)

16. One day before the midpoint of her menstrual cycle, a healthy 17-year-old girl suddenly develops pain in the right lower quadrant of her abdomen. Abdominal examination reveals tenderness in the right lower quadrant, and rectal examination also reveals right-sided tenderness. Her temperature is 37.2°C (99°F), and her leukocyte count is 10,000/mm$^3$. The most likely diagnosis is
    A. Acute appendicitis
    B. Pelvic inflammatory disease
    C. Infection of the urinary tract
    D. Ruptured graafian follicle

**Answer: D**
Although nothing in the case presented in the question is inconsistent with a diagnosis of acute appendicitis, the fact that symptoms developed during the midpoint of the girl's menstrual cycle makes mittelschmerz ("middle pain") the probable diagnosis. In this setting, to operate for appendicitis without first performing a pelvic examination or observing for a period of time would be premature. Pelvic inflammatory disease would be expected to be associated with a pelvic discharge, exquisite rectal tenderness, and a much higher temperature than is the case described. Infections of the urinary tract also tend to be associated with a high fever, as well as with suprapubic or costovertebral-angle tenderness. Epiploic appendicitis usually produces steady, progressive pain along the course of the colon. (See Schwartz 7th ed.)

1. The ligamentum teres hepaticus (round ligament of the liver) is the vestigial remains of the
   A. Umbilical artery
   B. Umbilical vein
   C. Ductus venosus
   D. Ductus arteriosus

**Answer: B**
The round ligament is the vestigial remnant of the umbilical vein, and is an external marker for the location of the intrahepatic portion of the left portal vein. (See Schwartz 8th ed., p 1140.)

2. The ligamentum teres hepaticus (round ligament of the liver) divides
   A. The right and left lobes of the liver
   B. The right medial and lateral segments of the liver
   C. The right superior and inferior segments of the liver
   D. The left medial and lateral segments of the liver

**Answer: D**
The gross anatomic landmarks of the liver include the falciform ligament and the ligamentum teres hepaticus (round ligament of the liver) separating the left lateral segment of the liver (segments II and III) from the remaining liver (Fig. 30-1). (See Schwartz 8th ed., p 1140.)

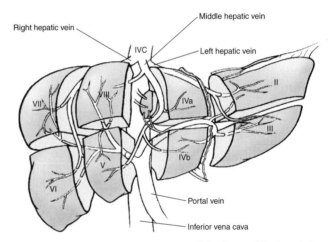

**FIG. 30-1.** Segmental anatomy of the liver with the eight segments based on portal vein blood supply and hepatic venous outflow as designated by Couinaud. Segment I is also known as the caudate lobe; segments II and III comprise the lateral segment of the left lobe; segment IV is the medial segment of the left lobe; and segments V to VIII comprise the right lobe. (Adapted from www.ahpba.org, the website of The American Hepato-Pancreato-Biliary Association.)

3. The ligamentum venosum is a marker for
   A. The main portal vein
   B. The bifurcation of the portal vein
   C. The right portal vein
   D. The left portal vein

**Answer: D**
The ligamentum venosum is the vestigial remnant of the ductus venosus. It runs from the intrahepatic portal vein to the vena cava. It marks the border between the caudate lobe (segment I) and the left lateral sector. (See Schwartz 8th ed., p 1140.)

4. What percentage of blood flow to the liver is provided by the portal vein?
   A. 30%
   B. 50%
   C. 75%
   D. 90%

**Answer: C**

The portal vein is a valveless structure that is formed by the confluence of the superior mesenteric vein and the splenic vein. The portal vein provides approximately 75% of the total liver blood supply by volume. In the hepatoduodenal ligament, the portal vein is found most commonly posterior to the bile duct and hepatic artery. The normal pressure in the portal vein is between 3 and 5 mm Hg. Since the portal vein and its tributaries are without valves, increases in venous pressure are distributed throughout the splanchnic circulation. In the setting of portal venous hypertension, portosystemic collaterals develop secondary to the increased pressure (see portal hypertension below). The most clinically important portosystemic connections include those fed through the coronary (left gastric) and short gastric veins through the fundus of the stomach and distal esophagus to the azygos vein, resulting in gastroesophageal varices. Recanalization of the round ligament/umbilical vein leads to a caput medusa around the umbilicus. Portal hypertension through the inferior mesenteric veins and hemorrhoidal plexuses can lead to engorged external hemorrhoids. (See Schwartz 8th ed., p 1141.)

5. A replaced right hepatic artery usually arises directly from
   A. The gastroduodenal artery
   B. The superior mesenteric artery
   C. The right renal artery
   D. The right gastric artery

**Answer: B**

The extrahepatic arterial anatomy can be highly variable (Fig. 30-8). In roughly half of the population, the common hepatic artery arises from the celiac trunk, giving off the gastroduodenal artery followed by a right gastric artery. The proper hepatic artery gives rise to the right and left hepatic arteries. However, there is great variation in hepatic artery anatomy that is important to understand and detect in performing cholecystectomies, portal dissections, and liver resections. Replaced hepatic arteries are lobar vessels that arise from either the superior mesenteric artery (replaced right hepatic artery) or left gastric artery (replaced left hepatic artery). The replaced right hepatic artery travels posterior to the portal vein in close proximity to the posterior aspect of the pancreas and bile duct. A replaced right hepatic artery is felt behind both the bile duct and the portal vein when palpating the portal triad structures through the foramen of Winslow. The left hepatic artery, regardless of its origin, enters the liver at the base of the round ligament. A replaced or accessory left hepatic artery will run in the lesser omentum anterior to the caudate lobe and is typically very easily identified. In contrast to a replaced hepatic artery, an accessory hepatic artery is one that exists in addition to an anatomically typical originating vessel. Accessory right hepatic arteries often supply the posterior sector of the right lobe (segment VI and VII). An accessory left hepatic artery will typically supply the left lateral segment. The cystic artery most commonly arises from the right hepatic artery, but has a variety of common anomalies as well. (See Schwartz 8th ed., p 1142.)

6. Appropriate treatment for a hepatic adenoma smaller than 4 cm in size is
   A. Cessation of oral contraceptives and serial imaging
   B. Treatment with tamoxifen and serial imaging
   C. Cryoablation
   D. Resection

**Answer: A**
The management of patients with hepatic adenomas is evolving. Cessation of oral contraceptive pills (OCPs) in patients with lesions less than 4 cm in diameter is prudent. Regression of the lesion is commonly seen and such a regression may obviate or facilitate liver-directed intervention. Surgical intervention is recommended in patients with lesions larger than 4 cm in diameter, in patients whose lesions do not shrink after cessation of OCP use, those who medically cannot stop OCP use, or in patients who plan to become pregnant. Radiofrequency ablation (RFA) is another potentially effective treatment option in managing hepatic adenomas, especially in patients with multiple adenomas. However, until further follow-up data of this technology are available, resection remains the standard therapy. A number of patients with large adenomas undergoing resection have been found to have foci of well-differentiated hepatocellular carcinoma, although large longitudinal studies have not supported a strong association between OCP use and hepatocellular carcinoma. (See Schwartz 8th ed., p 1160.)

7. Findings on computed tomography scan suggestive of focal nodular hyperplasia include
   A. Rupture of the lesion
   B. Central location in the liver
   C. Central scarring
   D. Large size (>12 cm)

**Answer: C**
In contrast to hepatic adenomas, focal nodular hyperplasia typically is not associated with symptoms and does not pose any risks of rupture or malignant degeneration. These lesions intensely enhance on the arterial vascular phase of axial imaging studies. Characteristically, up to two thirds of lesions will demonstrate a central scar. The lesions are often peripherally located and histologically composed of regenerative nodules with hyperplastic bile ducts and connective tissue septae. The etiology is thought to be a result of an early embryologic vascular injury and the histologic findings are a response to this event. (See Schwartz 8th ed., p 1161.)

8. What is the largest percentage of the liver (by volume) that can safely be resected without causing liver failure?
   A. 15%
   B. 35%
   C. 55%
   D. 75%

**Answer: D**
Patients with normal hepatic parenchyma and serum liver tests can tolerate resection of as much as 80% of their liver volume. The remaining 20% of normal, perfused liver has the metabolic capacity to provide adequate hepatic function while liver regeneration occurs. However, patients with abnormal liver function related to extensive fatty infiltration or cirrhosis, most commonly caused by chronic ethanol ingestion or chronic hepatitis B or C viral infections, may not tolerate resection of a significant proportion of the liver and are at increased risk for postoperative liver insufficiency or liver failure and death. (See Schwartz 8th ed., p 1164.)

9. The most appropriate initial treatment for a symptomatic simple (congenital) hepatic cyst is
   A. Nothing (observation only)
   B. Aspiration alone
   C. Aspiration with sclerotherapy
   D. Surgical resection

**Answer: C**
Congenital cysts include simple hepatic cysts, which are the most common benign lesions found in the liver. Simple cysts result from excluded hyperplastic bile duct rests and they are commonly identified on imaging studies as unilocular, homogeneous fluid-filled structures with a thin wall without projections. The epithelium of the cyst secretes clear fluid that does not contain bile, and they rarely are

symptomatic unless they are large, in which case patients may complain of pain, epigastric fullness or a mass, or early satiety related to gastric compression. Often these cysts are aspirated prior to surgical referral, but the recurrence rate after simple percutaneous aspiration is extremely high. Simple aspiration is not recommended as an initial therapy; however, useful information about symptom resolution is often obtained. Percutaneous aspiration, instillation of absolute alcohol, and reaspiration (PAIR) has a success rate as high as 80%. In patients with easily accessible lesions and appropriate interventional radiology support, PAIR is an excellent first line of therapy in the management of simple, congenital, hepatic cysts. (See Schwartz 8th ed., p 1159.)

10. Which of the following decreases the risk of an *initial* upper gastrointestinal bleed from varices in a patient with portal hypertension?
    A. Transjugular intrahepatic portocaval shunt (TIPS)
    B. Splenorenal shunt
    C. Sclerotherapy
    D. Beta-blockade

**Answer: D**

Esophageal varices are the most common cause of massive bleeding in patients with cirrhosis, and result from shunting of blood through the coronary (left gastric) vein into the submucosal plexus of the esophagus. When the pressure in these veins rises above 12 mm Hg, spontaneous rupture will occur in up to 30% of patients. In addition to increased pressure in the varix, mucosal ulceration can precipitate bleeding. Prevention of the first bleeding event with prophylactic beta-adrenergic blockade is more effective than placebo, and the addition of a systemic vasodilator agent is slightly more efficacious, but at the expense of increased peripheral edema. Sclerotherapy, TIPS, or surgical shunts have not been associated with a reduction in first bleeding risk in Western, alcoholic-cirrhotic patients. Prophylaxis is important since variceal bleeding in cirrhotic patients is a grave prognostic event with 70% of patients dying within 1 year. Indeed, patients with Child class C cirrhosis and variceal bleeding have a 70% mortality rate at 6 weeks (most in the hospital setting). (See Schwartz 8th ed., p 1154.)

11. Upper gastrointestinal bleeding in patients with portal hypertension
    A. Can be managed in approximately 85% of patients with banding
    B. Occurs when the pressure in the esophageal veins exceeds 25 mm Hg
    C. Is only rarely (<5%) due to a source other than esophageal varices
    D. Is unaffected by paracentesis in patients with ascites

**Answer: A**

The most critical treatment for acute hemorrhage in cirrhotic patients is prompt endoscopic intervention and therapy. Acute esophageal variceal bleeding can be managed with endoscopic variceal banding in 85% of patients. Sclerotherapy is being performed much less frequently. Administration of intravenous vasopressin or octreotide can decrease splanchnic blood flow, and are useful in reducing bleeding from esophageal varices in the acute phase of management. The systemic effects of vasopressin make it a less favorable drug in patients with concomitant cardiac problems. Paracentesis will reduce portal venous pressures in patients with tense ascites. Minnesota or Sengstaken-Blakemore tubes have inflatable reservoirs that serve to compress the lower esophagus, stomach, and gastroesophageal junction, and are reserved for control of rebleeding from documented esophageal varices. These tubes have a limited duration of safety and effectiveness, and should be considered as temporary methods to use while planning more definitive therapy. Patients should be endotracheally intubated when these tubes are used. (See Schwartz 8th ed., p 1155.)

12. Ito cells
    A. Are the primary mediators of fibrosis in the liver
    B. Are suppressed by hepatic necrosis
    C. Are the precursor to nodular hyperplasia
    D. Are of biliary tract origin

**Answer: A**
Liver stellate cells (Ito cells) are the principal mediators of fibrosis in the liver, and are stimulated by hepatocyte necrosis and cytokines (tumor necrosis factor-α, interleukin-1, interleukin-6), growth factors (epidermal growth factor, platelet-derived growth factor, transforming growth factor β₁) released by platelets, and Kupffer and endothelial cells. (See Schwartz 8th ed., p 1152.)

13. Computed tomography (CT) findings of cirrhosis include
    A. Hepatomegaly
    B. Decreased portal vein caliber
    C. Caudate lobe hypertrophy
    D. Portal lymphadenopathy

**Answer: C**
Grossly, cirrhosis can be described as micronodular, macronodular, or mixed. The CT findings of cirrhosis can be subtle, but include right lobe atrophy, ascites, caudate lobe hypertrophy, recanalization of the umbilical vein, enlargement of the portal vein caliber, and splenomegaly. (See Schwartz 8th ed., p 1152.)

14. Etiologies of presinusoidal portal hypertension include
    A. Alcoholism
    B. Budd-Chiari syndrome
    C. Hepatitis C
    D. Schistosomiasis

**Answer: D**
Portal hypertension may be classified as presinusoidal, sinusoidal, or postsinusoidal. Sinusoidal causes are the most common in the Western Hemisphere due to alcoholic cirrhosis that results from fibrous replacement in the space of Disse. Chronic liver insufficiency is common. Postsinusoidal portal hypertension often has a vascular etiology and also is associated with some degree of liver dysfunction. In contrast, patients with presinusoidal portal hypertension may have well-preserved hepatic function. Etiologies include schistosomiasis, extrahepatic portal vein thrombosis, and congenital hepatic fibrosis (most commonly seen in children). The sequelae of portal hypertension are varied, and the long-term outcomes are related most strongly to the underlying degree of hepatic dysfunction. Upregulation of nitric oxide synthase has been shown to play an important role in augmented blood flow in portal hypertension. Although excessive splanchnic blood flow is rarely a sole cause of portal hypertension, many cirrhotic patients have some increased splanchnic flow that may be attributed to nitric oxide. (See Schwartz 8th ed., p 1153.)

15. Budd-Chiari syndrome
    A. Causes presinusoidal portal hypertension
    B. Can be associated with a lupus anticoagulant
    C. Is more common in men
    D. Does not involve hepatic veins

**Answer: B**
Budd-Chiari syndrome, which is a rare cause of postsinusoidal liver failure and cirrhosis, can occur as a spectrum of presentations that range from asymptomatic disease to fulminant liver failure. The pathophysiology is related to thrombosis of the three major hepatic veins at the level of the inferior vena cava. In patients from Asia, there may also be an associated web in the vena cava, but this is not commonly seen in patients from Western countries. The disease is more common in women and is associated with a variety of hypercoagulable states: protein C, S, or antithrombin III deficiency; polycythemia vera; lupus anticoagulant; estrogen exposure; myeloproliferative disorders; and Behçet's disease. Patients will often present with jaundice, ascites, and hepatomegaly. Transcutaneous Doppler-flow ultrasound will show thrombosed hepatic veins and may demonstrate large collaterals into the retrohe-

patic inferior vena cava. Computed tomography (CT) findings include striking caudate lobe hypertrophy and inhomogeneous contrast enhancement. Anticoagulation is the standard immediate therapy. Treatment of acute decompensated Budd-Chiari includes placement of a transjugular intrahepatic portosystemic shunt (TIPS) or a nonselective shunt. The surgical shunt options include a side-to-side portocaval shunt or interposition mesocaval shunt. The latter procedure may be technically easier, as the side-to-side shunt may require resection of a portion of the hypertrophied caudate lobe. Liver transplantation is appropriate for patients with advanced liver disease, but is plagued by potential failure resulting from the underlying disorder. (See Schwartz 8th ed., p 1153.)

16. The stent placed during transjugular intrahepatic portosystemic shunt (TIPS)
    A. Is dilated until a gradient of less than 20 mm Hg is obtained
    B. Has a stenosis rate of more than 50%
    C. Is not covered (is bare metal) because it is placed through liver parenchyma
    D. Should be followed with computed tomography scan every 6 months after placement

**Answer: B**
The TIPS has revolutionized the management of the complications of portal hypertension. The procedure is minimally invasive and creates the equivalent of a nonselective surgical shunt. The indications for TIPS include bleeding refractory to endoscopic and medical management, refractory ascites, Budd-Chiari syndrome, and hepatopulmonary syndromes. The procedure involves the placement of an expandable wire mesh stent between the middle hepatic vein and region of the portal bifurcation using ultrasound and radiographic direction. The stent is expanded to a diameter that reduces the portosystemic gradient to less than 12 mm Hg (Fig. 30-27). TIPS is associated with postprocedure encephalopathy rates of approximately 25%, and patients with renal insufficiency are at risk for worsened renal function. The long-term problem with TIPS is stenosis of the shunt, which occurs in as many as two thirds of patients. Most centers advocate an aggressive Doppler ultrasound monitoring program with prompt balloon dilation for identified stenosis of the stent. The advent of new covered stents may improve the primary patency rates of this procedure. (See Schwartz 8th ed., p 1156.)

17. The preferred initial treatment of choice for cystic hydatid disease of the liver is
    A. Observation
    B. Albendazole orally
    C. PAIR (percutaneous aspiration, instillation of alcohol, and reaspiration)
    D. Cyst aspiration and sclerotherapy

**Answer: C**
Hydatid cysts can be uncomplicated and asymptomatic. However, these lesions may rupture, can become secondarily infected, or may infect other organs. The diagnosis is based on an enzyme-linked immunosorbent assay (ELISA) test for echinococcal antigens, which is positive in over 85% of infected patients. Ultrasound and computed tomography (CT) scanning will typically demonstrate either simple or complex cysts with a cyst wall of varying thickness. The treatment of hydatid disease involves the use of oral anthelmintics such as albendazole. Albendazole therapy is the mainstay of treatment in the majority of patients with hydatid disease. It is given alone and for prolonged periods of time in patients who are poor candidates for cyst-directed intervention. However, liver-directed treatment is preferred. In patients with anatomically appropriate lesions PAIR is the preferred initial treatment. The efficacy of PAIR in managing hydatid cysts is greater than 75%. For patients whose disease is refractory to PAIR, laparoscopic or open com-

plete cyst removal with instillation of a scolicidal agent generally is curative (see Fig. 30-36B). If surgical cystectomy with removal of the germinal laminated layers is not technically feasible, then formal liver resection can be employed. During aspiration or surgical treatment of hydatid cysts, extreme caution must be taken to avoid rupture of the cyst with release of protoscolices into the peritoneal cavity. (See Schwartz 8th ed., p 1164.)

18. Which of the following statements concerning patients with an amebic liver abscess is true?
    A. More than 50% of patients will have blood cultures positive for *Entamoeba coli*.
    B. More than 50% of patients will report diarrhea in the preceding 1–2 weeks.
    C. More than 50% will be diagnosed by serum antibodies.
    D. More than 50% will require percutaneous drainage.

**Answer: C**

*Entamoeba histolytica* enters into humans in a cyst form but transforms into a trophozoite in the colon. It enters into the colonic mucosa and invades the portal venous system, infecting the liver. Amebic abscesses result from local proteolytic destruction of the liver parenchyma with focal infarction. Amebiasis is a disease found in subtropical climates, especially in areas with poor sanitation. Although resulting from a colonic infection, a recent history of severe diarrhea is uncommon. Patients typically present with sweating and chills, usually of at least 1 week duration. Fevers can be high and patients typically have right upper quadrant abdominal pain and tenderness. The majority of patients have a positive fluorescent antibody test for *E. histolytica* as well as mild abnormalities in liver enzymes; hyperbilirubinemia is relatively uncommon. (See Schwartz 8th ed., p 1164.)

19. Which of the following patients should be considered for a surgical portocaval shunt?
    A. Child class C patient with liver transplant anticipated in less than 1 year
    B. Child class C patient with liver transplant anticipated in more than 1 year
    C. Child class B patient with liver transplant anticipated in less than 1 year
    D. Child class B patient with liver transplant anticipated in more than 1 year

**Answer: D**

The advent of liver transplantation and transjugular intrahepatic portosystemic shunt (TIPS) has markedly reduced the need for surgical shunts in the management of portal hypertension and its complications of bleeding and ascites. Indeed, patients who are being considered for a surgical shunt should also be evaluated as potential liver transplant candidates. Surgical shunts are best used in patients with relatively well-preserved liver function (Child class A and B) who are not candidates for liver transplantation or who have limited access to the medical surveillance necessary for TIPS monitoring. Patients who may require liver transplant in the future (>1 year) are also candidates for surgical shunts since surgical shunt patency is superior to that of TIPS. (See Schwartz 8th ed., p 1156.)

20. The most common benign lesion in the liver is
    A. Simple (congenital) hepatic cyst
    B. Hamartoma
    C. Hepatic adenoma
    D. Focal nodular hyperplasia

**Answer: A**

Congenital cysts include simple hepatic cysts, which are the most common benign lesions found in the liver. Simple cysts result from excluded hyperplastic bile duct rests and they are commonly identified on imaging studies as unilocular, homogeneous fluid-filled structures with a thin wall without projections. The epithelium of the cyst secretes clear fluid that does not contain bile, and they rarely are symptomatic unless they are large, in which case patients may complain of pain, epigastric fullness or a mass, or early satiety related to gastric compression. Often these cysts are aspirated prior to surgical referral, but the recurrence rate after simple percutaneous aspiration is extremely high. Simple aspiration is not recommended as an initial therapy; however, useful information about symptom resolution is often obtained. Percutaneous aspiration, instillation of absolute alcohol, and reaspiration (PAIR) has a success rate as high as 80%. In patients with easily accessible lesions and appropriate interventional radiology support, PAIR is an excellent first line of therapy in the management of simple, congenital, hepatic cysts. (See Schwartz 8th ed., p 1159.)

21. Perioperative management of the cirrhotic patient undergoing routine elective abdominal surgery includes
    A. Avoidance of sodium-containing solutions during surgery
    B. Avoidance of nonsteroidal anti-inflammatory drugs
    C. Placement of peritoneal dialysis catheters for drainage of ascites
    D. Placement of peritoneal-vascular shunts for drainage of ascites

**Answer: A**
A dysregulation of the compensatory blood flow response (e.g., increased hepatic arterial flow in response to decreased portal vein flow) is seen in cirrhosis. A variety of studies have shown that American Society of Anesthesiologists (ASA) score, renal insufficiency, and higher Child scores are adverse prognostic factors that predict an increased probability of complications and mortality after an operation. Laparoscopic cholecystectomy is safe in Child class A and B patients. In elective procedures, attention to preoperative control of ascites, electrolyte abnormalities, and coagulopathy are critical to the success of elective surgery. Prevention of postoperative ascites begins with restriction of sodium-containing intravenous fluids in the operating room. As ascites accumulates, continued fluid restriction, diuretic therapy, bedrest, and intermittent paracentesis may be needed. Chronic peritoneal catheter drainage should be avoided due to the risk of retrograde contamination of the peritoneal cavity. Ascites in this setting is highly morbid, especially if complicated by bacterial infection. Encephalopathy should also be anticipated. Administration of narcotic pain medicines and sedatives should be limited when possible, as the hepatic metabolism of most drugs is compromised. (See Schwartz 8th ed., p 1153.)

22. The H-type portocaval shunt
    A. Is performed with a 12-mm Dacron graft
    B. Prevents rebleeding in approximately 75% of patients
    C. Has a primary patency rate of 80%
    D. Decreases survival in patients who subsequently undergo liver transplantation

**Answer: C**
Surgical shunts can be divided into two general categories: selective and nonselective (Table 30-6). Nonselective shunts are associated with a high risk of encephalopathy, especially in patients with marginal liver function. Selective shunts are associated with a lower incidence of encephalopathy, as they maintain hepatopetal flow while lowering portal pressure. Currently, the most useful surgical shunts are the small-diameter portacaval H graft shunt and distal splenorenal shunt (DSRS). The small-diameter portacaval H graft shunt uses an 8-mm, ringed GoreTex graft anastomosed between the portal vein and the vena cava (Fig. 30-28). The portal vein and vena cava are approached from the right lateral side, where control of these vessels is easier and avoids dissection through omental and retroperitoneal varices. The success rate of the small-diameter portacaval H graft shunt at preventing rebleeding is 90% and the primary patency rate is near 80%. In patients who may require liver transplantation, the presence of this shunt increases the complexity of the transplant, but survival is not altered. (See Schwartz 8th ed., p 1156.)

23. Cystic hydatid disease of the liver is caused by
    A. *Echinococcus granulosus*
    B. *Echinococcus multilocularis*
    C. *Entamoeba histolytica*
    D. *Entamoeba coli*

**Answer: A**
Cystic hydatid disease is caused by the larval/cyst stage of *Echinococcus granulosus*, in which humans are an intermediate host (Fig. 30-36A). Humans are infected by oral ingestion of excrement from animals (most commonly canines). This form of hydatid disease occurs throughout the world, predominantly in the Southern Hemisphere, Europe, Russia, and China. (See Schwartz 8th ed., p 1163.)

24. The liver is divided into anatomic segments based on
    A. Bile duct drainage
    B. Hepatic arterial supply
    C. Hepatic venous drainage
    D. Portal vein distribution

**Answer: C**
The liver is divided into eight segments according to hepatic venous drainage into the inferior vena cava. The right lobe contains segments V through VIII, whereas the left lobe contains segments I through IV. The umbilical fissure divides the left anterior sector into segment IV, which contains the quadrate lobe and section III. (See Schwartz 7th ed.)

25. Appropriate maneuvers in a patient with hepatic encephalopathy include all of the following EXCEPT
    A. Addition of glucose to the diet
    B. Administration of lactulose
    C. Construction of a side-to-side portacaval shunt
    D. Limiting dietary protein

**Answer: C**
Hepatic encephalopathy has been related to hyperammonemia with ammonia intoxication. Ammonia is produced when intestinal bacteria break down blood in the gastrointestinal tract. Active bleeding should be controlled, and dietary protein should be reduced to reduce ingested blood. Glucose in the diet inhibits ammonia production by bacteria. Lactulose acts as a mild cathartic, and its breakdown products interfere with transfer across the colonic mucosa. Cleansing enemas remove any residual blood from the colon. Portosystemic shunts may interfere with ammonia metabolism in the liver. A side-to-side portacaval shunt is indicated when the patient has hepatic venous outflow obstruction. (See Schwartz 7th ed.)

26. Possible complications of umbilical hernia repair in a cirrhotic patient with marked ascites include all of the following EXCEPT
    A. Hepatic encephalopathy
    B. Leakage of ascitic fluid
    C. Necrosis of the abdominal wall
    D. Variceal bleeding

**Answer: A**
Umbilical herniorrhaphy in a cirrhotic patient with ascites is a risky undertaking. Leakage of ascitic fluid must be anticipated, and this increases the risk of wound infection. Necrosis of the abdominal wall may result from pressure on the incision from reforming ascites. Variceal bleeding may result from interruption of collateral veins. Hepatic encephalopathy should not be a problem unless it occurs secondary to massive variceal bleeding. (See Schwartz 7th ed.)

27. In the absence of secondary infection, the treatment for amebic abscess of the liver should consist of
    A. Injection of amebicidal drugs into the abscess and open drainage
    B. Injection of amebicidal drugs into the abscess and closed aspiration
    C. Systemic administration of amebicidal drugs and open drainage
    D. Systemic administration of amebicidal drugs and closed aspiration

**Answer: D**
To be effective, the treatment of amebic abscess of the liver must involve eradication of the parasite from the intestinal tract and the liver, as well as from the abscess itself. In uncomplicated cases, eradication usually can be accomplished by the administration of an amebicidal drug (i.e., metronidazole) combined with closed-needle aspiration of the abscess. Drug therapy usually is instituted several days before aspiration, and there is no indication for injection of any drug directly into the abscess cavity. Once an abscess is known to be secondarily infected, open surgical drainage is necessary. (See Schwartz 7th ed.)

28. A 17-year-old boy is admitted to the hospital after an automobile accident. Except for a quiet abdomen, he has no localizing physical findings. After receiving 2000 mL of lactated Ringer's solution intravenously, his pulse rate is 90 beats per minute, and his blood pressure is 110/70 mm Hg. Abdominal computed tomography (CT) scan reveals a laceration of the left lobe of the liver extending from the dome more than halfway through the parenchyma. Appropriate management at this time would be
    A. Bed rest and observation
    B. Abdominal exploration and ligature of intrahepatic blood vessels
    C. Abdominal exploration and packing of the hepatic wound
    D. Abdominal exploration and left hepatectomy

**Answer: A**

In a hemodynamically stable patient with an isolated liver injury, even one that appears alarming on CT scan, there is growing appreciation that careful observation allows restoration of the hepatic anatomy without loss of hepatic function. In an unstable patient, or in one with multiple injuries, surgical intervention is appropriate. In most instances, hemorrhage can be controlled by ligating vessels within the parenchyma, removing devitalized tissue, and establishing external drainage. With uncontrolled bleeding, packing of the liver injury can be life-saving; the packing is removed in the operating room several days later. Further débridement and packing may be required. Ligature of a main hepatic artery is rarely appropriate. Although it may control bleeding in certain instances, it is not physiologically innocuous and does not deal with the major cause of massive hepatic bleeding, hepatic vein injury. Formal lobectomy is done only when the injury demands it for removal of devitalized tissue. (See Schwartz 7th ed.)

# CHAPTER 31

# Gallbladder and Extrahepatic Biliary System

1. Mucus is secreted in the gallbladder by cells in the
   A. Infundibulum and neck
   B. Infundibulum and body
   C. Neck and fundus
   D. Infundibulum, neck, and fundus

**Answer: A**

The gallbladder is lined by a single, highly-folded, tall columnar epithelium that contains cholesterol and fat globules. The mucus secreted into the gallbladder originates in the tubuloalveolar glands found in the mucosa lining the infundibulum and neck of the gallbladder, but are absent from the body and fundus. The epithelial lining of the gallbladder is supported by a lamina propria. The muscle layer has circular longitudinal and oblique fibers, but without well-developed layers. The perimuscular subserosa contains connective tissue, nerves, vessels, lymphatics, and adipocytes. It is covered by the serosa except where the gallbladder is embedded in the liver. The gallbladder differs histologically from the rest of the gastrointestinal tract in that it lacks a muscularis mucosa and submucosa. (See Schwartz 8th ed., p 1188.)

2. The triangle of Calot is defined by the
   A. Cystic duct, common bile duct, and liver
   B. Cystic duct, common hepatic duct, and liver
   C. Common hepatic duct, common bile duct, and liver
   D. Cystic artery, common hepatic duct, and common bile duct
   E. Cystic artery, cystic duct, and common hepatic duct

**Answer: B**

The cystic artery that supplies the gallbladder is usually a branch of the right hepatic artery (>90% of the time). The course of the cystic artery may vary, but it nearly always is found within the hepatocystic triangle, the area bound by the cystic duct, common hepatic duct, and the liver margin (triangle of Calot). (See Schwartz 8th ed., p 1188.)

3. In what percentage of patients is the classic anatomy of the extrahepatic biliary tree present?
   A. 25%
   B. 33%
   C. 50%
   D. 66%

**Answer: B**

The classic description of the extrahepatic biliary tree and its arteries applies only in about one third of patients. The gallbladder may have abnormal positions, be intrahepatic, be rudimentary, have anomalous forms, or be duplicated. Isolated congenital absence of the gallbladder is very rare, with a reported incidence of 0.03%. Before the diagnosis is made, the presence of an intrahepatic bladder or anomalous position must be ruled out. Duplication of the gallbladder with two separate cavities and two separate cystic ducts has an incidence of about one in every 4000 persons. This occurs in two major varieties: the more common form in which each gallbladder has its own cystic duct that empties independently into the same or different parts of the extrahepatic biliary tree, and as two cystic ducts that merge before they enter the common bile duct. Duplication is only clinically important when some pathologic processes affect one or both organs. A left-sided gallbladder with a cystic duct emptying into the left hepatic duct or the common bile duct and a retrodisplacement of the gallbladder are both extremely rare. A partial or totally intrahepatic gallbladder is associated with an increased incidence of cholelithiasis. (See Schwartz 8th ed., p 1190.)

4. What percentage of conjugated bile is absorbed in the terminal ileum?
   A. 10%
   B. 30%
   C. 50%
   D. 80%

**Answer: D**
Bile is mainly composed of water, electrolytes, bile salts, proteins, lipids, and bile pigments. Sodium, potassium, calcium, and chlorine have the same concentration in bile as in plasma or extracellular fluid. The pH of hepatic bile is usually neutral or slightly alkaline, but varies with diet; an increase in protein shifts the bile to a more acidic pH. The primary bile salts, cholate and chenodeoxycholate, are synthesized in the liver from cholesterol. They are conjugated there with taurine and glycine, and act within the bile as anions (bile acids) that are balanced by sodium. Bile salts are excreted into the bile by the hepatocyte and aid in the digestion and absorption of fats in the intestines. In the intestines, about 80% of the conjugated bile acids are absorbed in the terminal ileum. The remainder is dehydroxylated (deconjugated) by gut bacteria, forming secondary bile acids deoxycholate and lithocholate. These are absorbed in the colon, transported to the liver, conjugated, and secreted into the bile. Eventually, about 95% of the bile acid pool is reabsorbed and returned via the portal venous system to the liver, the so-called enterohepatic circulation. Five percent is excreted in the stool, leaving the relatively small amount of bile acids to have maximum effect. (See Schwartz 8th ed., p 1191.)

5. Which of the following best describes the etiology of hydrops of the gallbladder?
   A. Secretion of abnormal bile by the liver
   B. Stone obstruction of the cystic duct
   C. Stone obstruction of the common bile duct
   D. Cancer of the common hepatic duct

**Answer: B**
When the pain lasts more than 24 hours, an impacted stone in the cystic duct or acute cholecystitis (see Acute Cholecystitis in Schwartz 8th ed., p 1199) should be suspected. An impacted stone will result in what is called hydrops of the gallbladder. The bile gets absorbed, but the gallbladder epithelium continues to secrete mucus and the gallbladder becomes distended with mucinous material. The gallbladder may be palpable, but usually is not tender. Hydrops of the gallbladder may result in edema of the gallbladder wall, inflammation, infection, and perforation. Although hydrops may persist with few consequences, early cholecystectomy is generally indicated to avoid complications. (See Schwartz 8th ed., p 1198.)

6. Which of the following is the primary stimulus for the gallbladder to empty?
   A. Motilin
   B. Somatostatin
   C. Migrating myenteric motor complex
   D. Cholecystokinin

**Answer: D**
Gallbladder filling is facilitated by tonic contraction of the sphincter of Oddi, which creates a pressure gradient between the bile ducts and the gallbladder. During fasting the gallbladder does not simply fill passively. In association with phase II of the interdigestive migrating myenteric motor complex in the gut, the gallbladder repeatedly empties small volumes of bile into the duodenum. This process is mediated at least in part by the hormone motilin. In response to a meal, the gallbladder empties by a coordinated motor response of gallbladder contraction and sphincter of

Oddi relaxation. One of the main stimuli to gallbladder emptying is the hormone cholecystokinin (CCK). CCK is released endogenously from the duodenal mucosa in response to a meal. When stimulated by eating, the gallbladder empties 50 to 70% of its contents within 30 to 40 minutes. Over the following 60 to 90 minutes the gallbladder gradually refills. This is correlated with a reduced CCK level. Other hormonal and neural pathways also are involved in the coordinated action of the gallbladder and the sphincter of Oddi. Defects in the motor activity of the gallbladder are thought to play a role in cholesterol nucleation and gallstone formation. (See Schwartz 8th ed., p 1191.)

7. Choledocholithiasis is associated with
   A. Elevation of conjugated bilirubin
   B. Elevation of unconjugated bilirubin
   C. Decrease in alkaline phosphate
   D. Increase in white blood cell count

**Answer: A**
Cholestasis, an obstruction to bile flow, is characterized by an elevation of bilirubin (i.e., the conjugated form), and a rise in alkaline phosphatase. Serum aminotransferases may be normal or mildly elevated. (See Schwartz 8th ed., p 1192.)

8. What is the sensitivity of ultrasound in the diagnosis of cholelithiasis?
   A. <80%
   B. 80–85%
   C. 85–90%
   D. >90%

**Answer: D**
An ultrasound will show stones in the gallbladder with sensitivity and specificity of over 90%. Stones are acoustically dense and reflect the ultrasound waves back to the ultrasonic transducer. Because stones block the passage of sound waves to the region behind them, they also produce an acoustic shadow (Fig. 31-6). Stones also move with changes in position. Polyps may be calcified and reflect shadows, but do not move with change in posture. Some stones form a layer in the gallbladder; others a sediment or sludge. A thickened gallbladder wall and local tenderness indicate cholecystitis. The patient has acute cholecystitis if a layer of edema is seen within the wall of the gallbladder or between the gallbladder and the liver. When a stone obstructs the neck of the gallbladder, the gallbladder may become very large, but thin walled. A contracted, thick-walled gallbladder indicates chronic cholecystitis. (See Schwartz 8th ed., p 1192.)

9. Which of the following is NOT a clear indication for cholecystectomy?
   A. Porcelain gallbladder
   B. Gallstones
   C. First bout of biliary colic
   D. Cholecystitis

**Answer: B**
Since few patients develop complications without previous biliary symptoms, prophylactic cholecystectomy in asymptomatic persons with gallstones is rarely indicated. For elderly patients with diabetes, for individuals who will be isolated from medical care for extended periods of time, and in populations with increased risk of gallbladder cancer, a prophylactic cholecystectomy may be advisable. Porcelain gallbladder, a rare premalignant condition in which the wall of the gallbladder becomes calcified, is an absolute indication for cholecystectomy. (See Schwartz 8th ed., p 1194.)

10. Cholesterol stones
    A. Are radiopaque
    B. Are caused by a decrease in phospholipids in bile salts
    C. Do not cause biliary obstruction
    D. Arise from cholesterol hypersecretion

**Answer: D**
Pure cholesterol stones are uncommon and account for less than 10% of all stones. They usually occur as single large stones with smooth surfaces. Most other cholesterol stones contain variable amounts of bile pigments and calcium, but are always more than 70% cholesterol by weight. These stones are

usually multiple, of variable size, and may be hard and faceted or irregular, mulberry-shaped and soft (Fig. 31-11). Colors range from whitish yellow and green to black. Most cholesterol stones are radiolucent; less than 10% are radiopaque. Whether pure or of mixed nature, the common primary event in the formation of cholesterol stones is supersaturation of bile with cholesterol. Therefore high bile cholesterol levels and cholesterol gallstones are considered as one disease. Cholesterol is highly nonpolar and insoluble in water and bile. Cholesterol solubility depends on the relative concentration of cholesterol, bile salts, and lecithin (the main phospholipid in bile). Supersaturation almost always is caused by cholesterol hypersecretion rather than by a reduced secretion of phospholipid or bile salts. (See Schwartz 8th ed., p 1196.)

11. Brown gallstones
    A. Are mainly cholesterol stones
    B. Are caused by infection
    C. Arise from an increase in conjugated bilirubin
    D. Are mainly found in South America

**Answer: B**

Brown stones are usually less than 1 cm in diameter, brownish-yellow, soft, and often mushy. They may form either in the gallbladder or in the bile ducts, usually secondary to bacterial infection caused by bile stasis. Precipitated calcium bilirubinate and bacterial cell bodies compose the major part of the stone. Bacteria such as *Escherichia coli* secrete beta-glucuronidase that enzymatically cleaves bilirubin glucuronide to produce the insoluble unconjugated bilirubin. It precipitates with calcium, and along with dead bacterial cell bodies, forms soft brown stones in the biliary tree.

   Brown stones are typically found in the biliary tree of Asian populations and are associated with stasis secondary to parasite infection. In Western populations, brown stones occur as primary bile duct stones in patients with biliary strictures or other common bile duct stones that cause stasis and bacterial contamination. (See Schwartz 8th ed., p 1197.)

12. Which of the following can be given to improve the success of surgery for choledocholithiasis?
    A. Somatostatin
    B. Cholecystokinin
    C. Glucagon
    D. Vasoactive intestinal polypeptide

**Answer: C**

If the stones in the duct are small, they may sometimes be flushed into the duodenum with saline irrigation via the cholangiography catheter after the sphincter of Oddi has been relaxed with glucagon. If irrigation is unsuccessful, a balloon catheter may be passed via the cystic duct and down the common bile duct, where it is inflated and withdrawn to retrieve the stones. The next attempt is usually made with a wire basket passed under fluoroscopic guidance to catch the stones (Fig. 31-20). If needed, a flexible choledochoscope is the next step. The cystic duct may have to be dilated to allow its passage. Once in the common bile duct, the stones may be caught into a wire basket under direct vision or pushed into the duodenum. When the duct has been cleared, the cystic duct is ligated and cut and the cholecystectomy completed. Occasionally a choledochotomy, an incision into the common bile duct itself, is necessary. The flexible choledochoscope is then passed into the duct for visualization and clearance of stones. The choledochotomy is sutured with a T tube left in the common bile duct with one end taken out through the abdominal wall for decompression of the bile ducts. By managing common bile duct stones at the time of the cholecystectomy, the patients can have all of their gallstone disease treated with one invasive procedure. It does, however, depend on the available surgical expertise. (See Schwartz 8th ed., p 1206.)

13. A choledochocele is what type of choledochal cyst?
    A. Type I
    B. Type II
    C. Type III
    D. Type IV

**Answer: C**
Type I, fusiform or cystic dilations of the extrahepatic biliary tree, are the most common type, making up over 50% of all choledochal cysts. Type II, saccular diverticulum of an extrahepatic bile duct, is rare, comprising less than 5% of choledochal cysts. Type III, bile duct dilatations within the duodenal wall (choledochoceles), make up about 5% of choledochal cysts. Types IVa and IVb, multiple cysts, make up 5 to 10% of choledochal cysts. Type IVa affects both extrahepatic and intrahepatic bile ducts, while type IVb cysts affect the extrahepatic bile ducts only. Type V, intrahepatic biliary cysts, are very rare and make up only about 1% of choledochal cysts. (See Schwartz 8th ed., p 1210.)

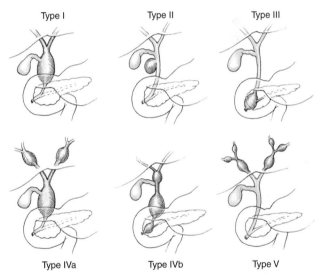

**FIG. 31-1.** Classification of choledochal cysts. Type I, fusiform or cystic dilations of the extrahepatic biliary tree, are the most common type, making up over 50% of all choledochal cysts. Type II, saccular diverticulum of an extrahepatic bile duct, is rare, comprising less than 5% of choledochal cysts. Type III, bile duct dilations within the duodenal wall (choledochoceles), make up about 5% of choledochal cysts. Types IVa and IVb, multiple cysts, make up 5 to 10% of choledochal cysts. Type IVa affects both extrahepatic and intrahepatic bile ducts, while type IVb cysts affect the extrahepatic bile ducts only. Type V, intrahepatic biliary cysts, are very rare and make up only about 1% of choledochal cysts. (See Schwartz 8th ed., p 1210.)

14. Which of the following improves outcome in patients with sclerosing cholangitis and advanced liver disease?
    A. Steroids
    B. Resection of extrahepatic biliary tree and hepaticojejunostomy
    C. Serial dilatation of bile duct strictures
    D. Liver transplantation

**Answer: D**

There is no known effective medical therapy for primary sclerosing cholangitis and no known curative treatment. Corticosteroids, immunosuppressants, ursodeoxycholic acid, and antibiotics have been disappointing. Biliary strictures can be dilated and stented either endoscopically or percutaneously. These measures have given short-term improvements in symptoms and serum bilirubin levels, and long-term improvements in only less than one half of the patients. Surgical management with resection of the extrahepatic biliary tree and hepaticojejunostomy has produced reasonable results in patients with extrahepatic and bifurcation strictures, but without cirrhosis or significant hepatic fibrosis. In patients with sclerosing cholangitis and advanced liver disease, liver transplantation is the only option. It offers excellent results with overall 5-year survival as high as 85%. Primary sclerosing cholangitis recurs in 10 to 20% of patients and may require retransplantation. (See Schwartz 8th ed., p 1211.)

15. The next diagnostic test in a jaundiced patient when ultrasonography suggests common duct dilatation is
    A. Computed tomography
    B. Biliary scintigraphy
    C. Endoscopic retrograde cholangiopancreatography
    D. Percutaneous transhepatic cholangiography

**Answer: C**

Endoscopic retrograde cholangiopancreatography may provide direct diagnosis of distal common duct pathology, and with common duct stones or ampullary stricture, it may be therapeutic as well. (See Schwartz 7th ed.)

16. In Western culture, the major element present in gallstones is
    A. Calcium
    B. Cholesterol
    C. Iron
    D. Pigment

**Answer: B**

Cholesterol, bile pigment, and calcium are the main components of gallstones, with cholesterol content averaging 71% of stone weight. Calcium bilirubinate stones are the most common types found in Asia. (See Schwartz 7th ed.)

17. When gallstone ileus occurs, obstruction is most frequent in
    A. The duodenum
    B. The jejunum
    C. The proximal ileum
    D. The terminal ileum

**Answer: D**

Gallstone ileus occurs after a stone erodes from the gallbladder into the gastrointestinal tract. The stone usually lodges in the terminal ileum, which is the narrowest part of the small intestine. (See Schwartz 7th ed.)

18. A biliary-enteric fistula most frequently connects the gallbladder with the
    A. Duodenum
    B. Jejunum
    C. Stomach
    D. Hepatic flexure of the colon

**Answer: A**

Although fistulization from the gallbladder into any part of the gastrointestinal tract can occur, more than half of the fistulas involve the duodenum. (See Schwartz 7th ed.)

19. The most common cause of acute cholecystitis is
    A. Cystic duct obstruction
    B. *Escherichia coli* infection
    C. Multiple gallstones
    D. *Salmonella* infection

**Answer: A**

Acute cholecystitis is an obstructive, not an infectious process. It develops when a stone becomes impacted in the cystic duct, preventing flow of bile from the gallbladder into the common bile duct. (See Schwartz 7th ed.)

20. The best initial procedure in defining the cause of obstructive jaundice in a 75-year-old man is
    A. Endoscopic retrograde cholangiopancreatography
    B. Percutaneous transhepatic cholangiography
    C. Ultrasonography
    D. Computed tomography scanning

**Answer: C**

When jaundice is believed to be due to ductal obstruction rather than hemolysis or hepatocellular disease, the first diagnostic procedure should be ultrasonography. Computed tomography scanning, which will yield similar information, is more expensive. If no ductal dilatation is found, endoscopic retrograde cholangiopancreatography (ERCP) should be the next step. With intrahepatic ductal dilatation only, percutaneous transhepatic cholangiography (PTC) is indicated. With both intra- and extrahepatic ductal dilatation, PTC is the procedure of choice, but ERCP is an acceptable alternative, especially with ascites or abnormal coagulation. (See Schwartz 7th ed.)

21. In the most common anomaly of extrahepatic bile duct anatomy, the cystic duct
    A. Inserts into the right hepatic duct
    B. Lies parallel to the common duct and enters it close to the duodenum
    C. Passes anterior to the common duct and enters its left side
    D. Passes posterior to the common duct and enters its left side

**Answer: B**

There may be a long cystic duct separate from or fused with the wall of the common duct. All of the described abnormalities occur, and the important issue is for the surgeon to define the anatomy correctly before dividing any structures in the biliary area. (See Schwartz 7th ed.)

22. Reabsorption of gallbladder fluid is largely determined by
    A. Concentration of bilirubin in gallbladder bile
    B. Concentration of cholesterol in gallbladder bile
    C. Transport of potassium ions
    D. Transport of sodium ions

**Answer: D**

Sodium leaves gallbladder bile by an active transport across the gallbladder membrane down an electromechanical gradient. Absorption of water and chloride follows sodium, and potassium passes in the opposite direction. Bilirubin and cholesterol are involved in stone formation when biliary stasis is present. (See Schwartz 7th ed.)

23. The presence of chronic liver disease, rather than extrahepatic biliary obstruction, is suggested by the presence on physical examination of each of the following EXCEPT
    A. Ascites
    B. Cutaneous xanthomas
    C. Intense jaundice
    D. Spider hemangiomas

**Answer: C**

Intense jaundice can develop in the presence of either chronic liver disease or extrahepatic biliary obstruction. The other physical findings listed are characteristic of advanced cirrhosis. (See Schwartz 7th ed.)

24. All of the following statements regarding cancer of the gallbladder are true EXCEPT
    A. Most affected patients are females.
    B. Most affected patients have associated gallstones.
    C. The liver is the most frequent site of metastases.
    D. Treatment should include right hepatic lobectomy.

**Answer: D**

Carcinoma of the gallbladder is the fifth most common cancer of the gastrointestinal tract, and approximately 80% of affected patients are females. Approximately 90% of patients who have carcinoma of the gallbladder have cholelithiasis, and 5–10% of patients older than the age of 65 years who have symptomatic cholelithiasis have carcinoma of the gallbladder. In patients who have metastases, the liver is involved in approximately two-thirds of cases, and the regional lymph nodes in about one-half. Spread to the liver occurs early, either along the lymphatics or by direct invasion. The prognosis for 5-year survival is extremely poor, approximately 2%, and most long-term survivors are patients in whom an incidental microscopic focus of cancer has been unexpectedly detected in a gallbladder specimen after surgery for acute or chronic cholecystitis. In patients who have grossly visible cancer, the best results have been achieved with cholecystectomy and regional lymph node dissection. Removal of the wedge of liver tissue containing the gallbladder bed also should be performed, but a formal right hepatic lobectomy does not improve the 5-year survival rate and has a high operative mortality and morbidity rate. (See Schwartz 7th ed.)

25. Abdominal ultrasonography is carried out during evaluation for a possible abdominal aortic aneurysm. The presence of stones in the gallbladder is identified on this study. The patient's only abdominal symptom is a sense of fullness after eating. The appropriate first step in managing the gallstones is
    A. Observation
    B. Laparoscopic cholecystectomy
    C. Open cholecystectomy
    D. Ursodeoxycholic acid therapy

**Answer: A**

Although gallstones have been managed successfully by medications such as ursodeoxycholic acid or by extracorporeal shockwave lithotripsy, laparoscopic cholecystectomy is the standard method today for dealing with most patients with symptomatic cholelithiasis. Open cholecystectomy remains a viable approach when there is some contraindication to a laparoscopic procedure, and it is mandatory when the biliary anatomy cannot be well appreciated through the laparoscope. In a patient who has asymptomatic cholelithiasis as an incidental finding, however, there are no data to suggest that any therapeutic intervention is justified. Fewer than 25% of patients with asymptomatic cholelithiasis will develop symptoms that require intervention over a 5-year follow-up period. (See Schwartz 7th ed.)

26. A higher than average incidence of gallstones is associated with all of the following hematologic disorders EXCEPT
    A. Hereditary spherocytosis
    B. Hereditary elliptocytosis
    C. Idiopathic autoimmune hemolytic anemia
    D. Primary hypersplenism

**Answer: D**

All hematologic disorders characterized by a hemolytic component are associated with a higher-than-average incidence of gallstone formation. Not unexpectedly, the gallstones are primarily of the pigmented variety and consist of crystals of pure bilirubin pigment or varying proportions of calcium bilirubinate. In the hemolytic diseases listed in the question, the reported incidence of cholelithiasis varies between 25 and 60% and correlates with the severity of the hemolytic process. Because the anemia that occurs with primary hypersplenism is due to the splenic sequestration of red blood cells and does not involve a hemolytic process, increased gallstone formation is not a feature of this condition. (See Schwartz 7th ed.)

1. Insulinomas
   A. Usually require selective venous sampling for localization
   B. Are more common in the head of the pancreas
   C. Are usually benign
   D. Are treated with an anatomic pancreatectomy

**Answer: C**

Insulinomas are the most common pancreatic endocrine neoplasms and present with a typical clinical syndrome known as Whipple's triad. The triad consists of symptomatic fasting hypoglycemia, a documented serum glucose level less than 50 mg/dL, and relief of symptoms with the administration of glucose. Patients will often present with a profound syncopal episode and will admit to similar less severe episodes in the recent past. They also may admit to palpitations, trembling, diaphoresis, confusion or obtundation, and seizure, and family members may report that the patient has undergone a personality change. Routine laboratory studies will uncover a low blood sugar, the cause of all these symptoms. The diagnosis is clinched with a monitored fast in which blood is sampled every 4 to 6 h for glucose and insulin levels until the patient becomes symptomatic. Elevated C-peptide levels rule out the unusual case of surreptitious administration of insulin or oral hypoglycemic agents, because excess endogenous insulin production leads to excess C-peptide. Insulinomas are usually localized with computed tomography (CT) scanning and endoscopic ultrasound (EUS). Technical advances in EUS have led to preoperative identification of more than 90% of insulinomas. Visceral angiography with venous sampling is rarely required to accurately localize the tumor. Insulinomas are evenly distributed throughout the head, body, and tail of the pancreas. Unlike most endocrine pancreatic tumors, the majority (90%) of insulinomas are benign and solitary, with only 10% malignant. They are typically cured by simple enucleation. However, tumors located close to the main pancreatic duct and large (>2 cm) tumors may require a distal pancreatectomy or pancreaticoduodenectomy. Intraoperative ultrasound is useful to determine the tumor's relation to the main pancreatic duct and guide intraoperative decision making. Enucleation of solitary insulinomas and distal pancreatectomy for insulinoma can be performed using minimally-invasive technique.

Ninety percent of insulinomas are sporadic and 10% are associated with the MEN-1 syndrome. Insulinomas associated with the MEN-1 syndrome are more likely to be multifocal and have a higher rate of recurrence. (See Schwartz 8th ed., p 1274–1275.)

2. Which of the following is the most common presenting symptom in patients with a somatostatinoma?
   A. Cholelithiasis
   B. Constipation
   C. Hypoglycemia
   D. Hypocalcemia

**Answer: A**

Because somatostatin inhibits pancreatic and biliary secretions, patients with a somatostatinoma present with gallstones due to bile stasis, diabetes due to inhibition of insulin secretion, and steatorrhea due to inhibition of pancreatic exocrine secretion and bile secretion. Most somatostatinomas originate in the proximal pancreas or the pancreatoduodenal groove, with the ampulla and periampullary area as the most common site (60%). The most common presentations are abdominal pain (25%), jaundice (25%), and cholelithiasis (19%). This rare type of pancreatic endocrine tumor is diagnosed by confirming elevated serum somatostatin levels, which are usually above 10 ng/mL. Although most reported cases of somatostatinoma involve metastatic disease, an attempt at complete excision of the tumor and cholecystectomy is warranted in fit patients. (See Schwartz 8th ed., p 1276.)

3. Which of the following imaging studies is the most accurate in identifying endocrine tumors of the pancreas?
   A. Ultrasound
   B. Dynamic computed tomography scan
   C. Magnetic resonance imaging
   D. Metaiodobenzylguanidine scan

**Answer: B**

The current diagnostic and staging test of choice for pancreatic cancer is a dynamic contrast-enhanced spiral computed tomography (CT) scan, and techniques are constantly improving. The accuracy of CT scanning for predicting unresectable disease is 90 to 95%. CT findings that indicate a tumor is unresectable include invasion of the hepatic or superior mesenteric artery, enlarged lymph nodes outside the boundaries of resection, ascites, distant metastases (e.g., liver), and distant organ invasion (e.g., colon). Invasion of the superior mesenteric vein or portal vein is not in itself a contraindication to resection as long as the veins are patent. In contrast, CT scanning is less accurate in predicting resectable disease. CT scanning will miss small liver metastases and predicting arterial involvement is sometimes difficult. (See Schwartz 8th ed., p 1280.)

4. What percentage of patients with a gastrinoma have multiple endocrine neoplasia (MEN-1) syndrome?
   A. 5%
   B. 10%
   C. 25%
   D. 40%

**Answer: C**

Only one fourth of gastrinomas occur in association with the MEN-1 syndrome. One half of patients with gastrinomas will have solitary tumors, while the remainder will have multiple gastrinomas. Multiple tumors are more common in patients with MEN-1 syndrome. Aggressive surgical treatment is justified in patients with sporadic gastrinomas. If patients have MEN-1 syndrome, the parathyroid hyperplasia is addressed with total parathyroidectomy and implantation of parathyroid tissue in the forearm. (See Schwartz 8th ed., p 1276.)

5. Which of the following is a cause of elevated serum gastrin?
   A. Renal failure
   B. Insulinoma
   C. Islet cell hyperplasia
   D. Pancreatic hypertrophy after pancreatectomy

**Answer: A**

Common causes of hypergastrinemia include pernicious anemia, treatment with proton pump inhibitors, renal failure, G-cell hyperplasia, atrophic gastritis, retained or excluded antrum, and gastric outlet obstruction. (See Schwartz 8th ed., p 1275.)

6. Which of the following statements about metastatic gastrinoma is true?
   A. Five-year survival for patients with liver metastases is <10%.
   B. Metastases limited to lymph nodes do not decrease survival.
   C. Debulking of liver metastases decreases symptoms.
   D. Lymph node metastases occur more commonly when the primary tumor is in the duodenum.

**Answer: B**

Unfortunately, a biochemical cure is achieved in only about one third of the patients operated on for Zollinger-Ellison syndrome (ZES). Despite the lack of success, long-term survival rates are good, even in patients with liver metastases. The 15-year survival rate for patients without liver metastases is about 80%, while the 5-year survival rate for patients with liver metastases is 20 to 50%. Pancreatic tumors are usually larger than tumors arising in the duodenum, and more often have lymph node metastases. In gastrinomas, liver metastases decrease survival rates, but lymph node metastases do not. The best results are seen after complete excision of small sporadic tumors originating in the duodenum. Large tumors associated with liver metastases, located outside of Passaro's triangle, have the worst prognosis. (See Schwartz 8th ed., p 1276.)

7. Which of the following is the most common pancreatic endocrine tumor?
   A. Gastrinoma
   B. Glucagonoma
   C. Insulinoma
   D. Vasoactive intestinal peptide-producing tumor (VIPoma)

**Answer: C**

Insulinomas are the most common pancreatic endocrine neoplasms and present with a typical clinical syndrome known as Whipple's triad. The triad consists of symptomatic fasting hypoglycemia, a documented serum glucose level less than 50 mg/dL, and relief of symptoms with the administration of glucose. Patients will often present with a profound syncopal episode and will admit to similar less severe episodes in the recent past. They also may admit to palpitations, trembling, diaphoresis, confusion or obtundation, and seizure, and family members may report that the patient has undergone a personality change. Routine laboratory studies will uncover a low blood sugar, the cause of all of these symptoms. (See Schwartz 8th ed., p 1274.)

8. Treatment of a 1-cm gastrinoma in the wall of the duodenum is best accomplished by
   A. Enucleation
   B. Full-thickness resection
   C. Duodenectomy
   D. Whipple procedure

**Answer: B**

Fifty percent of gastrinomas metastasize to lymph nodes or the liver, and are therefore considered malignant. Patients who meet criteria for operability should undergo exploration for possible removal of the tumor. Although the tumors are submucosal, a full-thickness excision of the duodenal wall is performed if a duodenal gastrinoma is found. All lymph nodes in Passaro's triangle are excised for pathologic analysis. If the gastrinoma is found in the pancreas and does not involve the main pancreatic duct, it is enucleated. Pancreatic resection is justified for solitary gastrinomas with no metastases. A highly-selective vagotomy can be performed if unresectable disease is identified or if the gastrinoma cannot be localized. This may reduce the amount of expensive proton pump inhibitors required. In cases in which hepatic metastases are identified, resection is justified if the primary gastrinoma is controlled and the metastases can be safely and completely removed. Debulking or incomplete removal of multiple hepatic metastases is probably not helpful, especially in the setting of multiple endocrine neoplasia (MEN-1). The application of new modalities such as radiofrequency ablation seems reasonable, but data to support this approach are limited. Postoperatively, patients are followed with fasting serum gastrin levels, secretin stimulation tests, octreotide scans, and computed tomography (CT) scans. In patients found to have inoperable disease, chemotherapy with streptozocin, doxorubicin, and 5-fluorouracil is used. Other approaches such as somatostatin analogs, interferon, and chemoembolization also have been used in gastrinoma with some success. (See Schwartz 8th ed., p 1276.)

9.  The majority of gastrinomas are found in which of the following?
    A.  Triangle of Calot
    B.  Passaro's triangle
    C.  Body of the pancreas
    D.  Tail of the pancreas

**Answer: B**

In 70 to 90% of patients, the primary gastrinoma is found in Passaro's triangle, an area defined by a triangle with points located at the junction of the cystic duct and common bile duct, the second and third portion of the duodenum, and the neck and body of the pancreas (Fig. 32-66). However, since gastrinomas can be found almost anywhere, whole-body imaging is required. The test of choice is somatostatin receptor (octreotide) scintigraphy in combination with computed tomography (CT) (Fig. 32-67). The octreotide scan is more sensitive than CT, locating about 85% of gastrinomas and detecting tumors smaller than 1 cm. With the octreotide scan, the need for tedious and technically demanding selective angiography and measurement of gastrin gradients has declined. Endoscopic ultrasound is another new modality that assists in the preoperative localization of gastrinomas. It is particularly helpful in localizing tumors in the pancreatic head or duodenal wall, where gastrinomas are usually less than 1 cm in size. A combination of octreotide scan and endoscopic ultrasound (EUS) detects more than 90% of gastrinomas. (See Schwartz 8th ed., p 1275.)

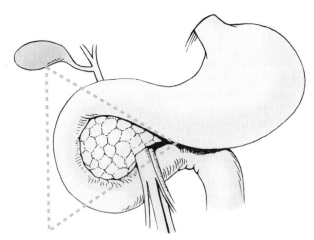

**FIG. 32-1.**   *Passaro's triangle. The typical location of a gastrinoma is described by this anatomic region, including the head of the pancreas, duodenum, and the lymphatic bed posterior and superior to the duodenum, as originally described by E. Passaro. (Reproduced with permission from Bell.) (See Schwartz 8th ed., p 1275.)*

10. Which of the following findings on physical examination in a diabetic patient should raise concern for a glucagonoma?
    A. Acanthosis nigricans
    B. Dermatitis
    C. Café au lait spots
    D. Axillary freckles

**Answer: B**
Diabetes in association with dermatitis should raise the suspicion of a glucagonoma. The diabetes usually is mild. The classic necrolytic migratory erythema manifests as cyclic migrations of lesions with spreading margins and healing centers typically on the lower abdomen, perineum, perioral area, and feet. The diagnosis is confirmed by measuring serum glucagon levels, which are usually over 500 pg/mL. Glucagon is a catabolic hormone and most patients present with malnutrition. The rash associated with glucagonoma is thought to be caused by low levels of amino acids. Preoperative treatment usually includes control of the diabetes, parenteral nutrition, and octreotide. Like vasoactive intestinal peptide-producing tumors (VIPomas), glucagonomas are more often in the body and tail of the pancreas and tend to be large tumors with metastases. Again, debulking operations are recommended in good operative candidates to relieve symptoms. (See Schwartz 8th ed., p 1276.)

11. When a patient is admitted with acute pancreatitis, signs present on admission or development within 48 h indicating poor prognosis include all of the following EXCEPT
    A. Serum amylase, 3500 U/L
    B. Change in blood urea nitrogen from 20 mg/dL to 30 mg/dL
    C. Change in hematocrit from 42% to 30%
    D. Leukocyte count, 25,000/mm$^3$

**Answer: A**
A very high-serum amylase level indicates a pancreas that is functional enough to respond to insult, and this change does not indicate a bad prognosis. Low arterial $Po_2$ and elevated leukocyte count are poor prognostic signs. A rise in blood urea nitrogen and a fall in hematocrit are ominous findings. Disease in a patient older than 55 years of age and a rising base deficit also are poor signs. (See Schwartz 7th ed.)

12. During abdominal exploration after an automobile accident, a deep laceration across the body of the pancreas with disruption of the pancreatic duct is discovered. The appropriate method of managing this injury is to carry out external drainage and
    A. A direct repair of the duct
    B. A distal pancreatectomy
    C. Implantation of the pancreas into the posterior wall of the stomach
    D. Lateral pancreaticojejunostomy

**Answer: B**
Minor injuries can be treated by débridement and drainage. This is not appropriate where duct injury is present. Lateral pancreaticojejunostomy is effective management for pain from chronic pancreatitis, but it is not appropriate when extensive tissue damage is present. (See Schwartz 7th ed.)

13. Symptoms and signs exhibited by a patient with a tumor secreting vasoactive intestinal polypeptide (VIP) include all of the following EXCEPT
    A. Diarrhea unresponsive to antidiarrheal agents
    B. Diarrhea that persists during fasting
    C. Hypokalemia
    D. Severe metabolic alkalosis

**Answer: D**
The patient with a vasoactive intestinal peptide-producing tumor (VIPoma), a pancreatic islet tumor, exhibits all of the listed symptoms except metabolic alkalosis. Severe metabolic acidosis occurs because of loss of bicarbonate in the stool. (See Schwartz 7th ed.)

14. To differentiate pancreatic ascites from ascites secondary to cirrhosis of the liver, the most important test is
    A. Abdominal paracentesis
    B. Computed tomography scan
    C. Endoscopic retrograde cholangiopancreatography
    D. Percutaneous transhepatic cholangiography

**Answer: A**
Pancreatic ascites usually occurs in male alcoholics, and confusion with ascites secondary to cirrhosis may be a problem. Paracentesis is diagnostic, returning fluid with a high protein content (>3 g/100 mL) and an amylase concentration greater than the serum amylase. The other tests listed may demonstrate the amount of fluid present or show ductal anatomy, but no other test defines pancreatic ascites as well as examination of the ascitic fluid. (See Schwartz 7th ed.)

15. In a patient suspected of having a pancreatic pseudo-cyst, the finding that suggests a cystadenoma is
    A. Calcification within the cyst
    B. Generalized weakness
    C. Severe anorexia
    D. Vague abdominal discomfort

**Answer: A**

The other symptoms can develop with either a pancreatic pseudocyst or a cystadenoma, but calcification within the sac on radiologic examination is unusual with a pseudocyst. Whenever a patient with a pseudocyst undergoes operation, the lining of the cyst should be inspected and biopsied to rule out an adenoma or an adenocarcinoma. (See Schwartz 7th ed.)

16. All of the following surgical procedures are appropriate for a patient who has a pseudocyst of the head of the pancreas EXCEPT
    A. Cystoduodenostomy
    B. Cystogastrostomy
    C. Removal of the involved segment of the pancreas
    D. Simple external drainage

**Answer: C**

Although simple external drainage is thought to be a poor choice for treatment of most patients who have uninfected pseudocysts, in patients who have evidence of infection or who are extremely ill but in whom a more extensive procedure might endanger life, external drainage is the treatment of choice. Internal drainage by means of cystogastrostomy, cystojejunostomy, or cystoduodenostomy, depending on the location of the cysts, can provide appropriate treatment for most pseudocysts. Removal of the head of the pancreas for a cyst is never indicated, as such an undertaking would necessitate a Whipple procedure; only the unusual, very small pseudocyst situated in the distal pancreas and unattached to vital structures lends itself in actuality to extirpation. Thus, in the vast majority of cases, removal of cysts is not practical, and adequate internal drainage of some type provides the best treatment. (See Schwartz 7th ed.)

17. The greatest effect of pancreatic insufficiency is decreased absorption of
    A. Calcium
    B. Carbohydrate
    C. Fat
    D. Fat-soluble vitamins

**Answer: C**

Pancreatic lipolytic hormones, such as lipase, are important in fat absorption. Protein digestion is aided by gastric pepsin and carbohydrate digestion by salivary amylase. Fat-soluble vitamins and calcium do not require pancreatic enzymes for absorption. (See Schwartz 7th ed.)

18. Pancreatography is performed on a 54-year-old alcoholic patient who has chronic pancreatitis. The study shows a "chain of lakes" pattern, with areas of ductal dilatation joined by areas of ductal stenosis. The patient's surgeon should
    A. Perform a cholecystectomy with exploration of the common bile duct
    B. Perform a cholecystectomy with sphincteroplasty
    C. Open the pancreatic duct longitudinally and perform a side-to-side pancreaticojejunostomy
    D. Resect the tail of the pancreas and perform a pancreaticojejunostomy

**Answer: C**

Areas of ductal dilatation alternating with areas of ductal stenosis are common findings in alcoholic patients who have severe chronic pancreatitis. Although gallstones frequently may be present, performing only a cholecystectomy and exploration of the common bile duct will not aid pancreatic drainage in these patients. Similarly, this type of duct obstruction cannot be relieved by a sphincteroplasty because of the multiple areas of stenosis along the duct, and resecting the tail of the pancreas and performing a Roux-en-Y anastomosis between the pancreatic duct and the jejunum would not be helpful. Although total pancreatectomy would be a beneficial approach, mortality and morbidity rate with this procedure are extremely high. Thus, the procedure of choice for the patient presented in the question should be a side-to-side pancreaticojejunostomy, in which the duct is opened longitudinally through the "chain of lakes." A Roux-en-Y limb of jejunum should then be brought up for anastomosis with the opened pancreas in side-to-side fashion, with either a one- or two-layer closure. If a two-layer closure is used, the inner layer is a mucosal anastomosis. (See Schwartz 7th ed.)

1. Which of the following is NOT a location where accessory spleens can be found?
   A. Gastrocolic ligament
   B. Gerota's fascia
   C. Large bowel mesentery
   D. Broad ligament

**Answer: B**
The most common anomaly of splenic embryology is the accessory spleen. Present in up to 20% of the population, one or more accessory spleen(s) may occur in up to 30% of patients with hematologic disease. Over 80% of accessory spleens are found in the region of the splenic hilum and vascular pedicle. Other locations for accessory spleens in descending order of frequency are: the gastrocolic ligament, the tail of the pancreas, the greater omentum, the greater curve of the stomach, the splenocolic ligament, the small and large bowel mesentery, the left broad ligament in women, and the left spermatic cord in men. (See Schwartz 8th ed., p 1297.)

2. Which of the following splenic ligaments is NOT an avascular plane?
   A. Gastrosplenic
   B. Splenocolic
   C. Phrenosplenic
   D. Splenorenal

**Answer: A**
Of particular clinical relevance, the spleen is suspended in position by several ligaments and peritoneal folds to the colon (splenocolic ligament); the stomach (gastrosplenic ligament); the diaphragm (phrenosplenic ligament); and the kidney, adrenal gland, and tail of the pancreas (splenorenal ligament) (Fig. 33-2). Whereas the gastrosplenic ligament contains the short gastric vessels, the remaining ligaments are usually avascular, with rare exceptions, such as in a patient with portal hypertension. The relationship of the pancreas to the spleen also has important clinical implications. In cadaveric anatomic series, the tail of the pancreas has been demonstrated to lie within 1 cm of the splenic hilum 75% of the time and to actually abut the spleen in 30% of patients. (See Schwartz 8th ed., p 1298.)

3. Which of the following is NOT produced in significant amounts by the spleen?
   A. Tuftsin
   B. Immunoglobulin A (IgA)
   C. Properdin
   D. Opsonic antibodies

**Answer: B**
The spleen plays a significant though not indispensable role in host defense, contributing to both humoral and cell-mediated immunity. As discussed in the previous section [see Schwartz, 8th ed., Embryology and Anatomy, pp. 1297–99], antigens are filtered in the white pulp and presented to immunocompetent centers within the lymphoid follicles. This gives rise to the elaboration of immunoglobulins (predominantly IgM). Following an antigen challenge, such an acute IgM response results in the release of opsonic antibodies from the white pulp of the spleen. Clearance of the antigen by the splenic and hepatic reticuloendothelial (RE) systems is then facilitated.

The spleen also produces the opsonins, tuftsin, and properdin. Tuftsin, a likely stimulant to general phagocytic function in the host, appears to specifically facilitate clearance of bacteria. It is circulating monocytes that are converted into fixed macrophages with the red pulp that account for the remarkable phagocytic activity of the spleen.

The spleen also appears to be a major source of the protein properdin, which is important in the initiation of the alternate pathway of complement activation. The splenic RE system is better able to clear bacteria that are poorly or inadequately opsonized from the circulation than is the hepatic RE system. Encapsulated bacteria generally fit such a profile, hence the risk posed by pneumococcus and *Haemophilus influenzae* to an asplenic patient. There appears to be sufficient physiologic capacity within the complement cascade to withstand the loss of tuftsin and properdin production without increasing patient vulnerability postsplenectomy. (See Schwartz 8th ed., p 1300.)

4. The initial treatment of autoimmune hemolytic anemia (AIHA) is
   A. Observation and transfusion
   B. Corticosteroids
   C. Splenic embolization
   D. Splenectomy

**Answer: B**
Treatment of AIHA depends on how severe it is and whether it is primary or secondary. Severe anemia (<4 g/dL), causing pulmonary edema, tachycardia, postural hypotension, dyspnea, and angina, demands red blood cell transfusion. Corticosteroids act as the mainstay of treatment for both primary and secondary forms of symptomatic, unstable AIHA. A dose of 1 to 2 mg/kg per day in divided doses is sufficient to start, and therapy should last until a response is noted by a rise in hematocrit and fall in reticulocyte count, which generally occurs within 3 weeks. Steroid therapy is more successful in producing a durable remission in children than in adults. Splenectomy is indicated for failure to respond to steroids, intolerance of steroid side effects, requirement for excessive steroid doses to maintain remission, or inability to receive steroids for other reasons. A favorable response to splenectomy can be expected in up to 80% of patients with warm-antibody AIHA. (See Schwartz 8th ed., p 1301.)

5. Which of the following proteins is not altered in hereditary spherocytosis (HS)?
   A. Pyruvate kinase
   B. Spectrin
   C. Ankyrin
   D. Band 3 protein

**Answer: A**
The underlying abnormality in HS is an inherited dysfunction or deficiency in one of the erythrocyte membrane proteins (spectrin, ankyrin, band 3 protein, or protein 4.2), which results in destabilization of the membrane lipid bilayer. This destabilization allows a release of lipids from the membrane, causing a reduction in membrane surface area and a lack of deformability, leading to sequestration and destruction of the spherocytic erythrocytes in the spleen.

Although less common than glucose-6-phosphate dehydrogenase (G6PD) deficiency overall, pyruvate kinase deficiency is the most common red blood cell enzyme deficiency to cause congenital chronic hemolytic anemia. (See Schwartz 8th ed., p 1302.)

6. The mortality rate of recurrent splenic sequestration in a patient with sickle cell anemia is
   A. 5%
   B. 20%
   C. 45%
   D. 70%

**Answer: B**
Sequestration occurs in the spleen with resultant splenomegaly early in the course of the disease. In most patients subsequent infarction of the spleen and autosplenectomy occur at some later time. The most frequent indications for splenectomy among patients with sickle cell disease are hyper-

splenism and acute sequestration crises, followed by splenic abscess. The occurrence of one major acute sequestration crisis, characterized by rapid painful enlargement of the spleen and circulatory collapse, is generally considered sufficient grounds for splenectomy, as subsequent attacks occur in 40 to 50% of patients, with a mortality rate of 20%. The incidence of acute sequestration crises is about 5% in children with sickle cell disease. Approximately 3% of children with sickle cell disease ultimately require splenectomy. Preoperative preparation includes special attention to adequate hydration and avoidance of hypothermia. (See Schwartz 8th ed., p 1302.)

7. Which of the following is an indication for splenectomy in a patient with thalassemia?
   A. >50 mL/kg year transfusion requirement
   B. Discomfort due to splenomegaly
   C. Recurrent sequestration crises
   D. Iron overload from transfusions

**Answer: B**
Treatment for thalassemia consists of red blood cell transfusions to keep the hemoglobin count greater than 9 mg/dL, along with intensive parenteral chelation therapy with deferoxamine. Splenectomy is indicated for patients with excessive transfusion requirements (>200 mL/kg per year), discomfort due to splenomegaly, or painful splenic infarction. A careful assessment of the risk:benefit ratio for splenectomy is essential, since infectious morbidity following splenectomy in patients with thalassemia is greater than in other patients undergoing splenectomy for hematologic indications. This increase in infectious complications is likely due to coexisting immune deficiency, precipitated in large part by iron overload associated both with thalassemia itself and transfusions. When indicated, in rare circumstances splenectomy should be delayed until absolutely necessary, if possible after the age of 4 years. (See Schwartz 8th ed., p 1303.)

8. Which of the following is appropriate initial therapy in a patient diagnosis with glucose-6-phosphate dehydrogenase (G6PD) deficiency?
   A. Total splenectomy
   B. Partial splenectomy
   C. Exchange transfusion
   D. Dietary counseling

**Answer: D**
G6PD is an enzyme that reduces nicotinamide adenine dinucleotide phosphate (NADP) to NADP plus hydrogen (NADPH) in the glutathione pathway. This helps to maintain the balance of reduced to oxidized glutathione and protects the red blood cell from oxidative damage. Depending on the variant of G6PD deficiency, the clinical manifestation may be chronic hemolytic anemia, acute intermittent hemolytic episodes, or no hemolysis. Although hundreds of millions of people worldwide are affected by G6PD deficiency, most experience only moderate health risks and no reduction in longevity. The diagnosis is established either by a fluorescent screening test or by spectrophotometric analysis of enzyme activity. Therapy consists of avoidance of drugs known to precipitate hemolysis in G6PD patients and transfusions in cases of symptomatic anemia. Splenectomy is not indicated in this disease. (See Schwartz 8th ed., p 1303.)

9. Which of the following is an indication for splenectomy in a patient with chronic myelogenous leukemia (CML)?
   A. Failure of chemotherapy to decrease splenomegaly
   B. Sequestration requiring transfusion
   C. Symptomatic relief of early satiety
   D. Presence of *bcr* gene mutation

**Answer: C**
CML is a disorder of the primitive pluripotent stem cell in the bone marrow, resulting in a significant increase in erythroid, megakaryotic, and pluripotent progenitors in the peripheral blood smear. The genetic hallmark is a transposition between the *bcr* gene on chromosome 9 and the *abl* gene on chromosome 22. CML accounts for 7 to 15% of all

leukemias, with an incidence of 1.5 in 100,000 in the United States. CML is frequently asymptomatic in the chronic phase, but symptomatic patients often present with the gradual onset of fatigue, anorexia, sweating, and left upper quadrant pain and early satiety secondary to splenomegaly. Enlargement of the spleen is found in roughly one half of patients with CML. Splenectomy is indicated to ease pain and early satiety. (See Schwartz 8th ed., p 1303.)

10. Patients with essential thrombocythemia present with
    A. Vasomotor symptoms
    B. Spontaneous mucosal bleeding
    C. Massive splenomegaly
    D. Lower extremity ulceration

**Answer: A**

Essential thrombocythemia (ET) represents abnormal growth of the megakaryocyte cell line, resulting in increased levels of platelets in the bloodstream. The diagnosis is made after the exclusion of other chronic myeloid disorders, such as chronic myelogenous leukemia (CML), polycythemia vera (PV), and myelofibrosis, that may also present with thrombocytosis. Clinical manifestations of ET include vasomotor symptoms, thrombohemorrhagic events, recurrent fetal loss, and the transformation to myelofibrosis with myeloid metaplasia or acute myeloid leukemia. Hydroxyurea reduces thrombotic events in high-risk patients, but does not alter transformation to myelofibrosis or leukemia. Splenomegaly occurs in one third to one half of patients with ET, and its presence may help to distinguish essential from secondary thrombocytosis. Splenectomy is not felt to be helpful in the early stages of ET, and is best reserved for the later stages of disease, in which myeloid metaplasia has developed. Even in these circumstances, candidates should be chosen selectively, since significant bleeding has been reported to complicate splenectomy. (See Schwartz 8th ed., p 1304.)

11. Which of the following is an indication for splenectomy in polycythemia vera?
    A. Failure of aspirin to prevent thrombotic complications
    B. Frequent need for phlebotomy
    C. Symptoms related to splenomegaly
    D. Prevention of progression to myeloid metaplasia

**Answer: C**

Polycythemia vera (PV) is a clonal, chronic, progressive myeloproliferative disorder characterized by an increase in red blood cell mass, frequently accompanied by leukocytosis, thrombocytosis, and splenomegaly. Patients affected by PV typically enjoy prolonged survival compared to others affected by hematologic malignancies, but remain at risk for transformation to myelofibrosis or acute myeloid leukemia (AML). The disease is rare, with an annual incidence of 5 to 17 cases per million population. Although the diagnosis may be discovered by routine screening laboratory tests in asymptomatic individuals, affected patients may present with any number of nonspecific complaints, including headache, dizziness, weakness, pruritus, visual disturbances, excessive sweating, joint symptoms, and weight loss. Physical findings include ruddy cyanosis, conjunctival plethora, hepatomegaly, splenomegaly, and hypertension. The diagnosis is established by an elevated red blood cell mass (>25% of mean predicted value), thrombocytosis, leukocytosis, normal arterial oxygen saturation in the presence of increased red blood cell mass, splenomegaly, low serum erythropoietin (EPO) stores, and bone marrow hypercellularity. Treatment should be tailored to the risk status of the patient and ranges from phlebotomy and aspirin to chemotherapeutic agents. As in ET, splenectomy is not helpful in the early stages of disease and is best reserved for late-stage patients in whom myeloid metaplasia has developed and splenomegaly-related symptoms are severe. (See Schwartz 8th ed., p 1304.)

12. The most common physical finding in a patient with hairy cell leukemia (HCL) is
    A. Massive splenomegaly
    B. Shortness of breath
    C. Abdominal pain
    D. Joint pain

**Answer: A**
HCL is an uncommon blood disorder, representing only 2% of all adult leukemias. HCL is characterized by splenomegaly, pancytopenia, and large numbers of abnormal lymphocytes in the bone marrow. These lymphocytes contain irregular hair-like cytoplasmic projections identifiable on the peripheral smear. Most patients seek medical attention because of symptoms related to anemia, neutropenia, thrombocytopenia, or splenomegaly. The most common physical finding is splenomegaly, which occurs in 80% of patients with HCL and is often palpable 5 cm below the costal margin. Many patients with HCL have few symptoms and require no specific therapy. Treatment is indicated for those with moderate to severe symptoms related to cytopenias, such as repeated infections or bleeding episodes, or to splenomegaly, such as pain or early satiety. Splenectomy does not correct the underlying disorder, but does return cell counts to normal in 40 to 70% of patients and alleviates pain and early satiety. Newer chemotherapeutic agents (the purine analogues 2′-deoxycoformycin [2′-DCF] and 2-chlorodeoxyadenosine [2-CdA]) are able to induce durable complete remission in most patients. (See Schwartz 8th ed., p 1305.)

13. In patients with immune thrombocytopenic purpura who successfully respond to steroids, a response is seen
    A. Within 2 days of starting therapy
    B. Within 3 weeks of starting therapy
    C. Within 3 months of starting therapy
    D. Within 6 months of starting therapy

**Answer: B**
Adults generally require treatment at the time of presentation, since up to one half will present with counts below 10,000/mm$^3$. The usual first line of therapy is oral prednisone at a dose of 1.0 to 1.5 mg/kg per day. No consensus exists as to the optimal duration of steroid therapy, but most responses occur within the first 3 weeks. Response rates range from 50 to 75%, but relapses are common. Intravenous immunoglobulin, given at 1.0 g/kg per day for 2 to 3 days, is indicated for internal bleeding when counts remain below 5000/mm$^3$ or when extensive purpura exists. Intravenous immunoglobulin is thought to impair clearance of immunoglobulin G (IgG)-coated platelets by competing for binding to tissue macrophage receptors. An immediate response is common, but a sustained remission is not. Splenectomy is indicated for failure of medical therapy, for prolonged use of steroids with undesirable effects, or for most cases of first relapse. Prolonged use of steroids can be defined in various ways, but a persistent need for more than 10 to 20 mg/d for 3 to 6 months in order to maintain a platelet count above 30,000/mm$^3$ generally prompts referral for splenectomy. Splenectomy provides a permanent response without subsequent need for steroids in 75 to 85% of the total number of patients undergoing splenectomy [see

Schwartz 8th ed., Splenectomy Outcomes, p 1311]. Responses usually occur within the first postoperative week. Patients with extremely low platelet counts (<10,000/mm$^3$) should have platelets available for surgery, but should not receive them preoperatively. Once the splenic pedicle is ligated, platelets are given to those who continue to bleed. (See Schwartz 8th ed., p 1306.)

14. The treatment of choice for splenic abscess is
    A. Antibiotics alone
    B. Percutaneous drainage
    C. Partial splenectomy
    D. Total splenectomy

**Answer: D**
Abscesses of the spleen are uncommon, with an incidence of 0.14 to 0.7%, based on autopsy findings. They occur more frequently in tropical locations, where they are associated with thrombosed splenic vessels and infarction in patients with sickle cell anemia. Five distinct mechanisms of splenic abscess formation have been described: (1) hematogenous infection; (2) contiguous infection; (3) hemoglobinopathy; (4) immunosuppression, including human immunodeficiency virus (HIV) and chemotherapy; and (5) trauma. The most common origins for hematogenous spread are infective endocarditis, typhoid fever, malaria, urinary tract infections, and osteomyelitis. Presentation is frequently delayed, with most patients enduring symptoms for 16 to 22 days prior to diagnosis. Clinical manifestations include fever, left upper quadrant pain, leukocytosis, and splenomegaly in about one third of patients. The diagnosis is confirmed by ultrasound or computed tomography (CT) scan, which has a 95% sensitivity and specificity. Upon discovery of a splenic abscess, broad-spectrum antibiotics should be started, with adjustment to more specific therapy based on culture results, and continued for 14 days. Splenectomy is the operation of choice, but percutaneous or open drainage are options for patients who cannot tolerate splenectomy. Percutaneous drainage is successful for patients with unilocular disease. (See Schwartz 8th ed., p 1307.)

15. Which of the following is NOT part of the triad seen with Felty's syndrome?
    A. Rheumatoid arthritis
    B. Splenomegaly
    C. Neutropenia
    D. Thrombocytopenia

**Answer: D**
The triad of rheumatoid arthritis (RA), splenomegaly, and neutropenia is called Felty's syndrome. It exists in approximately 3% of all patients with RA, two thirds of which are women. Immune complexes coat the surface of white blood cells, leading to their sequestration and clearance in the spleen with subsequent neutropenia. This neutropenia (<2000/mm$^3$) increases the risk for recurrent infections and often drives the decision for splenectomy. The size of the spleen is variable, from nonpalpable in 5 to 10% of patients, to massive enlargement in others. The spleen in Felty's syndrome is four times heavier than normal. Corticosteroids, hematopoietic growth factors, methotrexate, and splenectomy have all been used to treat the neutropenia of Felty's syndrome. Responses to splenectomy have been excellent, with over 80% of patients showing a durable increase in white blood cell count. More than one half of patients who had infections prior to surgery did not have any infections after splenectomy. Besides symptomatic neutropenia, other indications for splenectomy include transfusion-dependent anemia and profound thrombocytopenia. (See Schwartz 8th ed., p 1307.)

16. Which of the following is the most common etiology of splenic cyst worldwide?
    A. Bacterial infection
    B. Trauma
    C. Parasitic infection
    D. Congenital anomaly

**Answer: C**
Splenic cysts are rare lesions. The most common etiology for splenic cysts worldwide is parasitic infestation, particularly echinococcal. Symptomatic parasitic cysts are best treated with splenectomy, though selected cases may be amenable to percutaneous aspiration, instillation of protoscolicidal agent, and reaspiration. Nonparasitic cysts most commonly result from trauma and are called pseudocysts; however, dermoid, epidermoid, and epithelial cysts have been reported as well. The treatment of nonparasitic cysts depends on whether or not they produce symptoms. Asymptomatic nonparasitic cysts may be observed with close ultrasound follow-up to exclude significant expansion. Patients should be advised of the risk of cyst rupture with even minor abdominal trauma if they elect nonoperative management for large cysts. Small symptomatic nonparasitic cysts may be excised with splenic preservation, and large symptomatic nonparasitic cysts may be unroofed. Both of these operations may be performed laparoscopically. (See Schwartz 8th ed., p 1307.)

17. Which of the following is an indication for surgical treatment of a splenic aneurysm?
    A. Pregnancy
    B. Size >1.5 cm
    C. History of thrombocytopenia
    D. History of neutropenia

**Answer: A**
Although rare, splenic artery aneurysm (SAA) is the most common visceral artery aneurysm. Women are four times more likely to be affected than men. The aneurysm usually arises in the middle to distal portion of the splenic artery. The risk of rupture is between 3 and 9%; however, once rupture occurs, mortality is substantial (35 to 50%). According to a recent series, mortality is significantly higher in patients with underlying portal hypertension (>50%) than in those without it (17%). SAA is particularly worrisome when discovered during pregnancy, as rupture imparts a high risk of mortality to both mother (70%) and fetus (95%). Most patients are asymptomatic and seek medical attention based on an incidental radiographic finding. About 20% of patients with SAA have symptoms of left upper quadrant pain. Indications for treatment include presence of symptoms, pregnancy, intention to become pregnant, and pseudoaneurysms associated with inflammatory processes. For asymptomatic patients, size greater than 2 cm constitutes an indication for surgery. Aneurysm resection or ligation alone is acceptable for amenable lesions in the mid-splenic artery, but distal lesions in close proximity to the splenic hilum should be treated with concomitant splenectomy. An excellent prognosis follows elective treatment. Splenic artery embolization has been used to treat SAA, but painful splenic infarction and abscess may follow. (See Schwartz 8th ed., p 1308.)

18. The ideal time to give immunizations to patients undergoing elective splenectomy is
    A. A least 2 months before surgery
    B. At least 2 weeks before surgery
    C. In the holding area just prior to surgery
    D. On the day of discharge from the hospital after splenectomy

**Answer: B**
Splenectomy imparts a small (<1 to 5%) but definite lifetime risk of fulminant, potentially life-threatening infection [see Schwartz 8th ed., Overwhelming Postsplenectomy Infections, p 1312]. Therefore, when elective splenectomy is planned, vaccinations against encapsulated bacteria should be given at least 2 weeks before surgery to protect against

such infection. The most common bacteria to cause serious infections in asplenic hosts are *Streptococcus pneumoniae*, *Haemophilus influenzae* type B, and meningococcus. Vaccinations are available for these bacteria and should be given. Other potential infectious bacterial sources include group A streptococci, *Capnocytophaga canimorsus* (related to dog bites), group B streptococci, *Enterococcus* species, *Bacteroides* species, *Salmonella* species, and *Bartonella* species.

If the spleen is removed emergently (e.g., for trauma), vaccinations should be given as soon as possible following surgery, allowing at least 1 to 2 days for recovery. Booster injections of pneumococcal vaccine should be considered every 5 to 6 years regardless of the reason for splenectomy. In addition, annual influenza immunization is advisable. Splenectomized patients should maintain ongoing documentation and communication of immunization status. (See Schwartz 8th ed., p 1308.)

19. The lifetime risk of overwhelming post-splenectomy infection (OPSI) is approximately
    A. 1–5%
    B. 5–10%
    C. 15–20%
    D. 20–25%

**Answer: A**

Regardless of technique or indication, splenectomy imparts a lifetime risk of severe infection to the patient. The true incidence of postsplenectomy sepsis remains unknown, with estimates varying between less than 1 and 5% during a patient's lifetime. A 30-year review of the relevant literature in English (1966–96) revealed an incidence of 3.2%. Although the incidence of postsplenectomy infection was similar among children and adults, the mortality rate was higher for children (1.7 vs. 1.3%). The incidence and mortality rates were highest for patients with underlying hematologic conditions, such as thalassemia major (8.2% incidence rate and 5.1% mortality rate) and sickle cell disease (7.3% incidence rate and 4.8% mortality rate). However, much of the literature reporting OPSI and morbidity rates includes years before the widespread implementation of vaccinations, which occurred in the late 1970s and early 1980s. Substantial decreases in the incidence of OPSI among splenectomized children have been reported following the implementation of pneumococcal vaccine. (See Schwartz 8th ed., p 1312.)

# CHAPTER 34

# Abdominal Wall, Omentum, Mesentery, and Retroperitoneum

1. Persistence of the vitelline duct can lead to which of the following?
   A. Colonic diverticulum
   B. Urachal cyst
   C. Umbilical cord hernia
   D. Omphalomesenteric duct cyst

**Answer: D**

During the third trimester, the vitelline duct regresses. Persistence of a vitelline duct remnant on the ileal border results in a *Meckel's diverticulum*. Complete failure of the vitelline duct to regress results in a *vitelline duct fistula*, which is associated with drainage of small intestinal contents from the umbilicus. If both the intestinal and umbilical ends of the vitelline duct regress into fibrous cords, a central *vitelline duct (omphalomesenteric) cyst* may occur. Persistent vitelline duct remnants between the gastrointestinal tract and the anterior abdominal wall may be associated with small intestinal volvulus in neonates. When diagnosed, vitelline duct fistulas and cysts should be excised along with any accompanying fibrous cord. (See Schwartz 8th ed., p 1320.)

2. The appropriate treatment of rectus abdominis diastasis is
   A. Observation
   B. Resection and primary repair
   C. Reefing
   D. Patch repair

**Answer: A**

Rectus abdominis diastasis (or diastasis recti) describes a clinically evident separation of the rectus abdominus muscle pillars, generally as a result of decreased tone of the abdominal musculature. The characteristic bulging of the abdominal wall in the epigastrium is sometimes mistaken for a ventral hernia, despite the fact that the midline aponeurosis is intact and no hernia defect is present. Diastasis may be congenital, as a result of a more lateral insertion of the rectus muscles to the ribs and costochondral junctions, but is more typically an acquired condition with advancing age, obesity, or following pregnancy. In the postpartum setting, rectus diastasis tends to occur in women of advanced maternal age, after multiple or twin pregnancies, or in women who deliver high-birth-weight infants. Diastasis is usually easily identified on physical examination (Fig. 34-6). Computed tomography (CT) scanning provides an accurate means of measuring the distance between the rectus pillars and will differentiate rectus diastasis from a true ventral hernia if clarification is required. Surgical correction of a severe rectus diastasis by plication of the anterior rectus sheath may be undertaken for cosmetic indications, or if it is associated with disability of abdominal wall muscular function. (See Schwartz 8th ed., p 1320.)

3. Spigelian hernias occur
   A. On the lateral border of the rectus abdominis
   B. In the linea alba
   C. In the medial wall of the inguinal canal
   D. In the femoral triangle

**Answer: A**

*Spigelian* hernias can occur anywhere along the length of the Spigelian line or zone—an aponeurotic band of variable width at the lateral border of the rectus abdominus. However, the most frequent location of these rare hernias is at or slightly above the level of the arcuate line. These are not always clinically evident as a bulge, and may come to medical attention because of pain or incarceration. (See Schwartz 8th ed., p 1321.)

4. The blood supply to the omentum is
   A. Left gastroepiploic artery
   B. Left gastric artery
   C. Splenic artery
   D. Middle colic artery

**Answer: A**
The blood supply to the greater omentum is derived from the right and left gastroepiploic arteries. The venous drainage parallels the arterial supply to a great extent with the left and right gastroepiploic veins ultimately draining into the portal system. (See Schwartz 8th ed., p 1322.)

5. Which of the following statements concerning omental infarction is true?
   A. Patients present with nausea and vomiting.
   B. Most cases are diagnosed preoperatively by ultrasound or computed tomography scan.
   C. Most cases do not require surgery.
   D. Surgical resection is indicated in all cases.

**Answer: C**
Patients typically present with localized right lower quadrant, right upper quadrant, or left lower quadrant pain. Although a mild degree of nausea may be present, patients do not usually have concomitant intestinal symptoms. Physical examination typically reveals a mild tachycardia and a low-grade temperature elevation. Abdominal examination may demonstrate a tender, palpable mass associated with guarding and rebound tenderness. The diagnosis is rarely made before abdominal imaging studies are obtained. Either abdominal computed tomography or ultrasonography will show a localized, inflammatory mass of fat density. Treatment of omental infarction depends on the certainty with which the diagnosis is made. In patients who are not toxic and whose abdominal imaging is convincing, supportive care is sufficient. However, many cases will be indistinguishable from suppurative appendicitis, cholecystitis, or diverticulitis. In these instances, laparoscopy has provided a great advance, providing access to an accurate diagnosis as well as treatment. Resection of the infarcted tissue results in rapid resolution of symptoms. (See Schwartz 8th ed., p 1323.)

6. The most common presenting symptom in patients with sclerosing mesenteritis is
   A. Obstipation
   B. Vomiting
   C. Pain
   D. Fever

**Answer: C**
Sclerosing mesenteritis, also referred to as mesenteric panniculitis or mesenteric lipodystrophy, is a rare chronic inflammatory and fibrotic process that involves a portion of the intestinal mesentery. There is no gender or race predominance, but sclerosing mesenteritis is most commonly diagnosed in individuals older than 50 years of age.

The etiology of this process is unknown, but its cardinal features are a nonneoplastic mesenteric mass and varying relative quantities of fibrosis and chronic inflammation on histologic examination. The mass may be up to 40 cm in diameter. Accordingly, patients typically present with symptoms of a mass lesion. Abdominal pain is the most frequent presenting symptom, followed by the presence of a nonpainful mass or intestinal obstruction.

Computed tomography (CT) of the abdomen will verify the presence of a mass lesion emanating from the mesentery. CT cannot distinguish sclerosing mesenteritis from a primary or secondary mesenteric tumor (Fig. 34-10). Surgical intervention is usually necessary, if only to establish a diagnosis and rule out malignancy (Fig. 34-11). The extent of the disease process dictates the aggressiveness of the intervention, which may range from simple biopsy, to bowel and mesentery resection, to colostomy (in the cases of colonic obstruction). (See Schwartz 8th ed., pp 1323–24.)

7. The primary treatment for retroperitoneal fibrosis is
   A. Corticosteroids
   B. Cyclosporine
   C. Radiation therapy
   D. Surgery

**Answer: A**

Once malignancy, drug-induced, and infectious etiologies are ruled out, treatment of the retroperitoneal fibrotic process is instituted. Corticosteroids, with or without surgery, are the mainstay of medical therapy. Surgical debulking, ureterolysis, or ureteral stenting is required in patients who present with moderate or massive hydronephrosis. All patients with iliocaval thrombosis will require at least 6 months of oral anticoagulation. Medical therapy is initiated with prednisone (60 mg every other day, for 2 months). Following this initial therapy, prednisone is gradually tapered off over the next 2 months. Therapeutic efficacy is assessed on the basis of patient symptomatology, erythrocyte sedimentation rate, and diagnostic imaging. Cyclosporine, tamoxifen, or azathioprine may be used to treat patients who are recalcitrant to the above regimen. (See Schwartz 8th ed., p 1327.)

8. The first evidence of a rectus sheath hematoma is
   A. Anorexia and nausea without vomiting
   B. Bluish discoloration of the skin
   C. Development of an abdominal wall mass
   D. Sudden sharp abdominal pain

**Answer: D**

All of the listed items occur with a rectus sheath hematoma, but sudden, sharp abdominal pain is the first symptom. It is frequently confused with an intraabdominal cause for discomfort. (See Schwartz 7th ed.)

9. A desmoid tumor of the abdominal wall is best described as a
   A. Condensation of connective tissue
   B. Fibroma
   C. Fibrosarcoma
   D. Hemartoma

**Answer: C**

In the past, those tumors have been considered as fibromas. Because of their locally aggressive behavior, their tendency to recur, their lack of encapsulation, and the ultimate associated mortality, they are now considered low-grade fibrosarcomas. (See Schwartz 7th ed.)

10. A 16-year-old girl undergoes total colectomy for familial adenomatous polyposis. Two years later, there is a 4-cm, asymptomatic abdominal wall mass in the incision. The appropriate management is
    A. A course of dacarbazine and doxorubicin
    B. A course of vincristine, actinomycin D, and cyclophosphamide
    C. Radiation therapy to the area
    D. Wide resection of the mass

**Answer: D**

This young girl has a desmoid tumor. A significant number of patients with familial adenomatous polyposis develop desmoid tumors, and it is not necessary to biopsy this mass to establish a diagnosis. Under these circumstances, observation is contraindicated. The appropriate initial management is wide local resection. In the event of inoperable or recurrent disease, radiation therapy, chemotherapy, or pharmacologic management has been used. Vincristine, actinomycin D, and a cyclophosphamide have afforded some relief. Sulindac plus Coumadin or dacarbazine plus doxorubicin have also been recommended. (See Schwartz 7th ed.)

11. A 60-year-old woman is found to have a 6-cm mass in her greater omentum. The most likely diagnosis is
    A. Hemangiopericytoma
    B. Leiomyoma
    C. Lipoma
    D. Metastatic carcinoma

**Answer: D**

Any of the listed tumors can involve the omentum, but metastatic carcinoma is the most common. The primary tumor is usually in the colon, stomach, pancreas, or ovary. (See Schwartz 7th ed.)

12. Symptoms from a retroperitoneal sarcoma are usually produced by
    A. Bleeding into the tumor mass
    B. Compression of adjacent tissues
    C. Invasion of retroperitoneal organs
    D. Metastases to retroperitoneal lymph nodes

**Answer: B**

Retroperitoneal sarcomas grow along fascial planes and envelop rather than invade retroperitoneal organs. Lymph node metastases are unusual. The tumor does not usually grow rapidly enough to outgrow its blood supply, and major hemorrhage into the tumor mass is uncommon. (See Schwartz 7th ed.)

13. All of the following statements regarding rectus sheath hematomas are true EXCEPT
    A. They are more frequent in males than in females.
    B. They rarely occur in children.
    C. They occur in association with anticoagulant therapy.
    D. They occur in association with collagen diseases.

**Answer: A**

Rectus sheath hematomas are three times more frequent in females and have a peak incidence during the fifth decade of life. Diagnosis of the condition frequently is confused with other diagnoses of an acute abdomen, including appendicitis, cholecystitis, and incarcerated interstitial hernia. In addition to occurring in association with anticoagulant therapy, rectus sheath hematomas have been reported in collagen diseases and some infectious diseases, in blood dyscrasias, and in pregnancy and the puerperium. Whether the bleeding that causes the hematomas is arterial or venous is not known, but the bleeding presumably results because of the inelasticity of the vessels, which prevents them from accommodating to the marked variations in the length of the rectus muscle during contraction and relaxation. (See Schwartz 7th ed.)

14. Which of the following statements about idiopathic retroperitoneal fibrosis is correct?
    A. It occurs most frequently in males.
    B. The condition usually presents initially as an asymptomatic mass found during a routine physical examination.
    C. Duodenal obstruction is the most common complication of the process.
    D. Fine-needle biopsy under fluoroscopic control is the best study to confirm the diagnosis.

**Answer: A**

Idiopathic retroperitoneal fibrosis occurs most frequently in middle-aged men, and dull, noncolicky pain is the initial symptom. Ureteral obstruction with hydronephrosis is the most frequent symptom produced by compression from the fibrosis. Intravenous pyelography that demonstrates hydronephrosis, dilatation, and medial deviation of the ureter and external ureteral compression is the most definitive, noninvasive diagnostic test, and fine-needle aspiration is not recommended for diagnosis. The prognosis for the disease process is good unless irreversible renal damage occurs. Malignant change to fibrosarcoma does not occur. (See Schwartz 7th ed.)

# CHAPTER 35

# Soft Tissue Sarcomas

1. The primitive cell of origin for most soft tissue sarcomas is
   A. Ectoderm
   B. Mesoderm
   C. Endoderm
   D. Embryonic mesenchyme

**Answer: B**
Sarcomas are a heterogeneous group of tumors that arise predominantly from the embryonic mesoderm, but also can originate, as does the peripheral nervous system, from the ectoderm. (See Schwartz 8th ed., p 1329.)

2. Which of the following is NOT a soft tissue sarcoma?
   A. Rhabdomyosarcoma
   B. Angiosarcoma
   C. Chondrosarcoma
   D. Synovial sarcoma

**Answer: C**
Several distinct groups of sarcomas are recognized. Soft tissue sarcomas, the largest of these groups, is the focus of this chapter. Other groups include bone sarcomas (osteosarcomas and chondrosarcomas), Ewing's sarcomas, and peripheral primitive neuroectodermal tumors. (See Schwartz 8th ed., p 1329.)

3. The most common location for a soft tissue sarcoma is
   A. Head and neck
   B. Trunk
   C. Extremity
   D. Retroperitoneum

**Answer: C**
Most primary soft tissue sarcomas originate in an extremity (59%); the next most common sites are the trunk (19%), retroperitoneum (13%), and head and neck (9%). The most common histologic types of soft tissue sarcoma in adults (excluding Kaposi's sarcoma) are malignant fibrous histiocytoma (28%), leiomyosarcoma (12%), liposarcoma (15%), synovial sarcoma (10%), and malignant peripheral nerve sheath tumors (6%). (See Schwartz 8th ed., p 1329.)

4. The most common soft tissue sarcoma of childhood is
   A. Ewing's sarcoma
   B. Osteosarcoma
   C. Synovial sarcoma
   D. Rhabdomyosarcoma

**Answer: D**
Soft tissue sarcomas account for 7 to 8% of all pediatric cancers, totaling approximately 600 new cases per year. Associated with skeletal muscle, rhabdomyosarcomas are the most common soft tissue tumors among children younger than 15 years, and they can occur at any site that has striated muscle. These tumors generally present as a painless enlarging mass; about 30% arise in the head and neck region, 25% in the genitourinary system, and 20% in the extremities. About 15 to 20% of cases have metastasis at presentation, most commonly (40 to 50%) involving the lungs. Several staging systems for rhabdomyosarcoma are available; that of the Intergroup Rhabdomyosarcoma Study Group is based on surgical-pathologic groupings. (See Schwartz 8th ed., p 1343.)

5.  The most common method of metastases in most soft tissue sarcomas is
    A.  Seeding after biopsy
    B.  Hematogenous
    C.  Lymphatic
    D.  Direct extension

**Answer: B**
Overall the clinical behavior of most soft tissue sarcomas is similar and is determined by anatomic location (depth), grade, and size. The dominant pattern of metastasis is hematogenous. Lymph node metastases are rare (<5%) except for a few histologic subtypes such as epithelioid sarcoma, rhabdomyosarcoma, clear-cell sarcoma, and angiosarcoma. (See Schwartz 8th ed., p 1329.)

6.  The risk of developing a soft tissue sarcoma after radiation therapy is increased
    A.  2-fold
    B.  20-fold
    C.  100-fold
    D.  250-fold

**Answer: B**
External radiation therapy is a well-established risk factor for soft tissue sarcoma. An eight- to 50-fold increase in the incidence of sarcomas has been reported among patients treated for cancer of the breast, cervix, ovary, testes, and lymphatic system. In a review of 160 patients with postirradiation sarcomas, the most common histologic types were osteogenic sarcoma, malignant fibrous histiocytoma, angiosarcoma, and lymphangiosarcoma. In that study, the risk of developing a sarcoma increased with higher radiation doses, and the median latency period was 10 years. Postirradiation sarcomas are usually diagnosed at advanced stages and generally have a poor prognosis. (See Schwartz 8th ed., pp 1329–30.)

7.  Exposure to which of the following is considered a risk factor for hepatic angiosarcoma?
    A.  Arsenic
    B.  Phenoxyacetic acid
    C.  Chlorophenol
    D.  Asbestos

**Answer: A**
Exposure to some herbicides such as phenoxyacetic acids and wood preservatives containing chlorophenols has been linked to an increased risk of soft tissue sarcoma. Several chemical carcinogens, including thorium oxide (Thorotrast), vinyl chloride, and arsenic, have been associated with hepatic angiosarcomas. (See Schwartz 8th ed., p 1330.)

8.  Fine-needle biopsy of soft tissue sarcomas
    A.  Is contraindicated because of the risk of seeding tumor
    B.  Is the method of choice for biopsy of suspected soft tissue tumors
    C.  Should be used only to biopsy potential recurrences
    D.  Should always be performed by interventional radiology with ultrasound guidance

**Answer: B**
Fine-needle aspiration is an acceptable method of diagnosing most soft tissue sarcomas, particularly when the results correlate closely with clinical and imaging findings. However, fine-needle aspiration biopsy is indicated for primary diagnosis of soft tissue sarcomas only at centers where cytopathologists have experience with these types of tumors. Fine-needle aspiration biopsy is also the procedure of choice to confirm or rule out the presence of a metastatic focus or local recurrence. If tumor grading is essential for treatment planning, fine-needle aspiration biopsy is not the technique of choice.

Open biopsy is a reliable diagnostic method that allows adequate tissue to be sampled for definitive and specific histologic identification of bone or soft tissue sarcomas. When adequate tissue for diagnosis cannot be obtained by fine-needle aspiration biopsy or core biopsy, an incisional biopsy is indicated for deep tumors or for superficial soft tissue tumors larger than 3 cm. Because open biopsies may have complications, incisional biopsies are usually performed as a last resort when fine-needle aspiration or core biopsy specimens are nondiagnostic. (See Schwartz 8th ed., p 1331.)

9. Excisional biopsy of suspected soft tissue sarcomas <3 cm
   A. Should only be performed for superficial lesions
   B. Is the method of choice for lesions on the hand or feet
   C. Results in a 60–70% recurrence rate in all tumors
   D. Is contraindicated in all suspected soft tissue sarcomas

**Answer: A**

Excisional biopsy can be performed for easily accessible (superficial) extremity or truncal lesions smaller than 3 cm. Excisional biopsy should not be done for lesions involving the hands and feet because definitive reexcision may not be possible after the biopsy. Excisional biopsy results have a 30 to 40% rate of recurrence when margins are positive or uncertain. Excisional biopsies rarely provide any benefit over other biopsy techniques and may cause postoperative complications that could ultimately delay definitive therapy. (See Schwartz 8th ed., p 1333.)

10. Principles of operative resection of soft tissue sarcomas include
    A. Resection with a 4-cm margin of normal tissue
    B. Inclusion of the biopsy tract or incision
    C. Removal of all grossly obvious tumor with a 1-cm margin of normal tissue
    D. Amputation in all distal extremity lesions

**Answer: B**

Wide local excision is the primary treatment strategy for extremity sarcomas. The goal of local therapy for extremity sarcomas is to resect the tumor with a 2-cm margin of surrounding normal soft tissue. The tumors are generally surrounded by a zone of compressed reactive tissue that forms a pseudocapsule, which may mistakenly guide resection (enucleation) by an inexperienced surgeon. Extensions of tumor that go beyond the pseudocapsule must be considered in planning surgery and radiotherapy. In some anatomic areas, negative margins cannot be attained because of the tumor's proximity to vital structures. The biopsy site or tract (if applicable) should also be included en bloc with the resected specimen. (See Schwartz 8th ed., p 1335.)

11. The cell of origin of gastrointestinal stromal tumors is
    A. Goblet cell
    B. Submucosal fibroblast
    C. Interstitial cell of Cajal
    D. Smooth muscle cell

**Answer: C**

Gastrointestinal stromal tumors (GISTs), which constitute the majority of gastrointestinal sarcomas, have distinctive immunohistochemical and genetic features. They are thought to arise from a pacemaker cell within the gastrointestinal tract known as the interstitial cell of Cajal. The interstitial cells of Cajal and GIST cells express the hematopoietic progenitor cell marker CD34 and the growth factor receptor c-Kit (CD117). c-Kit is a transmembrane glycoprotein receptor with an internal tyrosine kinase component which when activated triggers a cascade of intracellular signals regulating cell growth and survival. (See Schwartz 8th ed., p 1342.)

# CHAPTER 36

# Inguinal Hernias

1. The overall ratio of indirect to direct inguinal hernias is
   A. 2:1 (indirect:direct)
   B. 1:1 (indirect:direct)
   C. 1:2 (indirect:direct)
   D. 1:3 (indirect:direct)

**Answer: A**

Seventy-five percent of all abdominal wall hernias occur in the groin. Indirect hernias outnumber direct hernias by about 2:1, with femoral hernias making up a much smaller proportion. Right-sided groin hernias are more common than those on the left. The male:female ratio for inguinal hernias is 7:1. There are approximately 750,000 inguinal herniorrhaphies performed per year in the United States, compared to 25,000 for femoral hernias, 166,000 for umbilical hernias, 97,000 for incisional hernias, and 76,000 for miscellaneous abdominal wall hernias. (See Schwartz 8th ed., p 1354.)

2. What percentage of children born weighing less than 1500 g will require hernia surgery before age 8 years?
   A. ~10%
   B. ~20%
   C. ~30%
   D. ~40%

**Answer: C**

The prevalence of inguinal hernias in males is clearly age dependent. Congenital inguinal hernias are common in low birthweight individuals with a preponderance on the right side. In a study of male children with birthweight less than 1500 grams, 32% required a hernia operation by age 8. For an adult male, the incidence increases steadily with age, and has been reported to approach 50% for men over the age of 75. Abramson and colleagues from Israel published a particularly helpful paper dealing with inguinal hernia epidemiology. Four hundred fifty-five men with inguinal hernias were identified in subjects who were members of a settlement community from the early 1950s. The population was uniquely suited for study because of its heterogenicity related to the political realities in that country at the time. In addition to native-born Israelis, the group included substantial numbers of immigrant Europeans, Americans, Asians, and Africans. The patients were interviewed using a strictly standardized technique and then examined by a physician. Abramson reported the current prevalence rates (which excludes repaired hernias) and the lifetime prevalence rates (which includes repaired hernias) for various ages, the results of which are reproduced in Table 36-1. The overall current risk for a male to have an inguinal hernia was 18% and the lifetime risk was 24%. The lifetime risk for the development of bilaterality was 39% (age 25 to 34 = 31%, age 65 to 74 = 45%, age 75+ = 59%). Although the Abramson data are felt to be among the most reliable and are often referenced, again it must be noted that there is considerable variance in the literature. For example, Akin and colleagues reviewed the files of 27,408 healthy adult male military recruits between 20 and 22 years of age who were examined to detect inguinal hernias.

Eight hundred eighty-five (3.2%) inguinal hernia cases were detected, which is substantially lower than that reported in the Abramson study. (See Schwartz 8th ed., p 1354.)

3. Approximately what percentage of men older than age 75 years has an inguinal hernia?
   A. ~10%
   B. ~30%
   C. ~50%
   D. ~70%

**Answer: C**

The prevalence of inguinal hernias in males is clearly age dependent. Congenital inguinal hernias are common in low birthweight individuals with a preponderance on the right side. In a study of male children with birthweight less than 1500 grams, 32% required a hernia operation by age 8. For an adult male, the incidence increases steadily with age, and has been reported to approach 50% for men over the age of 75. Abramson and colleagues from Israel published a particularly helpful paper dealing with inguinal hernia epidemiology. Four hundred fifty-five men with inguinal hernias were identified in subjects who were members of a settlement community from the early 1950s. The population was uniquely suited for study because of its heterogenicity related to the political realities in that country at the time. In addition to native-born Israelis, the group included substantial numbers of immigrant Europeans, Americans, Asians, and Africans. The patients were interviewed using a strictly standardized technique and then examined by a physician. Abramson reported the current prevalence rates (which excludes repaired hernias) and the lifetime prevalence rates (which includes repaired hernias) for various ages, the results of which are reproduced in Table 36-1. The overall current risk for a male to have an inguinal hernia was 18% and the lifetime risk was 24%. The lifetime risk for the development of bilaterality was 39% (age 25 to 34 = 31%, age 65 to 74 = 45%, age 75+ = 59%). Although the Abramson data are felt to be among the most reliable and are often referenced, again it must be noted that there is considerable variance in the literature. For example, Akin and colleagues reviewed the files of 27,408 healthy adult male military recruits between 20 and 22 years of age who were examined to detect inguinal hernias. Eight hundred eighty-five (3.2%) inguinal hernia cases were detected, which is substantially lower than that reported in the Abramson study. (See Schwartz 8th ed., p 1354.)

4. An 18-year-old patient refuses to have his inguinal hernia repaired and asks you what his risk is for incarceration and/or strangulation. The most accurate response would be
   A. Based on population data, the risk is 0.25–0.33% per year.
   B. The lifetime risk of incarceration is 4–6%.
   C. 1:1000 patients age 18 years will develop incarceration.
   D. 5% of patients develop an irreducible hernia at 10 years.

**Answer: A**

Some light can be shed on the subject by looking at patients with hernias from a time before inguinal herniorrhaphy was routinely performed. Records of patients from a Paris truss clinic (1880–1884) disclosed 242 episodes of hernia-related complications such as obstruction or strangulation in 8633 patients, for a probability of 0.0037 per patient per year. Hernia prevalence data are also available from Colombia, South America, due to a 1-year government initiative to aggressively examine a stratified random sample of the civilian population to determine the frequency of common conditions such as inguinal hernia. By examining records years later from the hospitals in the city of Cali the probability of a hernia-related complication was found to be 0.0029 per year. Using life table analyses and the average of these two probabilities the lifetime risk of a hernia accident for an 18-year-old man is 0.272% or 1:368 patients. For a 72-year-old, it is 0.034% or 1:2941 patients. (See Schwartz 8th ed., p 1355.)

5. Taxis
   A. Begins with distal traction on the hernia sac
   B. Refers to the method of securing mesh to the inguinal ligament
   C. Should not be repeated more than five times
   D. Are easier to get in Houston than New York

**Answer: A**

The initial treatment, in the absence of signs of strangulation, is taxis. Taxis is performed with the patient sedated and placed in the Trendelenburg position. The hernia sac neck is grasped with one hand, with the other applying pressure on the most distal part of the hernia. The goal is to elongate the neck of the hernia so that the contents of the hernia may be guided back into the abdominal cavity with a rocking movement. Mere pressure on the most distal part of the hernia causes bulging of the hernial sac around the neck that can occlude the neck and prevent its reduction (Fig. 36-1). Taxis should not be performed with excessive pressure. If the hernia is strangulated, gangrenous bowel might be reduced into the abdomen or perforated in the process. One or two gentle attempts should be made at taxis. If this is unsuccessful, the procedure should be abandoned. Rarely, the hernia together with its peritoneal sac and constricting neck may be reduced into the abdomen (reduction en masse). Reduction en masse of a hernia is defined as the displacement of a hernia mass without relief of incarceration or strangulation. This diagnosis must be considered in all cases of intestinal obstruction after apparent reduction of an incarcerated hernia. Laparoscopy can be both diagnostic and therapeutic and therefore is a particularly good option. Surgeon expertise may make laparotomy a better choice for some. (See Schwartz 8th ed., p 1355.)

6. Lipoma of the cord
   A. Is normal preperitoneal fat found adjacent to the cord structures
   B. Is histologically a benign tumor
   C. Should always be resected because of the small risk of degeneration into a liposarcoma
   D. Is never found in women

**Answer: A**

Excessive fatty tissue involving the cord or round ligament encountered by a surgeon during elective herniorrhaphy has traditionally been referred to as a lipoma of the cord. This term is unfortunate because it implies a neoplastic process, but a lipoma of the cord consists of normal fatty tissue. The reason for the term lipoma is that the fatty tissue can easily be separated from the cord structures and reduced into the preperitoneal space en masse, as if it were a tumor. A lipoma of the cord is important from a clinical standpoint for the following reasons: (1) it can cause hernia-type symptoms, although with less frequency than indirect hernias with a peritoneal sac; (2) it is often difficult to distinguish at physical examination from an indirect hernia with a peritoneal sac; and (3) it can be responsible for an unsatisfactory result because of an unchanged physical examination after elective inguinal herniorrhaphy, especially when a preperitoneal repair is utilized. For the purposes of the large clinical trials referred to in other parts of this chapter, a lipoma of the cord was classified as an indirect hernia. There is no peritoneal sac by definition, because the contents of the indirect hernia (i.e., preperitoneal fat) come from the preperitoneal space rather than the abdominal cavity. (See Schwartz 8th ed., p 1375.)

7. Which of the following anatomic structures contributes to the formation of a femoral hernia?
   A. Fossa ovalis
   B. Femoral vein
   C. Superior pubic ramus
   D. Iliopubic tract

**Answer: D**

The size and shape of the femoral ring and increased intra-abdominal pressure are factors that contribute to the development of a femoral hernia. The femoral vein and the superior pubic ramus are the borders of the femoral ring laterally and inferiorly. These two structures are more or less constant and therefore are not a factor in the development of this hernia. The iliopubic tract anteriorly and medially accounts for the variability that allows the development of the hernia. The iliopubic tract normally inserts for a distance of 1 to 2 cm along the pectinate line between the pubic tubercle and the midportion of the superior pubic ramus. A femoral hernia can result if the insertion is less than 1 to 2 cm or if it is medially shifted. The net effect of either anatomic subtlety is to widen the femoral ring, predisposing to the hernia. Femoral hernias are particularly dangerous because of the rigid structures that make up the femoral ring. The slightest amount of edema at the ring can produce gangrenous changes of the sac contents, continuing distally into the femoral canal and thigh. (See Schwartz 8th ed., p 1375.)

8. Which of the following makes up the myopectineal orifice of Fruchaud?
   A. Inguinal ligament
   B. Femoral vein
   C. Inferior epigastric artery
   D. Iliopsoas muscle

**Answer: D**

Fruchaud's contribution to inguinal herniology was to examine the common anatomic etiology of direct, indirect, and femoral hernias, rather than to look at each individually. He popularized the use of the term myopectineal orifice, an area bound superiorly by the internal oblique and transversus abdominis muscles, medially by the rectus muscle and sheath, laterally by the iliopsoas muscle, and inferiorly by Cooper's ligament (pecten pubis) (Fig. 36-2). Critical anatomic landmarks such as the inguinal ligament, spermatic cord, and the femoral vessels are contained within this area. This funnel-shaped orifice is lined in its entirety by the transversalis fascia. Fruchaud's concept is that the fundamental cause of all groin hernia is failure of the transversalis fascia to retain the peritoneum. Thus if the hernia surgeon concentrates his or her efforts on restoring the integrity of the transversalis fascia, whether a groin hernia is direct, indirect, or femoral becomes irrelevant, because the abdominal wall defect does not need to be addressed. Fruchaud was René Stoppa's mentor and his influence led Stoppa to develop "la grande prosthese de renforcement du sac visceral," that uses a large, permanent prosthesis that entirely replaces the transversalis fascia over Fruchaud's myopectineal orifice with a wide flap of surrounding tissue. The giant prosthetic reinforcement of the visceral sac (GPRVS) popularized by Wantz in the United States was the direct result. (See Schwartz 8th ed., p 1385.)

9. A sliding hernia
   A. Is easily reducible
   B. Is apparent only with a Valsalva maneuver
   C. Occurs in more than one orifice (e.g., inguinal and femoral)
   D. Has a viscus contained in the wall of the sac

**Answer: D**

A sliding inguinal hernia is defined as any hernia in which part of the sac is the wall of a viscus. Approximately 8% of all groin hernias present with this finding, but the incidence is age related. It is rarely found in patients less than 30 years of age, but increases to 20% after the age of 70. On the right, the cecum, ascending colon, or appendix are most commonly involved, and on the left, the sigmoid colon is involved. The uterus, fallopian tube, ovary, ureter, and bladder can be involved on either side. The sliding component is usually found on the posterolateral side of the internal ring. The importance of this condition has lessened considerably in the last several years with the realization that it is not necessary to resect hernia sacs, and that simple reduction into the preperitoneal space is sufficient. This eliminates the primary danger associated with sliding hernias, which is injury to the viscus during high ligation and sac excision. (See Schwartz 8th ed., p 1358.)

10. A Marcy repair
    A. Is the procedure of choice in Nyhus type IIIc hernias
    B. Is technically easier to perform laparoscopically
    C. Involves narrowing of the internal ring after high ligation of the sac
    D. Should not be performed in children

**Answer: C**

The Marcy repair is the simplest nonprosthetic repair performed today. Its main indication is in Nyhus type I indirect inguinal hernias where the internal ring is normal. It is appropriate for children and young adults in whom concern remains about the long-term effects of prosthetic material. The essential features of this operation are high ligation of the hernia sac plus narrowing of the internal ring. Displacing the cord structures laterally allows the placement of sutures through the muscular and fascial layers (Fig. 36-14). (See Schwartz 8th ed., p 1369.)

11. Chronic pain after inguinal hernia repair
    A. Occurs in approximately 25% of patients
    B. Is defined as pain persisting longer than 6 months
    C. Is rarely moderate or severe
    D. Is usually caused by nerve injury

**Answer: A**

Various groin pain syndromes may develop, usually from scar tissue, reaction to prosthetic material, or involvement of a nerve in staples or suture material during repair of the hernia. Chronic postherniorrhaphy groin pain, which is defined as pain lasting more than 3 months, occurs with greater frequency than was previously thought. The incidence in recent studies ranges from 0 to 53%. A critical review of studies published between the years 1987 and 2000 suggested the overall incidence to be about 25%, with 10% fitting a definition of moderate or severe (Table 36-10). There are predictors of the development of a postoperative groin pain syndrome (Table 36-11). However, it occurs without regard to the type of repair performed, and is difficult to categorize because patients' descriptions of their pain are so heterogeneous. The difficulty is magnified several fold if workman's compensation issues are involved. Nevertheless, an attempt should be made to assign patients to one of two types: (1) nociceptive pain that is caused by tissue damage and is further subdivided into somatic and visceral, and (2) neuropathic, which means direct nerve damage. Somatic pain is the most common and is usually caused by damage to ligaments, tendons, and muscles. Osteitis pubis and a new syndrome which includes various tendinitides involving the adductor mechanism of the hip called adductor tenoperiostitis (ATP) (formerly grouped under the heading of adductor strain) are part of this group. Visceral pain refers to that which is related to a specific visceral function such as urination or ejaculation (see dysejaculation syndrome section below). The principles for assessing and treating patients with nociceptive pain are similar to those used for patients who present with groin pain but do not have an obvious hernia. (See Schwartz 8th ed., p 1385.)

12. The most appropriate treatment for a "Sportsman's hernia" is
    A. Operative repair with open, anterior approach
    B. Operative repair with open, posterior approach
    C. Operative repair with laparoscopic approach
    D. Analgesics and rest

**Answer: D**
In the absence of a specifically correctable surgical lesion, conservative management consisting of rest, anti-inflammatory agents, ice, and specific stretching and strengthening exercises is used first. Other conservative measures such as pulsed radiofrequency, cryotherapy, and even acupuncture have been reported with varying degrees of success. Patients who fail conservative management will commonly come to surgery. Tenotomy of an adductor tendon is highly successful in the properly selected patient. Groin exploration is most rewarding when a specifically correctable lesion such as a torn external oblique aponeurosis with or without ilioinguinal nerve entrapment is found. More commonly, a nonspecific deficiency of the posterior wall of the inguinal canal that includes an occult hernia is found, and a variety of modified Bassini-type inguinal floor reconstructions have been proposed. Laparoscopic and prosthetic repairs have also been used. A consistent staging system to describe the pathology is lacking, and there is no consensus concerning the best procedure for patients with this difficult-to-treat condition. Given the level of discomfort endured by some of these patients, as well as the fact that many are high-profile athletes, there is significant potential for hucksterism in the treatment of this condition. (See Schwartz 8th ed., p 1390.)

13. The cremaster muscle is derived from
    A. External oblique aponeurosis
    B. Internal oblique muscle
    C. Transversus abdominis muscle
    D. Transversalis fascia

**Answer: B**
The cremaster muscle, which lies along the spermatic end, arises from the lowermost fibers of the internal oblique muscle. (See Schwartz 7th ed.)

14. The spermatic cord contains all of the following EXCEPT
    A. Autonomic nerve fibers
    B. Genital nerve
    C. Lymphatics
    D. Testicular artery

**Answer: B**
The genital nerve, a branch of the genitofemoral nerve, is motor to the cremaster muscle and sensory to the skin of the scrotum or labia. It lies on the iliopubic tract at the upper border of the femoral sheath. (See Schwartz 7th ed.)

15. A sliding hernia
    A. Has an abnormally high recurrence rate after repair
    B. Involves a retroperitoneal structure
    C. Is more common in the left groin
    D. Occurs almost exclusively in women

**Answer: B**
A sliding hernia is one in which a retroperitoneal organ makes up part of the posterior wall of an indirect hernia sac extending through the internal inguinal ring. Typically, the cecum is involved on the right where most sliding hernias occur. In the left groin, the sigmoid and sigmoid mesocolon may be involved. Sliding hernias are not more common in women. They should be repaired through a groin incision, and the retroperitoneal structure is merely replaced above the level of the internal ring closure. With a properly done operation, recurrences should be no more likely than in any other groin hernia operation. (See Schwartz 7th ed.)

16. When a sliding hernia is present in the right groin, the most common finding is
    A. A loop of ileum fixed in the sac by adhesions
    B. A loop of ileum that makes up part of the posterior wall of the sac
    C. A loop of ileum that makes up the anterior wall of the sac
    D. The cecum that makes up the posterior wall of the sac

**Answer: D**

A sliding component is present in only 3% of groin hernias. However, a surgeon should consider the possibility of a sliding component whenever a large indirect groin hernia is encountered, especially if the hernia is found in an elderly man and cannot be reduced or reduces with difficulty. As the sac enlarges in a long-standing direct hernia, parietal peritoneum is drawn into the groin through the internal inguinal ring to become part of the sac. As this process continues, retroperitoneal structures attached to the peritoneum enter the groin as part of the posterior wall of the sac. Thus, the cecum may form part of the posterior sac wall on the right side, and a sliding left inguinal hernia may involve either the sigmoid mesocolon or the colon itself. This situation must be recognized before removal of the hernia sac so that damage either to the colon or to its blood supply can be avoided. (See Schwartz 7th ed.)

# CHAPTER 37

# Thyroid, Parathyroid, and Adrenal

1. Which of the following is important to check before resection of a gastrinoma?
   A. Serum calcium
   B. Serum catecholamines
   C. Serum calcitonin
   D. Serum carcinoembryonic antigen

2. The substrate for catecholamine production is
   A. Arginine
   B. Glutamine
   C. Tyrosine
   D. Tryptophan

**Answer: A**

In patients with multiple endocrine neoplasia 1 (MEN-1), hypercalcemia should be treated prior to treatment of gastrinoma, because gastrin levels often decline in these patients following parathyroidectomy. (See Schwartz 8th ed., p 1444.)

**Answer: C**

Catecholamine hormones (epinephrine, norepinephrine, and dopamine) are produced both in the central and sympathetic nervous system and in the adrenal medulla. The substrate tyrosine is converted to catecholamines via a series of steps. (See Schwartz 8th ed., p 1452.)

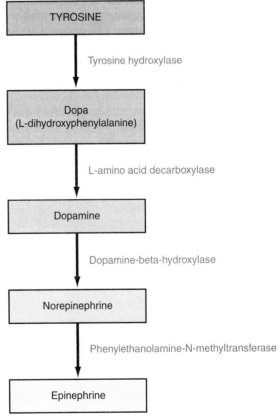

**FIG. 37-1.** Synthesis of catecholamines. (See Schwartz 8th ed., p 1452.)

3. Aldosterone
   A. Is secreted by the zona fascicularis of the adrenal cortex
   B. Secretion is regulated by the renin-angiotensin system
   C. Has a half-life of 3 h
   D. Functions mainly to decrease sodium reabsorption in the distal renal tubule

**Answer: B**

Aldosterone secretion is regulated primarily by the renin–angiotensin system Decreased renal blood flow, decreased plasma sodium and increased sympathetic tone, all stimulate the release of renin from juxtaglomerular cells. Renin, in turn, leads to the production of angiotensin I from its precursor angiotensinogen. Angiotensin I is cleaved by pulmonary angiotensin-converting enzyme (ACE) to angiotensin II, which is not only a potent vasoconstrictor, but also leads to increased aldosterone synthesis and release. Hyperkalemia is another potent stimulator of aldosterone synthesis, whereas adrenocorticotropic hormone (ACTH), pituitary pro-opiomelanocortin (POMC), and antidiuretic hormone (ADH) are weak stimulators. (See Schwartz 8th ed., p 1449.)

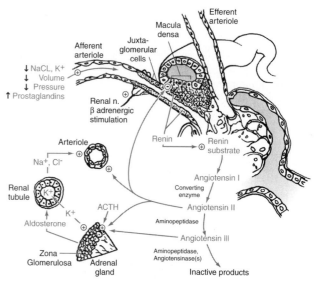

**FIG. 37-2.** The renin-angiotensin system. [Reproduced with permission from Hsueh W, et al: Endocrinology of hypertension, in Felig P Frohman L (eds): Endocrinology and Metabolism. McGraw-Hill, 2001, p 558.] (See Schwartz 8th ed., p 1451.)

4. Which of the following is the most sensitive test for a pheochromocytoma?
   A. 24-h urine vanillylmandelic acid
   B. 24-h urine metanephrine
   C. 24-h urine epinephrine
   D. 24-h urine norepinephrine

**Answer: B**

Pheochromocytomas are diagnosed by testing 24-hour urine samples for catecholamines and their metabolites, as well as by determining plasma metanephrine levels. Urinary metanephrines are 98% sensitive and are also highly specific for pheochromocytomas, whereas vanillylmandelic acid (VMA) measurements are slightly less sensitive and specific. False-positive VMA tests may result from ingestion of caffeine, raw fruits or medications (alpha-methyl dopa). Fractionated urinary catecholamines (norepinephrine, epinephrine, and dopamine) are also sensitive but less specific for pheochromocytomas. Because extra-adrenal sites lack phenylethanolamine-N-methyltransferase, these tumors secrete norepinephrine, whereas epinephrine is the main hormone secreted from adrenal pheochromocytomas. (See Schwartz 8th ed., p 1460.)

5. The most common cause of Cushing's syndrome is
   A. Pituitary adenoma
   B. Adrenal adenoma
   C. Ectopic adrenocorticotropic hormone production
   D. Adrenal hyperplasia

**Answer: A**

**Table 37-1.**
**Etiology of Cushing's Syndrome**

| |
|---|
| ACTH-dependent (70%) |
|    Pituitary adenoma or Cushing's disease (~70%) |
|    Ectopic ACTH production[a] (~10%) |
|    Ectopic CRH production (<1%) |
| ACTH-independent (20–30%) |
|    Adrenal adenoma (10–15%) |
|    Adrenal carcinoma (5–10%) |
|    Adrenal hyperplasia—pigmented micronodular cortical hyperplasia or gastric inhibitory peptide-sensitive macronodular hyperplasia (5%) |
| Other |
|    Pseudo-Cushing's syndrome |
|    Iatrogenic—exogenous administration of steroids |

ACTH = adrenocorticotropic hormone; CRH = corticotropin-releasing hormone.
[a]From small-cell lung tumors, pancreatic islet cell tumors, medullary thyroid cancers, pheochromocytomas, and carcinoid tumors of the lung, thymus, gut, pancreas, and ovary.
See Schwartz 8th ed., p 1455.

6. Which of the following should be the first drug administered in the preoperative preparation of a patient with a pheochromocytoma?
   A. Propanolol
   B. Phenoxybenzamine
   C. Nifedipine
   D. Captopril

**Answer: B**

The medical management of pheochromocytomas is aimed chiefly at blood pressure control and volume repletion. Alpha blockers such as phenoxybenzamine are started 1 to 3 weeks before surgery at doses of 10 mg twice daily, which may be increased to 300 to 400 mg/d. Patients who perspire are not adequately blocked and the dose should be increased. Other alpha blockers such as prazosin, and other classes of drugs, such as angiotensin-converting enzyme (ACE) inhibitors and calcium channel blockers, are also useful. Beta blockers, such as propranolol at doses of 10 to 40 mg every 6 to 8 hours, often need to be added preoperatively in patients who have persistent tachycardia and arrhythmias. Beta blockers should only be instituted after adequate alpha blockade and hydration in order to avoid the effects of unopposed alpha stimulation, i.e., hypertensive crisis and congestive heart failure. Patients should also be volume repleted preoperatively in order to avoid postoperative hypotension, which ensues with the loss of vasoconstriction after tumor removal. (See Schwartz 8th ed., p 1461.)

7. Which of the following is the most common etiology of an adrenal incidentaloma?
   A. Early adrenocortical cancer
   B. Adrenal adenoma
   C. Myelolipoma
   D. Past adrenal hemorrhage

**Answer: B**

The differential diagnosis includes a multitude of lesions that are listed in Table 37-2. Nonfunctional cortical adenomas account for the majority (36 to 94%) of adrenal incidentalomas in patients without a history of cancer. (See Schwartz 8th ed., p 1462.)

**Table 37-2.**
**Differential Diagnosis of Adrenal Incidentaloma**

| Functioning Lesions | Nonfunctioning Lesions |
| --- | --- |
| Benign | Benign |
|    Aldosteronoma |    Cortical adenoma |
|    Cortisol-producing adenoma |    Myelolipoma |
|    Sex-steroid-producing adenoma |    Cyst |
|    Pheochromocytoma |    Ganglioneuroma |
|  |    Hemorrhage |
| Malignant | Malignant |
|    Adrenocortical cancer |    Metastasis |
|    Malignant pheochromocytoma |  |

See Schwartz 8th ed., p 1462.

8. The computed tomography finding most suggestive of malignancy in an adrenal mass is
   A. Size larger than 6 cm
   B. Tumor heterogeneity
   C. Irregular margins
   D. Adjacent adenopathy

**Answer: A**

It is not necessary for asymptomatic patients whose imaging studies are consistent with obvious cysts, hemorrhage, myelolipomas, or diffuse metastatic disease to undergo additional investigations. All other patients should be tested for underlying hormonally active tumors by (1) low-dose (1 mg) overnight dexamethasone suppression test or 24-hour urine cortisol to rule out subclinical Cushing's syndrome; (2) a 24-hour urine collection for catecholamines, metanephrines, vanillylmandelic acid, or plasma metanephrine to rule out pheochromocytoma; and (3) in hypertensive patients, serum electrolytes, plasma aldosterone, and plasma renin to rule out an aldosteronoma. Confirmatory tests can be performed based on the results of the initial screening studies.

Determination of the malignant potential of an incidentaloma is more complicated. As discussed earlier, the risk of malignancy in an adrenal lesion is related to its size. Lesions greater than 6 cm in diameter have an approximate risk of malignancy of approximately 35%. However, this size cutoff is not absolute because adrenal carcinomas have also been reported in lesions smaller than 6 cm. (See Schwartz 8th ed., p 1463.)

9. The best screening test to evaluate a patient for possible Cushing's syndrome is
   A. Fasting a.m. cortisol
   B. 24-h urine cortisol
   C. Low-dose dexamethasone suppression test
   D. Serum adrenocorticotropic hormone levels

**Answer: C**

The secretion of cortisol is episodic and has a diurnal variation, therefore a single measurement of the plasma cortisol level is unreliable in diagnosing Cushing's syndrome. Cushing's syndrome is characterized by elevated glucocorticoid levels that are not suppressible by exogenous hormone administration and loss of diurnal variation. This phenomenon is used to screen patients using the overnight low-dose dexamethasone suppression test. In this test, 1 mg of a synthetic glucocorticoid (dexamethasone) is given at 11 p.m. and plasma cortisol levels are measured at 8 a.m. the following morning. Physiologically normal adults suppress cortisol levels less than 3 µg/dL, whereas most patients with Cushing's syndrome do not. False-negative results may be obtained in patients with mild disease, therefore some authors consider the test positive only if cortisol levels are suppressed to less than 1.8 µg/dL. False-positive results can occur in up to 3% of patients with chronic renal failure, depression, or those taking medications such as phenytoin, which enhance dexamethasone metabolism. In patients with a negative test, but a high clinical suspicion, the classic low-dose dexamethasone (0.5 mg every 6 hours for 8 doses, or 2 mg over 48 hours) suppression test or urinary cortisol measurement should be performed. Measurement of elevated 24-hour urinary cortisol levels is a very sensitive (95 to 100%) and specific (98%) modality of diagnosing Cushing's syndrome, and is particularly useful for identifying patients with pseudo-Cushing's syndrome. A urinary free cortisol excretion of less than 100 μg/dL (in most laboratories) rules out hypercortisolism. Recently, salivary cortisol measurements using commercially available kits also have demonstrated superior sensitivity in diagnosing Cushing's syndrome. However, they are not used routinely. (See Schwartz 8th ed., p 1456.)

10. The treatment of choice for Cushing's disease is
    A. Transsphenoidal hypophysectomy
    B. Laparoscopic adrenalectomy
    C. Open adrenalectomy
    D. Medical therapy

**Answer: A**

The treatment of choice in patients with Cushing's disease is transsphenoidal excision of the pituitary adenoma, which is successful in 80% of patients. Pituitary irradiation has been used for patients with persistent or recurrent disease after surgery. However, it is associated with a high rate of panhypopituitarism and some patients develop visual deficits. This has led to increased use of stereotactic radiosurgery, which uses computed tomography (CT) guidance to deliver high doses of radiotherapy to the tumor (photon or gamma knife). Patients who fail to respond to either treatment are candidates for pharmacologic therapy with adrenal inhibitors such as ketoconazole, metyrapone, or aminoglutethimide, or bilateral adrenalectomy. Several series have reported the safety and effectiveness of bilateral laparoscopic adrenalectomy in this setting. (See Schwartz 8th ed., p 1458.)

11. Adrenocortical carcinomas
    A. Are more likely to be functioning in women
    B. Are nonfunctioning in 90% of patients
    C. Most commonly secrete aldosterone if they are functioning
    D. Are usually the result of a specific gene mutation

**Answer: A**

Adrenal carcinomas are rare neoplasms with a worldwide incidence of 2 per 1 million. These tumors have a bimodal age distribution, with an increased incidence in children and in adults in the fourth and fifth decades of life. Functioning tumors are more common in women, whereas men are more likely to develop nonfunctioning carcinomas. The majority are sporadic, but adrenocortical carcinomas also occur in association with germline mutations of *p*53 (Li-Fraumeni syndrome) and MENIN (multiple endocrine neoplasia 1) genes. Loci on 11p (Beckwith-Wiedemann syndrome), 2p (Carney complex), and 9q have also been implicated. (See Schwartz 8th ed., p 1458.)

12. The primary androgens produced by the adrenal gland include
    A. Sulfated dehydroepiandrosterone
    B. 11-deoxycorticosterone
    C. Testosterone
    D. Estrogen

**Answer: A**

Adrenal androgens are produced in the zona fasciculata and reticularis from 17-hydroxypregnenolone in response to adrenocorticotropic hormone (ACTH) stimulation. The adrenal androgens include dehydroepiandrosterone (DHEA) and its sulfated counterpart (DHEAS), androstenedione, and small amounts of testosterone and estrogen. Adrenal androgens are weakly bound to plasma albumin. They exert their major effects by peripheral conversion to the more potent testosterone and dihydrotestosterone, but also have weak intrinsic androgen activity. Androgen metabolites are conjugated as glucuronides or sulfates and excreted in the urine. (See Schwartz 8th ed., p 1452.)

13. Which of the following predicts a good response after adrenalectomy for Conn's syndrome?
    A. Good preoperative control of hypertension with beta-blockers
    B. Diastolic blood pressure average less than 100 mm Hg
    C. Male gender
    D. Age younger than 50 years

**Answer: D**
After surgery for hyperaldosteronism (Conn's syndrome), some patients experience transient hypoaldosteronism requiring mineralocorticoids for up to 3 months. Rarely, acute Addison's disease may occur 2 to 3 days after unilateral adrenalectomy. Adrenalectomy is greater than 90% successful in improving hypokalemia and approximately 70% successful in correcting the hypertension. Patients who respond to spironolactone therapy, and those with a shorter duration of hypertension with minimal end-organ (renal) damage, are more likely to achieve improvement in hypertension, whereas male patients, those older than age 50 years, and those with multiple adrenal nodules are least likely to benefit from adrenalectomy. (See Schwartz 8th ed., p 1455.)

14. The multiple endocrine neoplasia (MEN) syndromes are caused by a mutation in which of the following?
    A. RET proto-oncogene
    B. *p*53
    C. 11q
    D. 2p

**Answer: A**
Pheochromocytomas occur in families with MEN-2A and MEN-2B, in approximately 50% of patients. Both syndromes are inherited in an autosomal dominant fashion and are caused by germline mutations in the RET proto-oncogene. (See Schwartz 8th ed., p 1460.)

15. The most common physical finding associated with Cushing's syndrome is
    A. Hirsutism
    B. Truncal obesity
    C. Striae
    D. Acne

**Answer: B**
Table 37-3 lists the classic features of Cushing's syndrome. Early diagnosis of this disease requires a thorough knowledge of these manifestations, coupled with a high clinical suspicion. In some patients, symptoms are less pronounced and may be more difficult to recognize, particularly given their diversity and the absence of a single defining symptom or sign. Progressive truncal obesity is the most common symptom, occurring in up to 95% of patients. This pattern results from the lipogenic action of excessive corticosteroids centrally and catabolic effects peripherally, along with peripheral muscle wasting. Fat deposition also occurs in unusual sites, such as the supraclavicular space and posterior neck region, leading to the so-called buffalo hump. Purple striae are often visible on the protuberant abdomen. Rounding of the face secondary to thickening of the facial fat leads to moon facies, and thinning of subcutaneous tissue leads to plethora. There is an increase in fine hair growth on the face, upper back, and arms, although true virilization is more commonly seen with adrenocortical cancers. Endocrine abnormalities include glucose intolerance, amenorrhea, and decreased libido or impotence. Large, purple striae on the abdomen or proximal extremities are most reliable for making the diagnosis. In children, Cushing's syndrome is characterized by obesity and stunted growth. Patients with Cushing's disease may also

present with headaches, visual field defects, and panhypopituitarism. Hyperpigmentation of the skin, if present, suggests an ectopic adrenocorticotropic hormone (ACTH)-producing tumor with high levels of circulating ACTH. (See Schwartz 8th ed., p 1456.)

**Table 37-3.**
**Features of Cushing's Syndrome**

| System | Manifestation |
| --- | --- |
| General | Weight gain—central obesity, buffalo hump, supraclavicular fat pads |
| Integumentary | Hirsutism, plethora, purple striae, acne, ecchymosis |
| Cardiovascular | Hypertension |
| Musculoskeletal | Generalized weakness, osteopenia |
| Neuropsychiatric | Emotional lability, psychosis, depression |
| Metabolic | Diabetes or glucose intolerance, hyperlipidemia |
| Renal | Polyuria, renal stones |
| Gonadal | Impotence, decreased libido, menstrual irregularities |

See Schwartz 8th ed., p 1456.

16. An adrenocortical carcinoma that is 4 cm in size with minimal local invasion into the diaphragm and negative nodes is what stage?
    A. Stage I
    B. Stage II
    C. Stage III
    D. Stage IV

**Answer: C**

**Table 37-4.**
**TNM Staging for Adrenocortical Cancer**

| Stage | TNM Class |
| --- | --- |
| I | T1, N0, M0 |
| II | T2, N0, M0 |
| III | T3, N0, M0 |
| | T1–2, N1, M0 |
| IV | T3–4, N1, M0 |
| | Any T, Any N, M1 |

Primary tumor (T): T1, size ≤5 cm without local invasion; T2 size >5 cm without local invasion; T3, any size with local invasion but no involvement of adjacent organs; T4, any size with involvement of adjacent organs.
Nodes (N): N0, no involvement of regional nodes; N1, positive regional lymph nodes.
Metastasis (M): M0, no known distal metastases; M1, distant metastases present.
Source: Reproduced with permission from *AJCC Cancer Staging Manual*, 6th ed. New York: Springer-Verlag, 2002.
See Schwartz 8th ed., p 1459.

17. Which of the following is a component of the multiple endocrine neoplasia 1 (MEN-1) syndrome?
    A. Pituitary tumors
    B. Medullary cancer of the thyroid
    C. Pheochromocytoma
    D. Pancreatitis

**Answer: A**
Although most cases of primary hyperparathyroidism (PHPT) are sporadic, PHPT does occur within the spectrum of a number of inherited disorders such as MEN-1, MEN-2A, isolated familial secondary hyperparathyroidism (HPT), and familial HPT with jaw-tumor syndrome. All of these syndromes are inherited in an autosomal dominant fashion. Primary HPT is the earliest and most common manifestation of MEN-1 and develops in 80 to 100% of patients by age 40 years. These patients are also prone to pancreatic neuroendo-

crine tumors and pituitary adenomas, and less commonly to adrenocortical tumors, lipomas, skin angiomas, and carcinoid tumors of the bronchus, thymus, or stomach. Approximately 50% of patients develop gastrinomas, which are often multiple and metastatic at diagnosis. Insulinomas develop in 10 to 15% of cases, whereas many patients have nonfunctional pancreatic endocrine tumors. Prolactinomas occur in 10 to 50% of MEN-1 patients and constitute the most common pituitary lesion. (See Schwartz 8th ed., p 1435.)

18. The zona glomerulosa of the adrenal gland is responsible for the production of
    A. Epinephrine
    B. Norepinephrine
    C. Aldosterone
    D. Androgens

**Answer: C**
The adrenal cortex appears yellow because of its high lipid content and accounts for approximately 80 to 90% of the gland's volume. Histologically, the cortex is divided into three zones: zona glomerulosa, zona fasciculata, and zona reticularis. The outer area of the zona glomerulosa consists of small cells and is the site of production of the mineralocorticoid hormone aldosterone. The zona fasciculata is made up of larger cells, which often appear foamy because of multiple lipid inclusions, whereas the zona reticularis cells are smaller. These latter zones are the site of production of glucocorticoids and adrenal androgens. The adrenal medulla constitutes up to 10 to 20% of the gland's volume and is reddish-brown in color. It produces the catecholamine hormones epinephrine and norepinephrine. The cells of the adrenal medulla are arranged in cords and are polyhedral in shape. They are often referred to as chromaffin cells because they stain specifically with chromium salts. (See Schwartz 8th ed., p 1449.)

19. Primary hyperaldosteronism
    A. Occurs most commonly in patients age 50–70 years
    B. May have associated hypokalemia
    C. Is usually caused by bilateral adrenal hyperplasia
    D. Is responsible for 8% of all primary hypertension

**Answer: B**
Hyperaldosteronism may be secondary to stimulation of the renin–angiotensin system from renal artery stenosis and to low-flow states such as congestive heart failure and cirrhosis. Hyperaldosteronism resulting from these conditions is reversible by treatment of the underlying cause. Primary hyperaldosteronism results from autonomous aldosterone secretion, which, in turn, leads to suppression of renin secretion. Primary aldosteronism usually occurs in individuals between the ages of 30 and 50 years and accounts for 1% of cases of hypertension. Primary hyperaldosteronism is usually associated with hypokalemia; however, more patients with Conn's syndrome are being diagnosed with normal potassium levels. Most cases result from a solitary functioning adrenal adenoma (approximately 70%) and idiopathic bilateral hyperplasia (30%). Adrenocortical carcinoma and glucocorticoid suppressible hyperaldosteronism are rare, each accounting for less than 1% of cases. (See Schwartz 8th ed., p 1453.)

20. Pheochromocytomas are associated with all of the following EXCEPT
    A. Congenital adrenal hyperplasia
    B. Tuberous sclerosis
    C. Carney's syndrome
    D. von Hippel Lindau syndrome

**Answer: A**
Pheochromocytomas occur in families with multiple endocrine neoplasia 2A (MEN-2A) and MEN-2B, in approximately 50% of patients. Both syndromes are inherited in an autosomal dominant fashion and are caused by germline mutations in the RET proto-oncogene. Another familial cancer

syndrome with an increased risk of pheochromocytomas includes von Hippel-Lindau disease, which also is inherited in an autosomal dominant manner. This syndrome also includes retinal angioma, hemangioblastomas of the central nervous system, renal cysts, and carcinomas, pancreatic cysts, and epididymal cystadenomas. The incidence of pheochromocytomas in the syndrome is approximately 14%, but varies depending on the series. The gene causing von Hippel-Lindau disease has been mapped to chromosome 3p and is a tumor-suppressor gene. Pheochromocytomas are also included within the tumor spectrum of neurofibromatosis type 1 and other neuroectodermal disorders (Sturge-Weber syndrome and tuberous sclerosis), Carney's syndrome (gastric epithelioid leiomyosarcoma, pulmonary chondroma, and extra-adrenal paraganglioma), and, rarely, in the MEN-1 syndrome. Familial pheochromocytomas may also rarely occur without other associated disorders. (See Schwartz 8th ed., p 1460.)

21. Steps in the synthesis of thyroid hormone include all of the following EXCEPT
    A. Coupling of iodotyrosines
    B. Ingestion of potassium iodide
    C. Linkage of iodine with tyrosine residues
    D. Oxidation of iodide to iodine

**Answer: B**
Thyroid hormone synthesis involves four steps: (1) active trapping and concentration of iodide in follicular cells, (2) rapid oxidation of iodide to iodine, (3) linkage of iodine with tyrosine residues in thyroglobulin, and (4) coupling of the iodotyrosines to form the active thyroid hormones triiodothyronine and thyroxine. Ingestion of potassium iodide blocks trapping of iodine in the thyroid gland. (See Schwartz 7th ed.)

22. The principal function of thyrotropin-releasing hormones is to
    A. Break down thyroxine to triiodothyronine at the cellular level
    B. Concentrate iodide in follicular cells
    C. Form active thyroxine by coupling iodotyrosines
    D. Stimulate thyroid-stimulating hormone release

**Answer: D**
Thyrotropin-releasing hormone formed in the hypothalamus reaches the anterior pituitary by the hypophyseal portal system to stimulate thyroid-stimulating hormone (TSH) release. TSH then initiates the cascade that leads to thyroxine and triiodothyronine. (See Schwartz 7th ed.)

23. The immediate cause of thyroid enlargement associated with chronic administration of thyroid-blocking agents or goitrogenic substances is
    A. Interference with the synthesis of iodotyrosine intermediates
    B. Increased production of thyroid-stimulating hormone by the pituitary gland
    C. Decreased production of thyroid hormone
    D. A reduction in the capacity of the thyroid gland to concentrate iodine

**Answer: B**
Nonneoplastic causes of thyroid enlargement include both idiopathic enlargement and excessive production of thyroid-stimulating hormone (TSH) by the pituitary gland. Enlargement of the thyroid gland can also be the result of interference with the synthesis of iodotyrosine intermediates, a fall in thyroid hormone production, or a rise in serum cholesterol concentration. However, it is the increased TSH secretion by the pituitary gland, which results from reduced plasma thyroid hormone levels, that is the immediate cause of the thyroid enlargement sometimes associated with chronic use of thyroid-blocking agents. (See Schwartz 7th ed.)

24. All of the following statements about Hashimoto's thyroiditis are true EXCEPT
    A. It is the most common kind of chronic thyroiditis.
    B. It affects women more often than men.
    C. It involves autoimmune mechanisms.
    D. Assessment of the state of thyroid function is diagnostically important in the condition.

**Answer: D**
The natural history of Hashimoto's disease, the most common type of chronic thyroiditis, begins with an autoimmune response to a thyroid autoantigen. Initial changes are those of hyperthyroidism, but as lymphocytic infiltration of the glands proceeds, the hyperfunctional state subsides and may eventually give way to myxedema. Thus, the state

of thyroid function, which may range from hyperthyroid to euthyroid to hypothyroid, is of no diagnostic importance. People who have Hashimoto's disease (women are affected more often than men) are more likely than other people to develop thyroid carcinoma. (See Schwartz 7th ed.)

25. A 30-year-old woman has had recurrent episodes of headache and sweating. Her mother had renal calculi and died of thyroid cancer. Physical examination reveals a thyroid nodule but no clinical signs of thyroid dysfunction. Before performing thyroid surgery, the woman's physician should order
   A. A thyroid scan
   B. Measurement of serum thyroid-releasing hormone and thyroid-stimulating hormone levels
   C. A 24-h urine test for 5-hydroxyindoleacetic acid excretion
   D. Serial 24-h urine tests for catecholamine, metanephrine, and vanillylmandelic acid excretion

**Answer: D**
The combination of medullary carcinoma of the thyroid gland, pheochromocytoma, and hyperparathyroidism defines Sipple's syndrome (multiple endocrine adenomatosis type II), which is associated with a familial predilection. Even minor surgery performed on a patient who has an unrecognized pheochromocytoma can lead to death from a hypertensive crisis or cardiac arrhythmia unless the patient is treated preoperatively with sympathetic-blocking agents. Pheochromocytoma is associated with excessive urinary excretion of catecholamines, metanephrines, and vanillylmandelic acid. (See Schwartz 7th ed.)

26. Twelve hours after having undergone a subtotal thyroidectomy, a 30-year-old woman develops agitation and difficulty breathing. Examination reveals tachycardia and anterior cervical swelling; the surgical dressing is dry. The most appropriate treatment at this point would be immediate
   A. Insertion of an orotracheal tube
   B. Re-opening of the cervical wound
   C. Determination of the serum calcium concentration
   D. Administration of morphine

**Answer: B**
Anterior cervical swelling in the first few hours after thyroid surgery suggests wound hemorrhage and formation of a hematoma, which could cause dyspnea and eventually asphyxia by tracheal compression. A true emergency, this condition should be managed by immediate opening of the incision. Vocal-cord paralysis resulting from damage to the recurrent laryngeal nerve would have caused dyspnea sooner than in the case described, and inadvertent total parathyroidectomy would have led to tetany later. (See Schwartz 7th ed.)

27. A 26-year-old woman presents with a palpable thyroid nodule, and needle biopsy demonstrates amyloid in the stroma of the lesion. A cervical lymph node is palpable on the same side as the lesion. The preferred treatment for this patient should be
   A. Removal of the involved lobe, the isthmus, and the enlarged lymph node
   B. Removal of the involved lobe, the isthmus, a portion of the opposite lobe, and the enlarged lymph node
   C. Removal of the involved lobe and the isthmus and neck dissection on the side of the enlarged lymph node
   D. Total thyroidectomy and modified neck dissection on the side of the enlarged lymph node

**Answer: D**
The finding of amyloid in the stroma of a thyroid nodule is diagnostic of medullary carcinoma because medullary carcinoma is the only thyroid tumor that contains this substance. Diagnosis of the condition can also be based on the finding of an increased serum calcitonin level in conjunction with a thyroid mass. Because medullary carcinomas are C-cell tumors, they do not respond to thyroxine therapy and do not concentrate radioiodine. They are relatively insensitive to external radiation, and surgery offers the only chance for cure. Total thyroidectomy should be performed because of frequent multicentricity; recurrences have occurred when thyroid tissue is left. More than 50% of patients have positive lymph nodes at the time of initial exploration, and single or bilateral neck dissection is the treatment of choice when nodes are clinically involved. With the appropriate operative approach, an overall survival rate of 80% at 5 years and 57% at 10 years has been reported. (See Schwartz 7th ed.)

28. On the fifth postoperative day after total thyroidectomy, a patient complains of tingling of the fingertips and is found to have a serum calcium level of 5.6 mg/dL. The next step in the treatment of this patient should be
    A. Careful observation until the calcium level increases
    B. Administration of vitamin $D_2$ or $D_3$, 50,000–100,000 U/day
    C. Administration of 1,25 $(OH)_2D_3$ (calcitriol), 1–2 µg/day
    D. Administration of calcium gluconate, 3–6 g/day, by slow intravenous drip

**Answer: D**

The most common cause of hypoparathyroidism is surgical removal of, trauma to, or devascularization of the parathyroids either during parathyroid surgical treatment, or, more commonly, during operations on the thyroid. When this condition occurs, the aim of treatment is to raise the calcium level toward normal by use of supplementary calcium and, when necessary, vitamin D and thus relieve symptoms of neuromuscular irritability. If postoperative hypocalcemia is mild, no treatment is needed other than careful observation. If, however, an affected patient develops symptoms, 3–6 g/day of calcium gluconate should be given by slow intravenous drip. For transient postoperative hypoparathyroidism, this type of calcium therapy usually can be stopped within a few days. If, however, hypocalcemia persists, oral calcium also should be administered; once a patient becomes asymptomatic, it usually can be discontinued within several weeks. If permanent hypoparathyroidism with persistent hypocalcemia is diagnosed, a vitamin D preparation should be given in addition to the oral calcium. Vitamin $D_2$ or $D_3$, dihydrotachysterol, or calcitriol can be given. Serum calcium concentrations should be checked frequently when vitamin D preparations are given. (See Schwartz 7th ed.)

1. The most common branchial cleft fistula originates from the
   A. 1st branchial cleft
   B. 2nd branchial cleft
   C. 3rd branchial cleft
   D. 4th branchial cleft

**Answer: B**

Paired branchial clefts and arches develop early in the fourth gestational week. The first cleft and the first, second, third, and fourth pouches give rise to adult organs. The embryologic communication between the pharynx and the external surface may persist as a fistula. A fistula is seen most commonly with the second branchial cleft, which normally disappears, and extends from the anterior border of the sternocleidomastoid muscle superiorly, inward through the bifurcation of the carotid artery, and enters the posterolateral pharynx just below the tonsillar fossa. The branchial cleft remnants may contain small pieces of cartilage and cysts, but internal fistulas are rare. A second branchial cleft sinus is suspected when clear fluid is noted draining from the external opening of the tract at the anterior border of the lower third of the sternocleidomastoid muscle. Rarely, branchial cleft anomalies occur in association with biliary atresia and congenital cardiac anomalies, an association that is referred to as Goldenhar's complex. (See Schwartz 8th ed., p 1475.)

2. The treatment of choice for cystic hygromas is
   A. Observation
   B. Antibiotics
   C. Intralesional sclerotherapy
   D. Surgical excision

**Answer: D**

The diagnosis of cystic hygroma by prenatal ultrasound (US) before 30 weeks' gestation has detected a "hidden mortality," as well as a high incidence of associated anomalies, including abnormal karyotypes and hydrops fetalis. Occasionally, very large lesions can cause obstruction of the fetal airway. Such obstruction can result in the development of polyhydramnios by impairing the ability of the fetus to swallow amniotic fluid. In these circumstances, the airway is usually markedly distorted, which can result in immediate airway obstruction unless the airway is secured at the time of delivery. Orotracheal intubation or urgent emergency tracheostomy while the infant remains attached to the placenta, the ex utero intrapartum technique (EXIT) procedure, may be necessary to secure the airway. (See Schwartz 8th ed., p 1476.)

3. The blood supply to an intralobar sequestration is primarily
   A. Pulmonary artery
   B. Pulmonary vein
   C. Bronchial artery
   D. Direct branch from the aorta

**Answer: D**

Pulmonary sequestration is uncommon and consists of a mass of lung tissue, usually in the left lower chest, occurring without the usual connections to the pulmonary artery or tracheobronchial tree, yet with a systemic blood supply from the aorta. There are two kinds of sequestration. Extralobar sequestration is usually a small area of nonaerated lung separated from the main lung mass, with a systemic blood supply, that is located immediately above the left diaphragm. It is commonly found in cases of congenital diaphragmatic hernia. Intralobar sequestration more commonly occurs within the parenchyma of the left lower lobe, but can occur on the right. There is no major connection to the tracheobronchial tree, but a secondary connection may be established, perhaps through infection or via adjacent intrapulmonary shunts. The blood supply is systemic from the aorta, is often multiple vessels, and frequently originates below the diaphragm (Fig. 38-7). Venous drainage of both types can be systemic or pulmonary. The cause of sequestration is unknown, but most probably involves an abnormal budding of the developing lung that picks up a systemic blood supply and never becomes connected with the bronchus or pulmonary vessels. Extralobar sequestration is asymptomatic and is usually discovered incidentally on chest X-ray (CXR). If the diagnosis can be confirmed (e.g., by computed tomography [CT] scan), resection is not necessary. Diagnosis of intralobar sequestration, on the other hand, is usually made after repeated infections manifested by cough, fever, and consolidation in the posterior basal segment of the left lower lobe. Increasingly the diagnosis is being made in the early months of life by ultrasound (US), and color Doppler often can be helpful in delineating the systemic arterial supply. Removal of the entire left lower lobe is usually necessary since the diagnosis often is made late after multiple infections. Occasionally the sequestered part of the lung can be removed segmentally. Prognosis is excellent. (See Schwartz 8th ed., p 1479.)

4. The most common form of esophageal atresia is
   A. Pure esophageal atresia (no fistula)
   B. Pure tracheoesophageal fistula (no atresia)
   C. Esophageal atresia with distal tracheoesophageal fistula
   D. Esophageal atresia with proximal tracheoesophageal fistula

**Answer: C**
The five major varieties of esophageal atresia (EA) and tracheoesophageal fistula (TEF) are shown in Fig. 38-8. The most commonly seen variety is EA with distal TEF (type C), which occurs in approximately 75–85% of the cases in most series. The next most frequent is pure EA (type A), occurring in 8 to 10% of patients, followed by TEF without EA (type E). This occurs in 5–8% of cases, and also is referred to as an H-type fistula, based on the anatomic similarity to that letter (Fig. 38-9). EA with fistula between both proximal and distal ends of the esophagus and trachea (type D) is seen in approximately 1–2% of cases, and type B, EA with TEF between proximal segments of esophagus and trachea, is seen in approximately 1% of all cases. (See Schwartz 8th ed., 1481.)

5. The initial treatment for a pure esophageal atresia (no fistula) is
   A. Repair of the esophageal atresia
   B. Repair of the esophageal atresia with placement of a gastrostomy
   C. Repair of the esophageal atresia, Nissen fundoplication, and placement of a gastrostomy
   D. Gastrostomy alone

**Answer: D**
Primary esophageal atresia (type A) represents a challenging problem, particularly if the upper and lower ends are too far apart for an anastomosis to be created. Under these circumstances, treatment strategies include placement of a gastrostomy tube and performing serial bougienage to increase the length of the upper pouch. Occasionally, when the two ends cannot be brought safely together, esophageal replacement is required, using either a gastric pull-up or colon interposition. (See Schwartz 8th ed., p 1485.)

6. Which of the following is most consistent with pyloric stenosis?
   A. Na 140 Cl 110 K 4.2 HCO$_3$ 26
   B. Na 142 Cl 90 K 5.2 HCO$_3$ 39
   C. Na 139 Cl 85 K 3.2 HCO$_3$ 36
   D. Na 140 Cl 95 K 4.0 HCO$_3$ 18

**Answer: C**
Infants with hypertrophic pyloric stenosis (HPS) develop a hypochloremic, hypokalemic metabolic alkalosis. The urine pH level is high initially, but eventually drops because hydrogen ions are preferentially exchanged for sodium ions in the distal tubule of the kidney as the hypochloremia becomes severe. The diagnosis of pyloric stenosis usually can be made on physical examination by palpation of the typical "olive" in the right upper quadrant, and the presence of visible gastric waves on the abdomen. When the olive cannot be palpated, ultrasound can diagnose the condition accurately in 95% of patients. Criteria for ultrasound diagnosis include a channel length of over 16 mm and pyloric thickness over 4 mm. (See Schwartz 8th ed., p 1486.)

7. The appropriate repair of duodenal obstruction from an annular pancreas is
   A. Division of the pancreatic ring
   B. Resection of the pancreatic ring
   C. Duodenoduodenostomy
   D. Duodenojejunostomy

**Answer: C**
An orogastric tube is inserted to decompress the stomach and duodenum and the infant is given intravenous fluids to maintain adequate urine output. If the infant appears ill, or if abdominal tenderness is present, a diagnosis of malrotation and midgut volvulus should be considered, and surgery should not be delayed. Typically, the abdomen is soft and the infant is stable. Under these circumstances, the infant should be evaluated thoroughly for other associated anomalies. Approximately one-third of newborns with duodenal atresia have associated Down syndrome (trisomy 21). Patients then should be evaluated for associated cardiac anomalies. Once the work-up is complete and the infant is stable, the patient is taken to the operating room and the abdomen is entered through a transverse right upper quadrant supraumbilical incision under general endotracheal anesthesia. Associated anomalies should be sought at the time of the operation. These include malrotation, anterior portal vein, a second distal web, and biliary atresia. The surgical treatment of choice for duodenal obstruction due to duodenal stenosis or atresia or annular pancreas is a duodenoduodenostomy. This procedure can be most easily performed using a proximal transverse-to-distal longitudinal (diamond-shaped) anastomosis. In cases in which the duodenum is extremely dilated, the lumen may be tapered using a linear stapler with a large Foley catheter ($\geq$24 F) in the duodenal lumen. It is important to emphasize that an annular pancreas is never divided. Treatment of duodenal web includes vertical duodenotomy, excision of the web, oversewing of the mucosa, and closing the duodenotomy horizontally. Gastrostomy tubes are not placed routinely. Recently reported survival rates exceed 90%. Late complications from repair of duodenal atresia occur in approximately 12 to 15% of patients, and include megaduodenum, intestinal motility disorders, and gastroesophageal reflux. (See Schwartz 8th ed., p 1488.)

8. A 9-month-old boy presents with two episodes of vomiting as well as episodes of colicky pain. The abdominal exam is normal. His stool is normal, but is 1+ guaiac positive. The next step is
   A. Ultrasound
   B. Barium enema
   C. Stool culture
   D. Exploratory laparotomy

**Answer: A**

Since intussusception is frequently preceded by a gastrointestinal viral illness, the onset may not be easily determined. Typically, the infant develops paroxysms of crampy abdominal pain and intermittent vomiting. Between attacks, the infant may act normally, but as symptoms progress, increasing lethargy develops. Bloody mucus ("currant-jelly" stool) may be passed per rectum. Ultimately, if reduction is not accomplished, gangrene of the intussusceptum occurs, and perforation may ensue. On physical examination, an elongated mass is detected in the right upper quadrant or epigastrium, with an absence of bowel in the right lower quadrant (Dance's sign). The mass may be seen on plain abdominal X-ray, but is more easily demonstrated on air or contrast enema. (See Schwartz 8th ed., p 1493.)

9. The defect in gastroschisis is
   A. Through the umbilicus
   B. Superior to the umbilicus
   C. To the right of the umbilicus
   D. To the left of the umbilicus

**Answer: C**

Gastroschisis represents a congenital defect characterized by a defect in the anterior abdominal wall through which the intestinal contents freely protrude. Unlike the omphalocele, there is no overlying sac and the size of the defect is much smaller (<4 cm). The abdominal wall defect is located at the junction of the umbilicus and normal skin, and is almost always to the right of the umbilicus (Fig. 38-31). The umbilicus becomes partly detached, allowing free communication with the abdominal cavity. The appearance of the bowel provides some information with respect to the in utero timing of the defect. The intestine may be normal in appearance, suggesting that the rupture occurred relatively late during the pregnancy. More commonly, however, the intestine is thick, edematous, discolored, and covered with exudate, implying a more long-standing process. (See Schwartz 8th ed., p 1503.)

10. Undescended testes are usually repaired at what age?
    A. When diagnosed
    B. In infancy
    C. Before 2 years of age
    D. Before 6 years of age

**Answer: C**

Males with bilateral undescended testicles are often infertile. When the testicle is not within the scrotum, it is subjected to a higher temperature, resulting in decreased spermatogenesis. Mengel and coworkers studied 515 undescended testicles by histology and demonstrated a decreasing presence of spermatogonia after 2 years of age. Consequently it is now recommended that the undescended testicle be surgically repositioned by 2 years of age. Despite orchidopexy, the incidence of infertility is approximately two times higher in men with unilateral orchidopexy compared to men with normal testicular descent. (See Schwartz 8th ed., p 1506.)

11. The predicted 4-year survival rate of a child with a Wilms' tumor that is confined to one kidney and is grossly excised is
    A. 24%
    B. 38%
    C. 68%
    D. 97%

**Answer: D**

Following nephroureterectomy for Wilms' tumor, the need for chemotherapy and/or radiation therapy is determined by the histology of the tumor and the clinical stage of the patient (Table 38-3). Essentially, patients who have disease confined to one kidney that is totally removed surgically receive a short course of chemotherapy, and can expect a 97% 4-year survival rate, with tumor relapse rare after that time. Patients with more advanced disease or with unfavorable histology receive more intensive chemotherapy and radiation. Even in stage IV, cure rates of 80% are achieved. The survival rates are worse in the small percentage of patients considered to have unfavorable histology. The major chemotherapeutic agents are dactinomycin and vincristine, with the addition of doxorubicin for more advanced stages. (See Schwartz 8th ed., p 1509.)

12. The major determinant of poor survival in infants after tracheoesophageal fistula repair is
    A. Esophageal anastomotic leak
    B. Low birth weight
    C. Pneumonia
    D. Presence of other anomalies

**Answer: D**
All of the listed problems may contribute to a poor outcome, but the presence of other severe anomalies is the most significant problem. Almost 20% of those infants have associated cardiac abnormalities. Low birth weight can be managed by proper nutritional support. Antibiotic therapy and fistula closure should permit control of pneumonia. If an anastomosis under tension is avoided by mobilizing the proximal esophageal segment, major anastomotic leaks should be avoided. Minor leaks are not unusual, and oral intake should be postponed until healing occurs spontaneously. Gastroesophageal reflux may be a problem, requiring an antireflux procedure such as a Nissen fundoplication. (See Schwartz 7th ed.)

13. A double bubble on an air contrast upper gastrointestinal series in an infant is characteristic of
    A. Duodenal atresia
    B. Jejunal atresia
    C. Meconium ileus
    D. Pyloric stenosis

**Answer: A**
The double bubble represents air in the stomach and in the duodenum proximal to the atretic urea in the duodenal loop. (See Schwartz 7th ed.)

14. An infant with duodenal atresia is also likely to have
    A. Aniridia
    B. Biliary atresia
    C. Down's syndrome
    D. Imperforate anus

**Answer: C**
Approximately one-third of newborns with duodenal atresia have Down's syndrome (trisomy 21). Aniridia is associated with Wilms' tumor. Biliary atresia is frequently accompanied with other malformations, especially polysplenia. Imperforate anus and ventricular septal defect are found in some patients with tracheoesophageal fistula anomaly. (See Schwartz 7th ed.)

15. A male infant with prune-belly syndrome will display all of the following abnormalities EXCEPT
    A. Bilateral intraabdominal testes
    B. Dilatation of the ureters
    C. Dilatation of the urinary bladder
    D. Malformed renal parenchyma

**Answer: D**
Prune-belly syndrome occurs almost exclusively in males. In addition to a lax abdominal wall, these babies show bilateral abdominal testes and impressive dilatation of the ureters and urinary bladder. However, renal parenchyma is functional, and the urinary tract dilatation does not require operative intervention unless there is a specific obstructive lesion present. Despite orchiopexy at age 6–12 months when the lax abdominal wall is reconstructed, late fertility is unlikely. (See Schwartz 7th ed.)

16. Before the removal of a fairly large mass from the base of the tongue in a 4-year-old child, which of the following procedures should be performed?
    A. Lateral X-ray of the neck
    B. Nasopharyngoscopy
    C. Measurement of radioactive iodine uptake
    D. Measurement of serum thyroxine concentration

**Answer: C**
When a mass of significant size is found at the base of the tongue of a young child, the presence of thyroid tissue in its normal anatomic position should be demonstrated before excision of the lesion to avoid the possibility of removing the child's ectopic but only functioning thyroid tissue from the base of the tongue. Therefore, before the removal of the mass, a radioactive iodine uptake scan should be carried out to determine whether other thyroid tissue is present. Neither measurement of thyroxine concentration nor thyrotropin studies can localize thyroid tissue, and neither nasopharyngoscopy nor lateral radiograms of the neck would be useful. (See Schwartz 7th ed.)

17. All of the following statements concerning Hirschsprung's disease in children are true EXCEPT
    A. An absence of ganglion cells in a dilated segment of the colon is the underlying problem.
    B. Constipation is a classic symptom and almost always begins in the early days of life.
    C. Fecal incontinence is unusual in older affected children.
    D. Rectal examination of affected patients usually reveals an empty rectal ampulla.

**Answer: A**
In Hirschsprung's disease, there is a congenital absence of ganglion cells in the rectum and rectosigmoid, and the aganglionic area of bowel is inert and acts as an obstructing lesion. Although the disease frequently is mild and thus may not be recognized until months or years after birth, careful questioning will almost always reveal a history of obstinate constipation from birth. In older affected children who have been toilet-trained, rectal incontinence is, however, an unusual historical finding. On rectal examination, an empty ampulla should be discovered, and the finding of stool pressing against the anal verge indicates a diagnosis of psychogenic constipation rather than Hirschsprung's disease. Although some surgeons carry out definitive surgery designed to eliminate aganglionic bowel in young infants, most surgeons prefer to perform a colostomy and then postpone the definitive operation until the distended bowel has returned to normal caliber. The hypertrophied, dilated portion of the intestine in Hirschsprung's disease contains normal ganglion cells, and it is in the narrow segment of the colon distal to the dilated portion that ganglion cells are absent. (See Schwartz 7th ed.)

18. A newborn with gastroschisis is at increased risk of
    A. Exstrophy of the cloaca
    B. Hepatomegaly
    C. Intestinal atresia
    D. Macroglossia

**Answer: C**
Because the bowel in patients with gastroschisis is frequently floating free in the amniotic cavity, bowel atresia and stenosis are frequent problems. The other conditions listed are found with another umbilical anomaly, omphalocele. Enlargement of the liver and kidneys, macroglossia, mild microcephaly, large size at birth, and intractable hypoglycemia along with omphalocele occur in Beckwith-Wiedemann syndrome. (See Schwartz 7th ed.)

19. All of the following statements concerning intussusception in infants are true EXCEPT
    A. The peak incidence occurs in infants 8–12 months of age.
    B. Characteristically, well-nourished, vigorous males are affected.
    C. The presence of a tubular mass in the right lower quadrant is the most frequent physical finding.
    D. Hydrostatic retrograde reduction by barium enema frequently is possible.

**Answer: C**
Intussusception occurs frequently in healthy infants in the latter third of the first year of life. Males are affected more frequently than females. The typical intussusception is of the ileocolic variety, and the pathognomonic physical finding is an absence of bowel in the right lower quadrant and the presence of a tubular mass in the right or middle upper part of the abdomen. Hydrostatic reduction of the intussusception by means of a barium enema is frequently successful, and the use of intravenous glucagon to relax the smooth

muscle of the intestinal wall is thought to facilitate the process. Hydrostatic reduction cannot be considered to have worked, however, until the retrograde flow of barium demonstrates that the ileal component as well as the cecal portion of the intussusception has been unequivocally reduced. When hydrostatic reduction fails, surgical exploration is mandatory. (See Schwartz 7th ed.)

1. Which of the following is NOT a common place for impaction of a kidney stone?
   A. Ureteral pelvic junction
   B. Pelvic brim
   C. Ureteral vesical junction
   D. Vesicourethral junction

**Answer: D**

Along the course of the ureter in the retroperitoneum, the ureteral lumen is relatively narrower at the ureteral pelvic junction, at the pelvic brim where the ureter crosses the common iliac vessels and at the ureteral vesical junction. In patients passing a kidney stone, these areas represent common sites of impaction. (See Schwartz 8th ed., p 1570.)

2. Urinary continence in women is maintained by
   A. Internal sphincter
   B. Middle circular layer of the bladder neck
   C. External sphincter
   D. Lower bladder pressure

**Answer: C**

In men, urinary continence is maintained by the internal and external sphincters. The internal sphincter, composed of smooth muscle, is formed by the middle circular layer of the bladder wall as it invests the prostate gland. Contraction of this sphincter during ejaculation prevents retrograde ejaculation by directing the semen toward the urethral meatus. The external sphincter surrounds the urethra at the level of the distal prostate gland and is composed of both smooth and striated muscle fibers.

In women, the continence mechanism is quite different. There is no internal sphincter and the middle circular layer of the bladder muscularis, which is prominent in the male bladder neck, is not found. Continence is maintained by the resistance provided by the coaptation of the urethral mucosa and the external striated sphincter surrounding the distal two-thirds of the urethra. (See Schwartz 8th ed., p 1521.)

3. Prostate cancer occurs most commonly in which zone of the prostate?
   A. Central zone
   B. Urethral zone
   C. Transitional zone
   D. Peripheral zone

**Answer: D**

Most prostate cancers form in the peripheral zone. The central zone surrounds the ejaculatory ducts as they empty into the urethra at the verumontanum. Benign prostatic hyperplasia (BPH) is caused by enlargement of the transition zone surrounding the urethra. BPH, which is common in the elderly population, can lead to increased urinary resistance and voiding symptoms. (See Schwartz 8th ed., p 1521.)

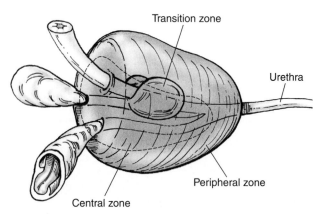

**FIG. 39-1.**    *Zonal anatomy of the prostate.*

4.  The function of the Leydig cells is
    A.  Testosterone production
    B.  Support of sperm maturation
    C.  Establishment of the blood-testis barrier
    D.  Production of sperm growth factors

5.  The tunica vaginalis corresponds to which layer of the abdominal wall?
    A.  External oblique
    B.  Internal oblique
    C.  Transversalis fascia
    D.  Peritoneum

**Answer: A**
The Leydig cells in the testis produce testosterone. The Sertoli cells support the maturation of spermatogenic cells into sperm. The Sertoli cells are also responsible for establishing a blood-testis barrier. (See Schwartz 8th ed., p 1521.)

**Answer: D**
The testicles are surrounded by several fascial layers that are embryologically derived from the same layers comprising the anterior abdominal wall (Fig. 39-2). The external spermatic fascia is analogous to the external oblique. The cremasteric muscle envelops the spermatic cord and is analogous to the internal oblique and transversus abdominis. The internal spermatic fascia is analogous to the transversalis fascia. The visceral and parietal layers of the tunica vaginalis testis represent peritoneum that surrounded the testicle during its descent into the scrotum. (See Schwartz 8th ed., pp 1521–22.)

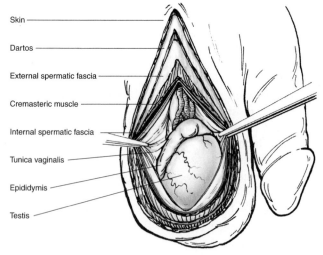

**FIG. 39-2.**    *The testicle and its surrounding layers.*

6. Which of the following is NOT part of the blood supply to the testicle?
   A. Gonadal artery
   B. Vasal artery
   C. Cremasteric artery
   D. Superior epigastric artery

**Answer: D**

The blood supply to the testicles is provided by three arteries: gonadal, cremasteric, and vasal. The gonadal artery branches directly from the aorta. The cremasteric artery branches from the inferior epigastric artery, and the vasal artery branches from the superior vesical artery. The venous drainage from the testicles forms the pampiniform plexus at the level of the spermatic cord. At the internal inguinal ring, the pampiniform plexus coalesces to form the gonadal vein, which drains into the inferior vena cava on the right and into the renal vein on the left. (See Schwartz 8th ed., p 1522.)

7. Appropriate treatment for a single episode of microscopic hematuria is
   A. Reassurance and serial urinalysis to confirm resolution
   B. Urine culture and intravenous pyelogram alone
   C. Cystoscopy alone
   D. Imaging of upper tract and cystoscopy

**Answer: D**

Patients with gross or microscopic hematuria, in the absence of obvious evidence of a urinary tract infection, need to be evaluated with upper and lower tract studies. On microscopic examination of the urine, more than five red blood cells per high power field in spun urine or more than two red blood cells per high power field in unspun urine is considered significant microscopic hematuria. Because hematuria can be intermittent, even a single documented episode of significant microscopic hematuria warrants a complete evaluation. The upper tract, which includes the kidney and ureter, should be evaluated with an intravenous pyelogram, computed tomography (CT) scan, or retrograde pyelogram. The CT scan should be performed with intravenous contrast and delayed images should be obtained once the excreted contrast has filled the upper tract collecting system. The lower tract, which includes the bladder and urethra, should be evaluated by cystoscopy.

The differential diagnosis for hematuria includes malignancies, infections, kidney stones, and trauma. Malignancies of the kidney and bladder classically present with painless hematuria. Patients with gross painless hematuria should be considered to have a urinary tract malignancy until proven otherwise. Infections involving the bladder or urethra are generally associated with symptoms of irritative voiding. Pyelonephritis is a clinical diagnosis based on findings of irritative voiding symptoms, fever, and flank pain. Kidney stones are associated with a colicky pain. The localization of the pain depends on the level of obstruction by the stone. An obstruction at the ureteropelvic junction will cause flank pain while obstruction of the lower ureter can produce colicky pain referred to the lower abdomen or groin. (See Schwartz 8th ed., p 1524.)

8. Kidney function in a preoperative patient is best measured by
   A. Serum blood, urea, nitrogen, and creatinine
   B. Creatinine clearance
   C. Renal ultrasound
   D. Computed tomography scan

**Answer: B**

The best measure of kidney function that does not involve infusion of exogenous substances is the endogenous creatinine clearance rate. Creatinine clearance is defined as the volume of plasma from which creatinine is completely removed per unit of time and is a clinical approximation of the glomerular filtration rate (GFR) and renal function. Creatinine clearance is calculated from a 24-hour urine collection according to the following formula:

$$Clearance = UV/P$$

In this formula, $U$ and $P$ represent the urine and plasma concentrations of creatinine, respectively, and $V$ represents the urine flow rate. Normal creatinine clearance is 90 to 110 mL/min. (See Schwartz 8th ed., p 1525.)

9. Which of the following studies is NOT useful in evaluating a patient with benign prostatic hypertrophy (BPH)?
   A. International prostate symptom score questionnaire
   B. Cystoscopy
   C. Pre-void ultrasound
   D. Pressure-flow study

**Answer: C**
The work-up for LUTS (lower urinary tract symptoms) should include a thorough voiding history. The symptoms can be quantified by having the patient fill out an international prostate symptom score (I-PSS) questionnaire (Table 39-1). This questionnaire has been validated as a useful means for assessing and following symptoms resulting from BPH. Treatment is recommended for an I-PSS greater than 7.

Other studies can be more selectively obtained in patients with voiding symptoms. Cystoscopy should be performed for patients who also present with hematuria or when a urethral stricture is suspected. For patients with a very poor stream, or for patients complaining of a sense of incomplete emptying, a postvoid residual should be measured by ultrasound or by catheterization. A renal ultrasound should be performed in patients with an elevated creatinine. For select patients, a pressure-flow study may be necessary. A decrease in urinary flow may result from bladder outlet obstruction or from failure of the bladder to effectively contract. To distinguish between the two, a small-diameter catheter can be inserted into the bladder to transduce bladder pressures during voiding. High bladder pressure and low flow rates are consistent with obstruction. Low bladder pressure and low flow rates suggest a neurogenic bladder that is unable to effectively contract. (See Schwartz 8th ed., p 1528.)

10. Which of the following is NOT a medication used for benign prostatic hypertrophy (BPH)?
    A. Terazosin
    B. Captopril
    C. Doxazosin
    D. Tamsulosin

**Answer: B**
The smooth muscles at the bladder outlet are under alpha$_1$-adrenergic innervation. The first line therapy for BPH is an alpha blocker, which targets the dynamic component of the bladder outlet obstruction. Three alpha blockers that are available in the United States for the treatment of BPH are terazosin, doxazosin, and tamsulosin. Terazosin and doxazosin are selective for alpha$_1$-adrenoceptors, which are found in the prostate, as well as in the vascular endothelium and central nervous system. Both terazosin and doxazosin significantly lower blood pressure, especially in men with clinical hypertension. Therefore, terazosin and doxazosin are good choices in the approximately 30% of men with BPH who also have clinical hypertension. The most common side effects with these two medications are dizziness and orthostatic hypertension. Both medications should be titrated up over 1 to 2 weeks to their target dose. (See Schwartz 8th ed., p 1529.)

11. Transurethral resection syndrome after endoscopic resection of the prostate occurs because of
    A. Air embolism during the procedure
    B. Blood loss from postoperative irrigation
    C. Absorption of irrigant
    D. Relaxation of the urethral sphincter from spinal anesthesia

**Answer: C**
The standard endoscopic procedure for benign prostatic hyperplasia (BPH) is a transurethral resection (TUR) of the prostate. TUR is performed with a nonhemolytic fluid such as 1.5% glycine. Saline cannot be used because electrolytes in the irrigation fluid will dissipate the electric current used to resect the prostate. During the resection some of the irrigation

fluid is absorbed through venous channels in the prostate. If enough fluid is absorbed, TUR syndrome may develop from the resulting hypervolemia and dilutional hyponatremia. Patients with TUR syndrome may experience hypertension, bradycardia, nausea, vomiting, visual disturbance, mental status changes, and even seizures. During the procedure and the postoperative period, patients should be monitored for evidence of TUR syndrome, which occurs in approximately 2% of patients. Patients with evidence of TUR syndrome should be treated with diuretics, and electrolyte imbalances should be corrected. (See Schwartz 8th ed., pp 1530–31.)

12. Which of the following can occur as a paraneoplastic manifestation of renal cell carcinoma?
    A. Hepatic dysfunction
    B. Hypocalcemia
    C. Thrombocytopenia
    D. Pulmonary edema

**Answer: A**

Patients with renal cell carcinoma also can present with paraneoplastic manifestations such as anemia, hepatic dysfunction (Stauffer syndrome), cachexia, polycythemia, and hypercalcemia. Paraneoplastic findings result from soluble substances released by the tumor or by immune cells in response to the tumor. Paraneoplastic findings resulting from localized disease resolve following a nephrectomy. (See Schwartz 8th ed., p 1531.)

13. Which of the following is NOT a treatment option for a localized, 2.5-cm renal cell carcinoma?
    A. Enucleation plus adjuvant therapy (chemotherapy)
    B. Partial nephrectomy
    C. Cryoablation
    D. Radical nephrectomy

**Answer: A**

The standard treatment for localized renal cell carcinoma remains a radical nephrectomy. The classic radical nephrectomy involves removal of the kidney, the ipsilateral adrenal gland, and all the fat contained within Gerota's fascia. However, it has been shown that if there is no evidence of adrenal involvement by the tumor on the computed tomography (CT) scan, the adrenal gland can be spared. A radical nephrectomy can be performed using either an open or a laparoscopic approach. The laparoscopic approach is associated with less postoperative pain and a more rapid return to normal activities. For a radical nephrectomy, a laparoscopic procedure is now the standard of care.

For tumors less than 4 cm in size, a partial nephrectomy is an equally effective option for cancer control. It is preferred in patients who are at risk for renal insufficiency secondary to conditions such as hypertension, recurrent stone disease, or diabetes. When performing a partial nephrectomy, meticulous attention needs to be paid to preventing bleeding and urine leaks, and this is most effectively accomplished by an open surgical approach (Fig. 39-15). Although laparoscopic partial nephrectomies have been reported, an open surgical procedure remains the standard of care when performing a partial nephrectomy.

Another option for a small renal lesion (less than 3 cm in diameter) is laparoscopic cryoablation. The tumor is mobilized laparoscopically and cryoprobes that deliver argon gas or liquid nitrogen are inserted into the tumor. Usually a double freeze-thaw cycle is used to ablate the tumor. Although follow-up is limited, early reports suggest that cryotherapy is an effective treatment for small, peripheral lesions. (See Schwartz 8th ed., p 1532.)

14. Appropriate treatment for a superficial bladder cancer is
    A. Endoscopic resection and fulguration
    B. Full-thickness resection with a 1-cm margin
    C. Full-thickness resection with a 3-cm margin (subtotal cystectomy)
    D. Total cystectomy

**Answer: A**

Most superficial bladder cancers are adequately treated by endoscopic resection and fulguration of the bladder tumor. No further metastatic work-up is indicated if the pathology confirms a low-grade, superficial transitional cell carcinoma (TCCa). However, bladder cancer is considered a polyclonal, field-change defect and continued surveillance is mandatory. In other words, the underlying genetic changes that resulted in the bladder cancer have occurred in the entire urothelium, making the entire urothelium susceptible to future tumor formation. The risk of recurrence following the treatment of superficial bladder cancer is approximately 70% within 5 years. (See Schwartz 8th ed., p 1534.)

15. Appropriate therapy for a woman with non-metastatic muscle invasive bladder cancer is
    A. Subtotal cystectomy (2-cm margin)
    B. Total cystectomy
    C. Total cystectomy with radical hysterectomy
    D. Anterior pelvic exenteration (removal of bladder, urethra, uterus, ovary, and anterior vaginal wall)

**Answer: D**

The gold standard for organ-confined, muscle-invasive bladder cancer (T2 and T3) is radical cystoprostatectomy in men and anterior pelvic exenteration in women. In men, radical cystectomy involves the removal of the bladder, prostate, and pelvic lymph nodes. A total urethrectomy also is performed if the urethral margin is positive. In women, a classic anterior pelvic exenteration includes the removal of the bladder, urethra, uterus, ovaries, and anterior vaginal wall. However, in a female patient, if the bladder neck margin is negative, the urethra and anterior vaginal wall may be spared. With treatment, the 5-year survival rates for pathologic T2, T3, T4a, and $N^+$ tumors are 63 to 80%, 19 to 57%, 0 to 36%, and 15 to 44% respectively. (See Schwartz 8th ed., p 1535.)

16. The most common urinary diversion after total cystectomy is
    A. End ureterostomy with external stoma
    B. Ureteroenterostomy (internal)
    C. Ileal conduit
    D. Colonic conduit

**Answer: C**

After cystectomy, the urine is diverted using segments of bowel. The various types of urinary diversions can be separated into continent and incontinent diversions. The most commonly performed incontinent diversion is the ileal conduit. A small segment of ileum is taken out of continuity with the gastrointestinal (GI) tract while maintaining its mesenteric blood supply. The ureters are anastomosed to one end of the conduit and the other end is brought out to the abdominal wall as a stoma. The urine continuously collects in an external collection device worn over the stoma. (See Schwartz 8th ed., p 1535.)

17. Initial therapy for metastatic prostate cancer is
    A. Total prostatectomy (sphincter-preserving)
    B. Radical prostatectomy
    C. Chemotherapy
    D. Bilateral orchiectomy

**Answer: D**

The first-line therapy for metastatic prostate cancer is androgen-ablative hormone therapy. Since Charles Huggins won the Nobel Prize in 1966 for discovering the therapeutic effects of androgen ablation on metastatic prostate cancer, the fundamental principles for treating metastatic prostate cancer have not changed. Androgen-ablation is accomplished by performing bilateral orchiectomies or by administering gonadotropin-releasing hormone (GnRH) agonist. Testosterone synthesis by the Leydig cell in the testicles is stimulated by luteinizing hormone (LH) from the pituitary. The release of LH requires a pulsatile discharge of GnRH. Therefore, a constant GnRH stimulation paradoxically results in inhibition of LH and testosterone. Nonsteroidal antiandrogens such as flutamide and bicalutamide are often added to block the low levels of androgens produced by the adrenal medulla. (See Schwartz 8th ed., p 1538.)

18. Appropriate treatment of a 30-year-old man with a solid testicular mass is
   A. Trans-scrotal needle biopsy
   B. Trans-scrotal open biopsy
   C. Inguinal open biopsy
   D. Radical orchiectomy

**Answer: D**

Any patient with a solid testicular mass, which has been confirmed on ultrasound, is considered to have testicular cancer until proven otherwise, and should undergo a radical orchiectomy to make a definitive diagnosis. Prior to surgery, serum markers for testicular cancer should be obtained. The two markers used in routine clinical practice are human chorionic gonadotropin (hCG) and follicle-stimulating hormone (FSH).

When performing a radical orchiectomy, the surgery should be performed by an inguinal approach rather than a scrotal approach. The metastatic spread of testicular cancer is ordered and predictable. The primary metastatic landing sites for left and right testicular cancers are the para-aortic and the interaortocaval nodes in the retroperitoneum, respectively. The lymphatic drainage of the scrotum, on the other hand, is to the inguinal nodes. If the scrotum is surgically violated by performing a scrotal orchiectomy, metastatic spread to both the retroperitoneal and the inguinal nodes becomes possible. (See Schwartz 8th ed., p 1538.)

19. A young man with a urinary tract infection (UTI) should be treated with antibiotics for
   A. 3 days
   B. 7 days
   C. 10 days
   D. 21 days

**Answer: B**

Symptoms of cystitis include urinary frequency, urgency, and dysuria. Uncomplicated cystitis does not generally cause fevers or leukocytosis. Patients with voiding symptoms can be worked up with a urinalysis. However, a urine culture provides a more definitive diagnosis of a UTI than a urinalysis. Important considerations when obtaining a urine culture have been previously discussed. Bacterial UTI in women should be treated with 3 days of antibiotics. In men, bacterial UTI should be treated for 7 days of antibiotics and younger men should be evaluated for correctable structural anomalies with an intravenous pyelogram (IVP) or computed tomography (CT) scan with IV contrast, and a cystoscopy. (See Schwartz 8th ed., p 1540.)

20. Patients with pyelonephritis require
   A. IV antibiotics for 7 days
   B. IV antibiotics for 14 days
   C. IV antibiotics until afebrile, then oral antibiotics for 7 days
   D. IV antibiotics until afebrile, then oral for a total of 14 days

**Answer: D**

Healthy adults with no significant comorbidities can be treated as an outpatient; however, most patients diagnosed with pyelonephritis are admitted to the hospital. Broad-spectrum IV antibiotics, such as ampicillin and gentamicin, should be started until the results of the urine culture are available and a more selective antibiotic can be identified. When patients are afebrile, they can be discharged on oral antibiotics. Uncomplicated pyelonephritis should be treated for a total of 14 days while pyelonephritis associated with structural or functional abnormalities should be treated for 21 days. (See Schwartz 8th ed., p 1540.)

21. Which of the following is an absolute indication for surgical treatment of a renal injury?
    A. Major urinary extravasation
    B. Vascular injury
    C. Expanding perirenal hematoma
    D. 20% devitalized renal parenchyma

**Answer: C**

The only absolute indications for surgical management of a renal injury are persistent bleeding resulting in hemodynamic instability or an expanding perirenal hematoma. Relative indications for surgical management include major urinary extravasation, vascular injury, and devitalized parenchymal tissue. Studies show that even large urinary extravasations will resolve with conservative management. Smaller vascular injuries resulting in devitalized tissue also can be managed without surgery; however, if the amount of devitalized tissue exceeds 20% of the renal tissue, surgical management leads to quicker resolution of the injury and to fewer subsequent complications. (See Schwartz 8th ed., p 1544.)

22. Extraperitoneal bladder rupture is usually treated by
    A. Placement of a Foley catheter and expectant management
    B. Suprapubic cystostomy
    C. Endoscopic repair
    D. Laparotomy

**Answer: A**

The management of bladder injury depends on the site of rupture. Extraperitoneal ruptures can usually be managed conservatively with prolonged catheter drainage; however, intraperitoneal ruptures should be explored and surgically repaired. (See Schwartz 8th ed., p 1545.)

# CHAPTER 40
# Gynecology

1. Skene's glands are located
   A. In the labia majora
   B. In the labia minora
   C. In the vaginal wall
   D. In the periurethral area

**Answer: D**
Skene's glands lie lateral and inferior to the urethral meatus and occasionally harbor pathogens such as *Neisseria gonorrhoeae*. Cysts, abscesses, and neoplasms may arise in these glands. (See Schwartz 8th ed., p 1562.)

2. Which of the following is NOT an avascular plane in the pelvis?
   A. Lateral pararectal space
   B. Prevesical space of Retzius
   C. Vaginourethral space
   D. Rectovaginal space

**Answer: C**
On transverse section several avascular, and therefore important, surgical planes, can be identified. These include the lateral paravesical and pararectal spaces, and, from anterior to posterior, the retropubic or prevesical space of Retzius and the vesicovaginal, rectovaginal, and retrorectal or presacral spaces. The pelvic brim demarcates the obstetric, or true, from the false pelvis contained within the iliac crests. (See Schwartz 8th ed., p 1563.)

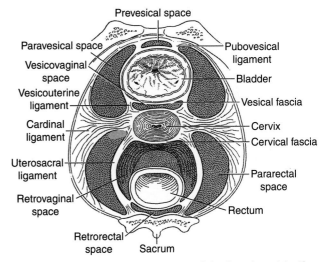

**FIG. 40-1.** *The avascular spaces of the female pelvis. (See Schwartz 8th ed., p 1563.)*

3. In a patient with a vaginal discharge, a pH of 4.9 of the fluid is indicative of
   A. Pregnancy
   B. Cervical cancer
   C. Infection
   D. Non-infectious vaginitis

**Answer: C**
The patient's complaint of abnormal vaginal discharge should be investigated. Vaginal secretions that appear abnormal or have a foul odor must be studied. The pH of the vagina, which is normally between 3.8 and 4.4, may be an aid to diagnosis. A vaginal pH of 4.9 or more indicates either a

bacterial or protozoal infection. The pH is obtained by dipping a pH tape in the vaginal secretions collected in the vaginal speculum. (See Schwartz 8th ed., p 1566.)

4. Appropriate treatment for candidal vulvovaginitis includes
   A. Avoiding baths
   B. Single dose of fluconazole
   C. Topical barrier cream
   D. Daily vaginal irrigation with saline

**Answer: B**

The most common cause of vulvar pruritus is candidal vulvovaginitis. The infection is most common in patients who are diabetic, pregnant, or on antibiotics. The majority of cases are caused by *C. albicans*, although other species may be incriminated. The most prominent symptom is itching; burning of the skin, dysuria, and dyspareunia are also common. Diagnosis is confirmed by examination of the vaginal secretions and recognition of the characteristic pseudomycelia. The condition is treated by the topical application of any one of a number of azole preparations. Intravaginal agents include a number of azole creams generally used over a 3- to 7-day period. Systemic treatment is possible through the oral use of fluconazole 150 mg tablet in a single dose. (See Schwartz 8th ed., p 1568.)

5. Appropriate treatment for vulvar infection with human papillomavirus includes
   A. IV ganciclovir for 1 week
   B. IV acyclovir for 1 week
   C. Oral ganciclovir for 2 weeks
   D. Ablation of superficial lesions

**Answer: D**

A number of viral infections affect the vulva and vagina, the most common of these being condyloma acuminatum. The causative organism is the human papillomavirus. This infection has increased dramatically in the past 20 years. The lesions are characteristic wart-like growths that begin as single lesions but can grow to huge confluent lesions that distort the normal structures. The lesions enlarge rapidly in pregnancy. Diagnosis is suspected on the basis of appearance and confirmed by biopsy. Treatment depends on the destruction of the lesions with caustic agents, cryocautery, laser ablation, or electrocautery. Some large lesions could require surgical removal. (See Schwartz 8th ed., p 1568.)

6. Which of the following is a recommended treatment for pelvic inflammatory disease?
   A. Metronidazole IV for 7 days
   B. Cefuroxime IV for 7 days
   C. Metronidazole orally for 7 days
   D. Levofloxacin orally for 14 days

**Answer: D**

Empiric antibiotic treatment of sexually active women who have even minimal symptoms of pelvic inflammatory disease is indicated if no other cause for the symptoms is found. Women with pelvic inflammatory disease can be treated as inpatients or outpatients, depending on the severity of their disease. Patients with evidence of peritonitis, high fever, or suspected tuboovarian abscess should be admitted to the hospital for observation and intravenous antibiotics. Some specialists believe that all women with pelvic inflammatory disease should be admitted to the hospital for more intensive care, which may preserve fertility.

The Centers for Disease Control (CDC) recommends one of the following oral regimens: ofloxacin 400 mg orally twice a day for 14 days or levofloxacin 500 mg orally once daily for 14 days with or without metronidazole 500 mg orally twice daily for 14 days.

Follow-up of patients treated on an ambulatory basis should be carried out within 48 to 72 hours. If there is no improvement in the patient, she should be admitted for intravenous antibiotics.

Recommendations from the CDC for parenteral treatment include cefotetan 2.0 g IV every 12 hours or cefoxitin 2 g IV every 6 hours plus doxycycline 100 mg orally or IV every 12 hours. This regimen is continued for at least 24 hours after the patient shows clinical improvement. Doxycycline 100 mg orally twice daily is given to complete a total of 14 days of therapy. (See Schwartz 8th ed., p 1569.)

7. Which of the following is NOT an indication for surgery in a woman with pelvic inflammatory disease?
   A. 3-cm tuboovarian abscess
   B. Persistent pelvic abscess
   C. Rupture of a tuboovarian abscess
   D. Chronic pain

**Answer: A**
Surgery becomes necessary under the following conditions: (1) the intraperitoneal rupture of a tuboovarian abscess; (2) the persistence of a pelvic abscess despite antibiotic therapy; and (3) chronic pelvic pain.

At one time, total abdominal hysterectomy with bilateral salpingo-oophorectomy was considered the procedure of choice when surgery for pelvic inflammatory disease was required. The availability of good antibiotics and a better understanding of the pathophysiology of the disease allow less-radical surgery. In young women whose reproductive goals have not been achieved, especially in the presence of unilateral disease, a unilateral salpingo-oophorectomy may be more appropriate than total hysterectomy with removal of both ovaries and fallopian tubes.

The rupture of a tuboovarian abscess is a true surgical emergency. Physical findings are frequently nonspecific. Rupture is most frequently associated with a sudden severe increase in abdominal pain. A shock-like state commonly accompanies rupture. Leukocyte counts are not necessarily increased, and some patients are afebrile. In the days before surgical intervention for this problem was common, mortality approached 100%. With prompt surgical intervention and intensive medical management, the mortality rate today is less than 5%. (See Schwartz 8th ed., p 1569.)

8. What percentage of women have physical findings of endometriosis at the time of laparotomy?
   A. <5%
   B. 10%
   C. 20%
   D. 30%

**Answer: C**
Endometriosis is one of the most common conditions encountered by the pelvic surgeon. It has been estimated that endometriosis will be demonstrated in approximately 20% of all laparotomies in women in the reproductive age group. Although the condition occurs in teenage women, it is found most often in the third and fourth decades of life. Endometriosis persists into the postreproductive years.

The exact cause of endometriosis is unknown, but the most common theory is that it is initiated by retrograde menstruation. The theory is supported by the fact that it is extremely common in women who have congenital anomalies of the lower reproductive tract that would favor menstrual reflux. The most common of these anomalies is an imperforate hymen.

The most common lesions of endometriosis can be recognized as bluish or black lesions, sometimes raised, sometimes puckered, giving them a "gunpowder burn" appearance. Some lesions are white or yellow, but these are less common. The disease is found most commonly on the ovary, and in many cases will involve both ovaries. Other involved organs can include the uterosacral ligaments, the peritoneal surfaces of the deep pelvis, the fallopian tubes, rectosigmoid, and a number of distant sites, including the skin or even the lungs, diaphragm, and nasopharynx. (See Schwartz 8th ed., p 1569.)

9. Appropriate treatment of a "chocolate cyst" (ovarian endometrioma) found at the time of surgery is
   A. Nothing
   B. Cyst removal with closure of defect
   C. Cyst removal without closure of the defect
   D. Oophorectomy

**Answer: C**
The approach to ovarian endometriomas deserves special consideration. These "chocolate cysts" cannot be treated effectively medically. In general, even large endometriomas can be drained and the cyst lining removed laparoscopically. Although it was recommended in the past to close the ovary with several layers of absorbable sutures, it appears that this approach tends to increase postoperative adhesion formation. For this reason, it is recommended that after hemostasis is achieved, the ovary should be left open to close spontaneously. Other methods to minimize adhesion formation include atraumatic handling of the tissues and the use of a cellulose-adhesion barrier (Interceed) over the surgical site. Several series document pregnancy rates of approximately 50% following conservative operation. (See Schwartz 8th ed., p 1570.)

10. The most common presenting symptom of a patient with an ectopic pregnancy is
    A. Pain
    B. Vomiting
    C. Shortness of breath
    D. Shock

**Answer: A**
The most common complaint of patients with ectopic pregnancy is pain, frequently associated with irregular vaginal bleeding. Approximately 80% of affected women will recall a missed menstrual period. Physical findings include abdominal tenderness on cervical motion and adnexal tenderness on bimanual pelvic examination. An adnexal mass may be palpated in approximately 50% of patients. As a result of the intraperitoneal bleeding, some patients present in shock.

The most helpful laboratory examination is measurement of the beta subunit of hCG (beta-hCG). Modern-day testing, with a sensitivity of 50 mIU/mL or less, enables the surgeon to confirm the pregnant state in almost all patients at risk for ectopic pregnancy. Once the physician is assured that the patient is pregnant, it must be determined that the pregnancy is in the uterus. Pelvic ultrasonography, particularly when performed with a vaginal transducer, is proving important in differentiating uterine gestations from ectopic gestations. (See Schwartz 8th ed., pp 1570–71.)

11. Which of the following is the treatment of choice in a stable woman with a 3.5-cm distal tubal pregnancy?
    A. Linear salpingostomy with removal of conceptus and reconstruction of the tube
    B. Linear salpingostomy with removal of conceptus without reconstruction of the tube
    C. Subtotal salpingectomy
    D. Total salpingectomy

**Answer: B**
The laparoscope has been an important diagnostic tool for the last several decades, but only recently has it become the standard approach for treatment. Linear salpingostomy is the treatment of choice for ectopic pregnancies less than 4 cm in diameter that occur in the distal third (ampullary) segment of the tube. To aid in hemostasis, the mesentery below the involved tubal segment is infiltrated with a dilute vasopressin solution. The tube may then be opened in its long axis along the antimesenteric side with either a laser or a unipolar cutting cautery. The conceptus is then aspirated, and any bleeding is electrocoagulated with bipolar cautery. Closing the tube is not necessary because the tube closes spontaneously in almost every case. If hemostasis cannot be achieved, coagulation of a portion of the mesosalpinx just below the segment

may be required. Partial or total salpingectomy is indicated when the pregnancy is located in the isthmic portion of the tube. Bipolar electrocoagulation is used to desiccate a short segment of fallopian tube on either side of the pregnancy, and the pregnancy and tubal segment are removed together. Larger ectopic pregnancies are managed by total salpingectomy because adequate hemostasis is difficult to achieve without extensive tubal damage. For this procedure, the mesosalpinx is serially coagulated with bipolar cautery and transected with scissors. When the uterotubal junction is reached, the tube is desiccated with bipolar cautery, and the entire tube and pregnancy are removed with the aid of a specimen bag and a large port. (See Schwartz 8th ed., p 1571.)

12. Which of the following is most likely to result in rupture with hemorrhagic shock?
    A. Follicular cyst
    B. Corpus luteum cyst
    C. Endometrium
    D. Wolffian duct remnants
    E. Müllerian duct remnants

**Answer: B**

**Follicular Cysts.** These are unruptured, enlarged graafian follicles. They grossly resemble true cystomas. They can rupture, causing acute peritoneal irritation, undergo torsion and infarction of the ovary or infarction of the tube and ovary, or spontaneously regress.

**Corpus Luteum Cysts.** These cysts may become as large as 10 to 11 cm. They can rupture and lead to severe hemorrhage and, occasionally, to vascular collapse from blood loss. The symptoms and physical findings of these cysts mimic those of ectopic pregnancy, and they are occasionally associated with delayed menses and spotting.

**Endometriomas.** These account for most "chocolate cysts" and are cystic forms of endometriosis of the ovary.

**Wolffian Duct Remnants.** These are not ovarian cysts but often cannot be distinguished clinically from tumors of the ovary. They are small unilocular cysts. Occasionally, they enlarge and can twist and infarct. In most instances, they are incidental findings at laparotomy and cause no difficulties or symptoms.

**Müllerian Duct Remnants.** These can appear as para-ovarian cysts or as small cystic swellings at the fimbriated end of the fallopian tube (hydatids of Morgagni). (See Schwartz 8th ed., p 1577.)

13. Which of the following is seen in a patient with Meigs' syndrome?
    A. Pleural effusion
    B. Malignant ovarian tumor
    C. Polycythemia
    D. Lower extremity edema

**Answer: A**

This pertains to ascites with hydrothorax, seen in association with benign ovarian tumors with fibrous elements, usually fibromas. It is more common to see fluid accumulation with ovarian fibromas that are more than 6 cm in size. The cause of the condition is unknown, but the ascitic fluid may originate from the tumor, as a result of lymphatic obstruction of the ovary. Frequently, this clinical picture is encountered with other ovarian tumors, especially ovarian malignancies, which can produce a cytologically benign pleural effusion; in such cases, it is termed a pseudo-Meigs' syndrome. Meigs' syndrome can be cured by excising the fibroma. (See Schwartz 8th ed., p 1577.)

14. Which of the following tumors can be associated with hyperthyroidism?
    A. Theca cell tumors
    B. Sertoli-Leydig cell tumor
    C. Struma ovarii
    D. Arrhenoblastoma

**Answer: C**
**Struma Ovarii.** This term refers to the presence of grossly detectable thyroid tissue in the ovary, usually as the predominant element in dermoid cysts. This tissue occasionally may produce the clinical picture of hyperthyroidism and is rarely malignant. (See Schwartz 8th ed., p 1578.)

15. Nabothian cysts are located in the
    A. Ovary
    B. Endometrium
    C. Cervix
    D. Labia minora

**Answer: C**
Nabothian cysts are mucous inclusion cysts of the cervix. They are occasionally associated with chronic inflammation and can be removed easily with a cautery. They are harmless, usually asymptomatic, and generally do not require surgery. (See Schwartz 8th ed., p 1579.)

16. Which of the following vulvar lesions is NOT premalignant?
    A. Leukoplakia
    B. Lichen sclerosis
    C. Hypertrophic dystrophy
    D. Epithelial dysplasia

**Answer: B**
The term leukoplakia is often used for any white patch of the vulva; it is properly reserved for areas that show histologically atypical epithelial activity. These alterations may precede the development of malignant changes. In many instances, chronically irritated and itchy white areas of the vulva will show sclerosing atrophy of the skin (lichen sclerosus). Lichen sclerosus is a pruritic lesion that does not appear to be premalignant. Hyperplastic lesions termed hypertrophic dystrophies are found that may be benign (epithelial hyperplasia) or that may show atypia, in which case dysplastic changes can be observed. The pruritic symptoms can be helped by topical application of corticosteroids. Testosterone or clobetasol ointment also has been beneficial, especially for the atrophic changes of lichen sclerosus. (See Schwartz 8th ed., p 1579.)

17. The most important predictor of survival after surgery for advanced ovarian cancer is
    A. Presence of ascites
    B. Histologic grade
    C. Type of chemotherapy used
    D. Volume of tumor remaining after surgery

**Answer: D**
Survival in advanced ovarian cancer is influenced by a number of factors, such as patient age, the histologic type and grade of the lesion, the presence or absence of ascites, and the type of chemotherapy employed. Of prime importance in advanced-stage disease, however, is the volume of tumor remaining after the initial surgical procedure. Many patients with stages III and IV ovarian cancer have diffuse peritoneal, retroperitoneal, diaphragmatic, and mesenteric metastases that resist complete surgical resection. It is often possible, however, to remove large amounts of peritoneal tumor by entering the retroperitoneal spaces and freeing the disease-laden surfaces from the underlying viscera. (See Schwartz 8th ed., p 1580.)

18. The most common ovarian malignancy diagnosed during pregnancy is
    A. Dysgerminoma
    B. Yolk sac tumor
    C. Immature teratoma
    D. Choriocarcinoma

**Answer: A**
Dysgerminoma, the female equivalent of testicular seminoma, is composed of pure, undifferentiated germ cells. It is bilateral in 10 to 15% of patients and is occasionally associated with elevated levels of human chorionic gonadotropin (hCG) or lactate dehydrogenase (LDH). It is the most common ovarian malignancy diagnosed during pregnancy. Patients bearing dysgerminomas should undergo appropriate staging at the time of the primary resection but need not un-

dergo hysterectomy (if fertility is to be preserved) or removal of the opposite ovary if it is normal in appearance. Secondary operations solely for staging purposes are unwarranted. Adjuvant therapy is unnecessary unless there is evidence of extraovarian spread. Either radiotherapy encompassing the whole abdomen or systemic chemotherapy can be given to patients with metastases. This tumor is exquisitely sensitive to either type of treatment, and the cure rate exceeds 90% even in patients with metastases. Chemotherapy has the advantage of preserving ovarian function, whereas radiotherapy results in ovarian failure. (See Schwartz 8th ed., p 1582.)

19. Which of the following tumors is associated with elevated levels of alpha-fetoprotein?
    A. Endodermal sinus tumor
    B. Yolk sac tumor
    C. Immature teratoma
    D. Choriocarcinoma

**Answer: A**

The other germ cell tumors, in order of frequency, are immature teratoma; endodermal sinus, or "yolk sac," tumor; mixed tumors; embryonal carcinomas; and choriocarcinomas. The first may be associated with elevated levels of alpha-fetoprotein (AFP). Elevated AFP levels are found in all patients with endodermal sinus tumors and mixed tumors that contain this component. Embryonal carcinomas are associated with abnormal levels of both AFP and human chorionic gonadotropin (hCG), and choriocarcinomas secrete hCG. (See Schwartz 8th ed., p 1582.)

20. The appropriate treatment for locally advanced carcinoma of the cervix (stages IIB to IVA) is
    A. Hysterectomy alone
    B. Hysterectomy and bilateral salpingo-oophorectomy
    C. Radiation therapy alone
    D. Combination radiation and chemotherapy

**Answer: D**

These cancers are treated primarily with radiotherapy, with cisplatin as a radiosensitizer. Treatment consists of a combination of external therapy to the pelvis (teletherapy) from a high-energy source such as a linear accelerator and a local dose delivered to the cervix and parametrial tissue (brachytherapy) using a cesium applicator such as a Fletcher-Suite tandem and ovoids (Fig. 40-14). Combination therapy is essential because doses adequate to control cervical tumors exceeding about 1 cm in diameter cannot be given using teletherapy alone. Bladder and rectal tolerances are approximately 6000 rads; higher doses can only be attained by combination therapy. The addition of cisplatin as a weekly radiosensitizer has resulted in improved survival with no apparent increase in toxicity when compared with radiation alone. (See Schwartz 8th ed., p 1584.)

21. Which of the following is NOT a complication of hysteroscopy?
    A. Gas embolism
    B. Hypernatremia
    C. Uterine perforation
    D. Fluid overload

**Answer: B**

**Gas Embolism.** Gas embolism has been reported when using $CO_2$ for distention after intrauterine surgery. It is recommended that $CO_2$ not be used for any operative procedure or after significant dilation of the cervix. If symptoms of massive gas embolism occur during diagnostic hysteroscopy, the procedure should be stopped and the patient treated as described [in Schwartz 8th ed., Risks of Laparoscopy, Gas Embolism].

**Fluid Overload and Hyponatremia.** During operative hysteroscopy, significant intravasation of distention medium can occur through venous channels opened during surgery or transperitoneally as a result of any fluid forced through the tubes. Symptomatic fluid overload has been reported with all fluid distention media, including 32% dextran 70 in dextrose. The volume of distention medium introduced through the operating hysteroscope or hysteroresectoscope should always be compared with the volume retrieved using a urologic collection drape. When using a balanced salt solution (e.g., Ringer's lactate), symptomatic fluid overload is treated effectively with diuretics.

**Uterine Perforation and Bowel Injury.** Uterine perforation is a common risk of uterine dilation prior to hysteroscopy. If it is not possible to distend the uterine cavity when the hysteroscope is placed in the uterus, perforation should be suspected. If no sharp instrument or power source has been placed through the defect, expectant outpatient management is appropriate.

Occasionally, perforation will occur during resection of a septum or leiomyoma or other operative procedures. If any chance of bowel injury exists, laparoscopy to evaluate contiguous bowel for injury is a reasonable precaution.

**Intrauterine Synechia.** The formation of adhesions between the anterior and posterior uterine walls, referred to as synechiae, is an uncommon complication after intrauterine surgery.

Although intrauterine devices, intrauterine catheters, and high-dose estrogen therapy have been advocated to decrease the risk of this complication, the efficacy of these treatments remains uncertain. (See Schwartz 8th ed., p 1598.)

# CHAPTER 41

# Neurosurgery

1. A patient who withdraws from pain, is mumbling inappropriate words and opens his eyes to pain has a Glasgow Coma Scale score of
   A. 3
   B. 6
   C. 9
   D. 12

**Answer: C**

**Table 41-1.**
**The Glasgow Coma Scale (GCS) Score[a]**

| Motor Response (M) | | Verbal Response (V) | | Eye-Opening Response (E) | |
|---|---|---|---|---|---|
| Obeys commands | 6 | Oriented | 5 | Opens sponta- | 4 |
| Localizes to pain | 5 | Confused | 4 | neously | |
| Withdraws from | 4 | Inappropriate | 3 | Opens to speech | 3 |
| pain | | words | | Opens to pain | 2 |
| Flexor posturing | 3 | Unintelligible | 2 | No eye opening | 1 |
| Extensor posturing | 2 | sounds | | | |
| No movement | 1 | No sounds | 1 | | |

[a]Add the three scores to obtain the Glasgow Coma Scale score, which can range from 3 to 15. Add "T" after the GCS if intubated and no verbal score is possible. For these patients, the GCS can range from 2T to 10T. See Schwartz 8th ed., p 1613.

2. The halo test is used
   A. To test for cerebrospinal fluid (CSF) leak
   B. To test for blood behind the tympanic membrane
   C. To determine if cervical fixation is needed
   D. To determine if pupil dilation is related to neurologic injury

**Answer: A**

Fractures of the skull base are common in head-injured patients, and they indicate significant impacts. They are generally apparent on routine head computed tomography (CT), but should be evaluated with dedicated fine-slice coronal-section CT scan to document and delineate the extent of the fracture and involved structures. If asymptomatic, they require no treatment. Symptoms from skull base fractures include cranial nerve deficits and CSF leaks. A fracture of the temporal bone, for instance, can damage the facial or vestibulocochlear nerve, resulting in vertigo, ipsilateral deafness, or facial paralysis. A communication may be formed between the subarachnoid space and the middle ear, allowing CSF drainage into the pharynx via the eustachian tube or from the ear (otorrhea). Extravasation of blood results in ecchymosis behind the ear, known as Battle's sign. A fracture of the anterior skull base can result in anosmia (loss of smell from damage to the olfactory nerve), CSF drainage from the nose (rhinorrhea), or periorbital ecchymoses, known as raccoon eyes.

Copious clear drainage from the nose or ear makes the diagnosis of CSF leakage obvious. Often, however, the drainage may be discolored with blood or small in volume if some drains into the throat. The halo test can help differentiate. Allow a drop of the fluid to fall on an absorbent surface such as a facial tissue. If blood is mixed with CSF, the drop will form a double ring, with a darker center spot containing blood components surrounded by a light halo of CSF. If this is indeterminate, the fluid can be sent to the lab for beta-transferrin testing. Beta-transferrin testing will only be positive if CSF is present. (See Schwartz 8th ed., p 1617.)

3. The use of high-dose steroids after spinal cord injury
   A. Is indicated in all patients
   B. Is indicated in all patients except if <14 years of age or pregnant
   C. Is controversial and dictated by local practice patterns
   D. Is never indicated

**Answer: C**

The National Acute Spinal Cord Injury Study (NASCIS) I and II papers provide the basis for the common practice of administering high-dose steroids to patients with acute spinal cord injury. A 30-mg/kg IV bolus of methylprednisolone is given over 15 minutes, followed by a 5.4-mg/kg per hour infusion begun 45 minutes later. The infusion is continued for 23 hours if the bolus is given within 3 hours of injury, or for 47 hours if the bolus is given within 8 hours of injury. The papers indicate greater motor and sensory recovery at 6 weeks, 6 months, and 1 year after acute spinal cord injury in patients who received methylprednisolone. However, the NASCIS trial data have been extensively criticized, as many argue that the selection criteria and study design were flawed, making the results ambiguous. Patients who receive such a large corticosteroid dose have increased rates of medical and ICU complications, such as pneumonias, which have a deleterious affect on outcome. A clear consensus on the use of spinal-dose steroids does not exist. A decision to use or not use spinal-dose steroids may be dictated by local or regional practice patterns, especially given the legal liability issues surrounding spinal cord injury. Patients with gunshot injuries or nerve root (cauda equina) injury, as well as those on chronic steroid therapy, who are pregnant, or who are less than 14 years old were excluded from the NASCIS studies, and should not receive spinal-dose steroids. (See Schwartz 8th ed., pp 1625–26.)

4. The most common malignant tumor of the brain is
   A. Ependymoma
   B. Astrocytoma
   C. Ganglioglioma
   D. Teratoma

**Answer: B**

Astrocytoma is the most common primary central nervous system (CNS) neoplasm. The term glioma is often used to refer to astrocytomas specifically, excluding other glial tumors. Astrocytomas are graded from I to IV. Grades I and II are referred to as low-grade astrocytoma, grade III as anaplastic astrocytoma, and grade IV as glioblastoma multiforme (GBM). Prognosis varies significantly between grades I/II, III, and IV, but not between I and II. Median survival is 8 years after diagnosis with a low-grade tumor, 2 to 3 years with an anaplastic astrocytoma, and roughly 1 year with a GBM. GBMs account for almost two-thirds of all astrocytomas, anaplastic astrocytomas account for two-thirds of the rest, and low-grade astrocytomas the remainder. Fig. 41-20 demonstrates the typical appearance of a GBM. (See Schwartz 8th ed., p 1633.)

5. A 25-year-old man is seen in the emergency department after he struck his head against the windshield in an automobile accident. He opens his eyes and withdraws his arm during painful stimulation of his hand. He responds verbally to questions with inappropriate words. His Glasgow Coma Scale score is
   A. 6
   B. 9
   C. 12
   D. 15

**Answer: B**
The Glasgow Coma Scale is a rough but reproducible evaluation of a patient's status following a head injury (see Table 41–1, p 299). It is made up of three components: motor response, verbal response, and eye opening. The score for a conscious adult is 15. The patient scores 4 out of 6 for his motor response—withdrawal, 3 out of 5 for his verbal response—unintelligible words, 2 out of 4 for his eye opening response—open with painful stimulation. (See Schwartz 7th ed.)

6. Complete transection of the spinal cord at the C7 level produces all of the following effects EXCEPT
   A. Limited respiratory effort
   B. Areflexia below the level of the lesion
   C. Flaccidity below the level of the lesion
   D. Hypotension

**Answer: A**
Because the phrenic nerves, which are the motor nerves to the diaphragm, arise from the 3rd, 4th, and 5th cervical roots, diaphragmatic respiration would not be disturbed by a cord transection at C7. Anesthesia, areflexia, and flaccidity below this level would be anticipated. Hypotension results from any transection above T5 because of the loss of sympathetic vascular tone. (See Schwartz 7th ed.)

7. A 60-year-old man has had recurrent episodes of amaurosis fugax and hemiparesis for the last year. Which of the following measures would be LEAST helpful in the workup of this man's disorder?
   A. Electrocardiography
   B. Cerebral blood flow studies
   C. Doppler flow studies
   D. Computed tomography scan of the head

**Answer: D**
Transient ischemic attacks are clear warning signals of a possible stroke, and all affected patients should be considered for surgery. Noninvasive studies such as Doppler and cerebral flow studies provide useful information in many cases. Electrocardiography may reveal abnormalities incriminating the heart as a possible source of emboli. Cerebral and arch angiography is necessary to define the presence and location of a stenotic or ulcerated lesion. Computed tomography scanning, though quite helpful in accurately defining mass lesions, may be normal in persons who have intermittent alterations of cerebral circulation. (See Schwartz 7th ed.)

8. A 35-year-old mother of two children, ages 5 and 6 years, has had amenorrhea and galactorrhea for the last 12 months. Her serum prolactin level is elevated, and radiographs of her skull show an "empty sella." The most likely diagnosis is
   A. Menopause
   B. Pregnancy
   C. Pituitary tumor
   D. Sheehan's syndrome

**Answer: C**
The combination of galactorrhea and amenorrhea in a woman whose serum prolactin concentration is elevated suggests the presence of a pituitary microadenoma. Supporting this diagnosis would be the radiographic finding of an idiopathically enlarged sella turcica, which would be likely to harbor a pituitary microadenoma. When a hypersecreting pituitary tumor is strongly suspected, even an "empty sella" should be explored because a moderate number of microadenomas have been removed from so-called empty sellas. Intraductal papillomas do not cause galactorrhea. Sheehan's syndrome, postpartum necrosis of the pituitary gland, produces amenorrhea together with an inability to lactate. (See Schwartz 7th ed.)

9. Disruption of the pituitary stalk can occur during head trauma caused by deceleration. A person with this injury would be expected to develop all the following EXCEPT
   A. Hypothyroidism
   B. Diabetes insipidus
   C. Acute onset of diabetes mellitus
   D. Inappropriate secretion of antidiuretic hormone

**Answer: C**
The adenohypophysis derives all of its blood supply from the pituitary portal vessels. It has no independent arterial supply. With pituitary necrosis, production of thyroid-stimulating hormone (TSH) and adrenocorticotropic hormone (ACTH) would be reduced and in turn cause decreased stimulation of the thyroid and adrenal cortex. Antidiuretic hormone is produced by the neurohypophysis, and its production can be disrupted in head trauma. The only connection between the pituitary and pancreas is a direct relationship between growth hormone and secretion of glucagon. (See Schwartz 7th ed.)

10. The most common level of cervical radiculopathy from cervical disc herniation is
    A. C4-C5
    B. C5-C6
    C. C6-C7
    D. C7-T1

**Answer: C**
See Table 41-2 on p 303.

**Table 41-2.**
**Cervical Disc Herniations and Symptoms by Level**

| Level | Frequency | Root Injured | Reflex | Weakness | Numbness |
|---|---|---|---|---|---|
| C4-C5 | 2% | C5 | — | Deltoid | Shoulder |
| C5-C6 | 19% | C6 | Biceps | Biceps brachii | Thumb |
| C6-C7 | 69% | C7 | Triceps | Wrist extensors (wrist drop) | Second and third digits |
| C7-T1 | 10% | C8 | — | Hand intrinsics | Fourth and fifth digits |

Source: Adapted with permission from Greenberg MS: *Handbook of Neurosurgery*, 4th ed: Greenberg Graphics, 1997, Chap. 10.2, p 199.
See Schwartz 8th ed., p 1641.

# CHAPTER 42

# Orthopaedics

1. The broadest segment of a long bone is the
   A. Epiphysis
   B. Metaphysis
   C. Diaphysis
   D. Primary growth center

**Answer: A**

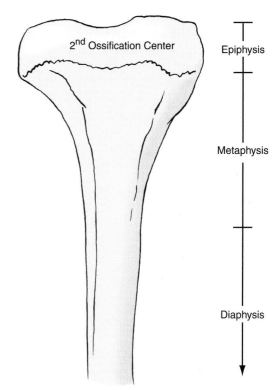

**FIG. 42-1.** Long bones have three sections. The end is the epiphysis or secondary ossification center, the adjacent area is the metaphysis, and the middle of the bone is the diaphysis. The metaphysis is broader than the diaphysis, has a thin cortex, and is composed of primarily cancellous bone. (See Schwartz 8th ed., p 1655.)

2. Which of the following statements concerning sprains is correct?
   A. The degree of injury cannot be predicted based on physical examination.
   B. Ligaments shorten if held in their shortest position.
   C. Surgical repair is limited to ligament rupture.
   D. Chronic arthritis is a frequent sequelae.

**Answer: B**
Joints are stabilized by a combination of ligaments and muscles that cross the joint. These ligaments are subject to injury when stretched, resulting in a sprain. The degree of the injury is usually reflected in the severity of the local swelling and pain. Ligaments heal as does other collagenous tissue. Often the ligaments need surgical repair to assure that they are properly tensioned. Otherwise, persistent joint laxity occurs, which leads to early degeneration of the joint.

Ligaments tend to shorten if held in their shortest position. This is especially true if they have been injured. This shortening accounts for the joint stiffness observed after prolonged immobilization. Proper positioning of joints to keep the major ligaments at their maximal length during prolonged immobilization produces the least amount of joint stiffness and allows the quickest return to function once the immobilization device is discontinued.

Ligaments alone cannot continuously keep a joint stable. If the muscles that cross the joint do not act to maintain joint stability (i.e., secondary to paralysis) the ligaments will be stretched and the joint will become lax. (See Schwartz 8th ed., p 1657.)

3. Which of the following is NOT a typical symptom in a patient with a musculoskeletal tumor?
   A. Nighttime pain
   B. Warmth over the lesion
   C. Distal edema
   D. Tenderness

**Answer: D**
Patients typically present with a history of pain that is often worse at night and usually is not activity related. A mass or swelling may be present, but constitutional symptoms (weight loss, fevers, night sweats, malaise) usually are absent, except in cases with disseminated disease. Lesions adjacent to joints can cause effusion, contractures, and pain with motion. Soft-tissue tumors often are painless unless there is involvement of neurovascular structures. Compression of veins or lymphatics in a limb can cause distal edema, and larger masses exhibit a pattern of overlying venous distention. Malignant soft-tissue masses can be firm and fixed to subcutaneous tissue, muscle, or bone, and usually are nontender. Local warmth is evident because malignant lesions induce local angiogenesis. Patients may also present with a pathologic fracture as a manifestation of benign or malignant intraosseous lesions, with bone destruction and subsequent mechanical failure. Pain on weight bearing is an ominous clinical symptom that often indicates an impending fracture. (See Schwartz 8th ed., pp 1660–61.)

4. Which of the following statements concerning osteoid osteoma is true?
   A. It occurs more frequently in males.
   B. It is a painless lesion.
   C. Radiographically, it can be diagnosed by a radiodense lesion.
   D. Resection is required to prevent progression.

**Answer: A**
Osteoid osteoma is a benign bone-forming lesion which primarily affects patients under 30 years of age and has a male preponderance. Patients present with local pain, which can be quite severe and is often relieved by aspirin. Radiographically, a small (less than 1 cm) lucent lesion (nidus) is seen, typically surrounded by marked reactive sclerosis (Fig. 42-17). Sometimes areas of radiodensity are seen within the lucent lesion, corresponding histologically to disorganized woven bone formation. The lesion gradually regresses over a period of 5 to 10 years, but most patients are unable to tolerate the symptoms and opt for surgical resection of the lesion, which usually is curative if the entire nidus is removed. (See Schwartz 8th ed., p 1664.)

5. Which of the following is the most common malignant lesion of the bone?
   A. Chondroblastoma
   B. Fibrosarcoma
   C. Ewing's sarcoma
   D. Osteosarcoma

**Answer: D**
Osteosarcoma is the most common primary bone malignancy apart from multiple myeloma, although it is nonetheless a rare disease (incidence 2.8/1,000,000). Patients 10 to 25 years of age are most often affected, and the most common sites are areas of maximal bone growth (distal femur—52%; proximal

tibia—20%; proximal humerus—9%). Usually the lesions are metaphyseal. Although any bone can be involved, the disease seldom occurs in the small bones of the distal extremities and in the spine. This disease has a number of variants: (1) "classic" central or medullary high-grade osteosarcoma; (2) periosteal osteosarcoma; (3) parosteal osteosarcoma; (4) osteosarcoma secondary to malignant degeneration of Paget's disease, fibrous dysplasia, or radiation; and (5) telangiectatic osteosarcoma. (See Schwartz 8th ed., p 1665.)

6. The most common location for an adamantinoma is
   A. Skull
   B. Jaw
   C. Spine
   D. Pelvis

**Answer: B**

Adamantinoma is a rare epithelial tumor occurring in the jaw and occasionally in the tibia or fibula of young adults. The tumor, although malignant, is slow growing and presents with pain and a lytic, multiloculated or bubbly radiographic appearance. The diaphyseal portion of the bone tends to be involved. Treatment is with wide resection or amputation, and adjuvant therapies have not been shown to be effective. Metastasis to the lungs occurs in about 50 percent of cases. (See Schwartz 8th ed., p 1671.)

7. Which of the following is thought to be the embryonic tissue of origin of a chordoma?
   A. Ectoderm
   B. Endoderm
   C. Germ cell
   D. Notochord

**Answer: D**

This rare, low-grade malignant neoplasm arises in the sacrococcygeal or occipitocervical area and is thought to develop from embryonic remnants of the notochord. Sixty percent of cases occur in the sacrum or coccyx (Fig. 42-28). Patients present with a mass, neurologic symptoms, or pain. The lesions are slow growing and occur usually in older adults. Differential diagnosis includes plasmacytoma, giant cell tumor, and metastatic carcinoma. The tumor is composed of cords and nests of cells resembling chondrocytes, with typical highly vacuolated "basket" or physaliferous cells. The stroma consists of a basophilic, mucoid, or myxoid ground substance. The location makes wide resection difficult and causes significant morbidity, but without treatment the lesion is uniformly fatal, with late pulmonary metastases. The lesions are not responsive to radiotherapy or chemotherapy, and surgical resection is the treatment of choice. Some recent evidence suggests that this tumor may be somewhat responsive to proton beam irradiation. (See Schwartz 8th ed., p 1671.)

8. Which of the following does NOT frequently metastasize to bone?
   A. Renal cell carcinoma
   B. Thyroid cancer
   C. Lung cancer
   D. Colon cancer

**Answer: D**

Carcinomas often metastasize to the skeleton, and metastatic lesions are much more common than primary bone lesions in general orthopaedic practice. The five primary cancers with a strong propensity to metastasize to bone are those originating in the breast, prostate, lung, kidney, and thyroid. Multiple myeloma, although technically a primary bone tumor, also must be considered in this group because of its similar age distribution (patients over age 50 years), radiographic presentation, and orthopaedic problems and treatment (pathologic fractures). Over 90% of patients with metastatic breast or prostate carcinoma have at least microscopic bone involvement. (See Schwartz 8th ed., p 1672.)

9. Which of the following is the most common causative organism in osteomyelitis?
   A. *Salmonella*
   B. *Pseudomonas*
   C. *Staphylococcus*
   D. *Escherichia coli*

**Answer: C**
Osteomyelitis is an infection of the bone that most commonly occurs secondary to an open wound with an associated or compound fracture. However, osteomyelitis also can occur spontaneously, presumably as a consequence of circulating bacteria in the bloodstream, and is known as hematogenous osteomyelitis. Hematogenous osteomyelitis is an infection that predominantly occurs in children. The most common causative organism is *Staphylococcus*, but any bacteria can produce osteomyelitis. Less-common infectious agents include viruses, fungi, and mycobacteria. (See Schwartz 8th ed., p 1677.)

10. The treatment of choice for septic arthritis of the hip is
    A. Antibiotic therapy alone and immobilization
    B. Antibiotic therapy alone and physical therapy
    C. Surgical drainage if no response to antibiotic therapy
    D. Surgical drainage

**Answer: D**
Controversy exists as to whether surgical drainage, arthroscopic drainage, or repeated daily aspiration represents the best treatment option. Generally it is agreed that for hip infections, which can result in rapid destruction and secondary osteonecrosis and can be difficult to aspirate, emergent surgical drainage is indicated. Chronic infections with loculation or thick purulence also require surgical drainage. In chronic infections removal of hypertrophic infected synovium can be advantageous. For the knee, arthroscopic drainage may be appropriate. Shoulder and ankle infections can be managed either by sequential aspiration or surgical drainage. In general, patients who undergo surgical drainage undergo defervescence and improve clinically more rapidly. Depending on the organism, intravenous antibiotic therapy is indicated for 2 to 4 weeks. If the septic arthritis results from extension from an adjacent osteomyelitis, intravenous antibiotic therapy for 6 weeks or longer is needed. Early joint motion is encouraged to restore nutrition to the articular cartilage and prevent stiffness. (See Schwartz 8th ed., p 1678.)

11. Positive HLA-B27 titer is associated with which of the following?
    A. Gout
    B. Systemic lupus erythematosus
    C. Calcium pyrophosphate deposition disease
    D. Ankylosing spondylitis

**Answer: D**
Ankylosing spondylitis predominantly affects males. The predominant feature is joint pain and restricted motion, with the spine usually having the most involvement. An early physical examination finding is restricted chest expansion. These patients usually have a positive HLA-B27 titer in their serum. (See Schwartz 8th ed., p 1680.)

12. Nondisplaced acetabular fractures are treated by
    A. Open surgery with pinning of the fracture
    B. Open surgery with plating of the fracture
    C. Closed reduction and casting
    D. Traction

**Answer: D**
Nondisplaced acetabular fractures may be treated with a period of traction followed by progressive weight bearing. An alternative treatment would be immediate nonweight bearing on that acetabulum fracture. A complication of this strategy would be displacement of the fracture. Healing of the joint surface with anatomic restoration has been shown to result in excellent long-term results. The amount of residual articular displacement affects the development of posttraumatic arthritis. Studies show that 2 mm of intra-articular displacement of fractures and incongruous hip reduction, marginal impaction greater than 2 mm, and intra-articular debris accelerate the development of arthritis. (See Schwartz 8th ed., p 1684.)

13. The appearance of the leg in a patient with a femoral neck fracture will be
    A. Shortened and externally rotated
    B. Shortened and internally rotated
    C. Lengthened and externally rotated
    D. Lengthened and internally rotated

**Answer: A**

Femoral neck fractures are most commonly related to falls. The patient most often complains of pain in the groin or thigh and is unable to bear weight on the injured extremity. The lower extremity appears shortened and externally rotated. Most attempts at motion, especially rotational motion, cause severe pain. The diagnosis is confirmed by anteroposterior and lateral radiographs of the hip. A careful physical examination is necessary to rule out other injuries to the patient. (See Schwartz 8th ed., p 1685.)

14. In the Salter classification, a fracture through the growth plate with extension into the epiphysis is a
    A. Type I
    B. Type II
    C. Type III
    D. Type IV

**Answer: C**

The Salter-Harris classification system groups fractures through the growth plate into five types. Type I is through the growth plate; type II is through the growth plate with extension into the metaphysis; type III is through the growth plate with extension into the epiphysis; type IV crosses the growth plate; and type V is a crush of the growth plate. The higher the type, the greater the risk of a growth abnormality. All growth plates can sustain fractures, but the most common site is the distal femur. (See Schwartz 8th ed., p 1688.)

15. The most common mechanism of injury in a distal fracture of the fibula is
    A. Supination with eversion
    B. Supination without eversion
    C. Pronation with eversion
    D. Pronation without eversion

**Answer: C**

The mechanism of injury can suggest what tissues may be injured. Almost all ankle sprains are caused by inversion of the ankle with axial loading. This means the ankle is turned in and the weight is placed on the lateral aspect of the foot. This leads to injuries to the lateral ligaments. Depending on the degree of injury, the patient can sustain a strain, sprain, or complete disruption of the lateral ligaments. The degree of swelling and ecchymosis is directly correlated with the degree of ligamentous injury and is a simple means of determining the significance of the injury. If there is concern that the ligaments are completely torn and that the ankle is unstable, stress radiographs can be taken to evaluate the stability of the ankle. When stress radiographs are taken, both ankles need to be examined because the amount of stability is variable. Injuries leading to completely torn lateral ligament are not common. When the degree of the ligamentous injury is in question the initial management should be immobilization in a cast with a reassessment after the swelling and acute pain has subsided.

The description of the injury that leads to an ankle fracture is a combination of the position the ankle was in and the direction of the force when the injury occurred, i.e., supination-eversion, supination-adduction, pronation-eversion, or pronation-abduction. When the ankle is in pronation, the medial malleolus fractures on the deltoid ligament tears, the tibiofibular syndesmosis fails, and the fibula fractures (Fig. 42-49). When the ankle is in supination, the fibula usually fails without disruption of the tibiofibular syndesmosis and the medial malleolar fractures on the deltoid ligament tears. When treating this injury with a closed procedure, it is important to reverse the direction of the injury and hold the ankle in the opposition position. (See Schwartz 8th ed., pp 1691–92.)

16. The risk of osteonecrosis of the talus in a patient with a subtalar, ankle, and talonavicular dislocation (type IV) is
    A. 10%
    B. 40%
    C. 70%
    D. 100%

**Answer: D**

The talus is at risk of sustaining a fracture. Fortunately these fractures are uncommon and are usually the result of major trauma. The most common fracture location is through the neck of the talus. The degree of displacement is both prognostically important and indicates the best treatment. The classification system used most commonly is that of Hawkins. There are four types of displacement in this classification system. Type I is a nondisplaced fracture, which can be treated nonoperatively with cast immobilization. In type I, the patient has less than a 10% risk of developing osteonecrosis of the talar head. The other types are all displaced fractures. Type II is associated with a subtalar dislocation; type III is associated with a subtalar and ankle dislocation; and type IV is associated with subtalar, ankle, and talonavicular dislocation. These fractures usually need internal fixation and the risk of osteonecrosis increases from approximately 35% for type II to 100% with type IV. Prolonged nonweight bearing until the talus has a chance to revascularize is the treatment for the osteonecrosis. (See Schwartz 8th ed., p 1692.)

17. The most common treatment of a fracture of the proximal phalanx of the 2nd toe is
    A. Nothing
    B. Taping to adjacent toe
    C. Closed reduction and casting
    D. Internal fixation (pins)

**Answer: B**

Fractures of the phalanges of the toes are very common. Treatment is almost always only taping to the adjacent toe. If the great toe has a displaced fracture, pin fixation may be indicated. (See Schwartz 8th ed., p 1693.)

18. The treatment of choice for a displaced fracture of the middle third of the clavicle is
    A. Figure-of-eight splint
    B. Arm sling
    C. Internal fixation with pins
    D. Internal fixation with plates

**Answer: B**

Fractures of the clavicle occur in adults and children. More than 80% occur in the middle third of the clavicle, and almost all of the remainder occur in the distal third of the clavicle (Fig. 42-52). The most common causes are a direct blow to the clavicle, a fall on the shoulder, or a fall on an outstretched arm. Clavicle fractures are often seen in patients with multiple injuries and should be specifically looked for in this situation because they can be easily missed. Swelling and tenderness are usually found at the fracture site and pain is associated with shoulder motion. Associated neurovascular injuries can occur, but are uncommon.

Fractures that occur in the middle third of the clavicle are treated by placing the injured arm in a sling. In the past, a "figure-of-eight" splint was used but it is uncomfortable and is no longer felt to be needed. The patient should start to move the shoulder as soon as pain allows, usually within a few days to a week, to reduce the risk of developing restricted shoulder motion. Healing usually occurs in about 6 to 8 weeks with return to full function in about 3 months. Children will heal the fracture faster and start using their arm earlier than an adult. Nonunion is rare. (See Schwartz 8th ed., p 1693.)

19. Which of the following is an indication for operative treatment of a midshaft humeral fracture?
    A. Displacement >15 degrees
    B. Shortening of the humerus >3 cm
    C. Associated fracture of the radius and ulna
    D. Profession with need for fine motor control

**Answer: C**

The vast majority of humeral shaft fractures can be treated nonoperatively. A U-shaped plaster coaptation splint is commonly used initially. This is frequently converted to a humeral functional brace after 1 to 2 weeks, allowing better early range-of-motion exercises of the shoulder and elbow. A large amount of fracture displacement can be tolerated because of the mobility of the shoulder. Acceptable limits of 30 degrees of varus, 20 degrees of anterior-posterior angulation, and 3 cm of shortening have been proposed. Operative stabilization of humeral shaft fractures is recommended in certain cases including inability to obtain an adequate alignment with a splint or brace, open fracture, floating elbow (fractures of humerus and radius/ulna), fracture with vascular injury, polytrauma, and pathologic fracture. Fracture fixation can be done with compression plate, intramedullary rod, or external fixation. (See Schwartz 8th ed., p 1696.)

20. A fracture to the ulna with associated dislocation of the radial head is called a
    A. Morgagni fracture
    B. Galeazzi fracture
    C. Monteggia fracture
    D. Sever fracture

**Answer: C**

A fracture of the ulna with an associated dislocation of the radial head was first described by Monteggia in 1814 (before radiographs were discovered) and is now known as a Monteggia fracture (Fig. 42-60). A fracture in the distal third of the radius with an associated dislocation of the distal radioulnar joint is called a Galeazzi fracture after the physician who, in 1934, described this combination of injuries (Fig. 42-61). An isolated fracture of the ulna is called a "nightstick" fracture because being hit by a nightstick was a common mechanism of injury. (See Schwartz 8th ed., p 1698.)

# CHAPTER 43

# Surgery of the Hand and Wrist

1. The maximum time continuous tourniquets can be used for hand surgery is
   A. 1 h
   B. 2 h
   C. 3 h
   D. 4 h

**Answer: C**

Pneumatic tourniquet pressures of 225 to 250 mm Hg for adults and 200 mm Hg in children are adequate. Patients with large or obese arms require higher pressures and larger cuffs, as do hypertensive patients, in whom tourniquet pressure should be 100 mm Hg over systolic blood pressure. Tourniquet time is limited by the most oxygen-sensitive extremity cells, muscle cells, and their most oxygen-sensitive organelles, the mitochondria. Continuous tourniquet application should not exceed 3 hours to avoid irreversible mitochondrial changes. In cases in which longer tourniquet times are required, the tourniquet should be deflated after the wound has been dressed temporarily, and left deflated for at least 10 minutes per hour of prior inflation. Tourniquet complications involve not only ischemia in labile distal tissues, but also ischemia and direct injury to skin, nerves, and muscles located immediately beneath tourniquets. Assuming operative tourniquet times greater than 30 minutes, at tourniquet deflation, tissues show reactive hyperemia driven by the tourniquet-induced hypoxia that is directly proportional to the time of tourniquet use. This hyperemia may complicate hemostasis if the surgeon tries to immediately close the skin. (See Schwartz 8th ed., p 1728.)

2. An articular, displaced radial fracture is treated with
   A. Cast immobilization only
   B. Percutaneous pins
   C. Closed reduction with external fixation
   D. Open reduction and pin fixation

**Answer: B**

**Table 43-1.**
**Classification and Treatment of Distal Radius Fractures**

| Classification of Radius Fracture | Treatment Preference |
|---|---|
| I. Nonarticular, nondisplaced | Cast immobilization |
| II. Nonarticular, displaced | |
|   A. Reducible, stable | Cast immobilization |
|   B. Reducible, unstable | Percutaneous pins |
|   C. Irreducible | Open reduction/external fixation |
| III. Articular, nondisplaced | Cast immobilization with or without percutaneous pins |
| IV. Articular, displaced | Closed reduction |
|   A. Reducible, stable | Percutaneous pins (Kirschner wires) with or without external fixation |
|   B. Reducible, unstable | Closed reduction/external fixation, with or without percutaneous pins, with or without bone graft |

*(continued)*

**Table 43-1.**
**Classification and Treatment of Distal Radius**
**Fractures (continued)**

| Classification of Radius Fracture | Treatment Preference |
|---|---|
| C. Irreducible | Open reduction/external fixation with percutaneous pins |
| D. Complex | Open reduction/external plate fixation with bone graft (with or without percutaneous pins) |

See Schwartz 8th ed., p 1730.

3. The next test to order if you suspect a scaphoid fracture that is not detectable on plain X-ray is
   A. Ultrasound
   B. Computed tomography scan
   C. Magnetic resonance imaging
   D. PET scan

**Answer: B**

Nearly two-thirds of all carpal fractures are of the scaphoid. This injury occurs most often in males aged 15 to 30 years. Scaphoid fractures occur most commonly through the middle third of the waist or at the juncture of the middle and proximal poles. Diagnosis requires clinical and imaging information. After a fall on the outstretched hand, the patient's wrist is tender at the anatomic snuffbox, the hollow between the thumb extensor tendons on the radial aspect of the wrist, just dorsal and distal to the styloid process of the radius. Pain is elicited and symptoms reproduced with direct pressure over the tuberosity of the scaphoid at the palmar base of the thenar eminence and with passive wrist motion. Routine radiographs in posteroanterior, lateral, and oblique views, along with a posteroanterior projection in ulnar deviation of the wrist to elongate the scaphoid, helps to visualize the fracture. If initial radiographs are normal but the history and physical examination suggest the possibility of scaphoid fracture, continuous immobilization in a thumb spica splint or cast is advised. Repeat radiographs in 2 to 3 weeks, magnetic resonance imaging (MRI) scan, or technetium bone scan after 72 hours, will make the diagnosis. (See Schwartz 8th ed., p 1734.)

4. The most common complication of scaphoid fractures is
   A. Osteomyelitis
   B. Nonunion
   C. Ischemic contracture
   D. Chronic wrist instability

**Answer: B**

Fracture configuration (Fig. 43-26) and location affect stability and lability of the fractured bone's blood supply. The proximal pole of the scaphoid is supplied from vessels entering the distal two-thirds. Fracture of the proximal one-third or a smaller fragment risks avascularity in the small proximal fragment, resulting in nonunion and secondary arthrosis. Nondisplaced scaphoid fractures treated with adequate immobilization have a union rate of 90 to 95%. Displaced fractures, defined as ≥1.0 mm displacement, are associated with avascular necrosis and nonunions in half of patients if not reduced and stabilized operatively. Scaphoid fracture fragment displacement of 2.0 mm or more should raise suspicion of an associated intercarpal ligament injury, such as transscaphoid perilunate instability, or subluxation. (See Schwartz 8th ed., pp 1734–35.)

5. Appropriate treatment of a nail bed injury associated with a tuft fracture is
   A. Nothing
   B. Splinting only
   C. Removal of the nail and repair of the nail bed
   D. Percutaneous pinning and repair of the nail bed

**Answer: C**
Distal phalangeal fractures, including bursting or tuft fractures, are frequently associated with crush trauma and nail bed disruption or lacerations. Nail bed injuries are not always obvious, and subungual hematoma may be the only sign of nail bed injury. Nail bed injuries should be repaired to prevent permanent late nail deformity. Nail bed repairs usually are done with fine, 6-0 absorbable suture. After repair, the nail that was removed is replaced beneath the cuticle to splint (stent) the bed (Figs. 43-51 and 43-52). (See Schwartz 8th ed., p 1743.)

6. Which of the following statements concerning digital block is true?
   A. No more than 4 cc of local anesthetic should be injected per digit.
   B. A ring block is more effective than a web block.
   C. Epinephrine is advantageous because it will prolong the anesthetic effect.
   D. The dorsal branch should be injected separately.

**Answer: D**
The fingers receive their sensory supply from the common digital nerve branches of the median and ulnar nerves. Digital anesthesia can be achieved by injecting the anesthetic into the looser web tissues about the common digital nerves, which is preferable to a ring block in the base of the finger. The so-called ring block technique risks vascular compromise from volume compression when a solution is injected circumferentially about the base of the finger. Digital anesthetic solution must not include epinephrine, because resulting digital vessel spasm may compromise finger circulation. Anesthetic is injected retrograde from the web, advancing about 1 cm proximally into the palm, where 2 mL of anesthetic is injected after aspiration. The needle can be withdrawn and turned into the dorsal subcutaneous tissues of the web to ensure anesthesia of the dorsal branch of the digital nerve with another 1 to 2 mL of anesthetic. The technique is repeated on the opposite side of the finger or sequentially in several digits as needed. No more than 5 to 7 mL total of anesthetic solution should be injected for any one finger with this technique (Fig. 43-13). (See Schwartz 8th ed., p 1727.)

7. Which carpal bone is most frequently fractured?
   A. Lunate
   B. Trapezium
   C. Capitate
   D. Scaphoid

**Answer: D**
Nearly two-thirds of all carpal fractures are of the scaphoid. This injury occurs most often in males aged 15 to 30 years. Scaphoid fractures occur most commonly through the middle third of the waist or at the juncture of the middle and proximal poles. (See Schwartz 8th ed., p 1734.)

8. Proper handling of an amputated digit or limb includes which of the following?
   A. Place dry in a waterproof bag
   B. Immerse in an antiseptic solution
   C. Prep and irrigate before packaging
   D. Place on dry ice

**Answer: C**
The amputated part should be scrub-prepped, then irrigated and cleansed under saline solution, wrapped in a saline-moistened gauze, and placed in a plastic bag. The plastic bag containing the part is then placed on (not packed in) a bed of ice in a suitable container. The part should never be immersed in nonphysiologic solutions such as antiseptics or alcohols. The amputated part is never put in dry ice, it is not perfused, and it must not be allowed to freeze. (See Schwartz 8th ed., p 1755.)

9. Appropriate treatment of a felon is
   A. Oral antibiotics and warm soaks
   B. Admission and IV antibiotics
   C. Surgical decompression of the compartment
   D. Incision and drainage of the nail bed

**Answer: C**
Felon is an expanding abscess within the finger pulp, and represents up to one-quarter of hand infections. Felons can be extremely painful, as the expanding abscess produces a localized compartment syndrome within the fibrous septae

that normally anchor the pulp and subcutaneous tissues to the distal phalanx. Felons usually are caused by penetrating direct trauma producing bacterial inoculation. Untreated felons, like other compartment syndromes, compromise local circulation and produce secondary tissue ischemia and necrosis (osteomyelitis and septic distal interphalangeal (DIP) arthritis), in addition to septic destruction. In surgical drainage, additional injury to the finger pulp should be avoided, but an abscess may already point to a superficial location. (See Schwartz 8th ed., p 1762.)

10. Which of the following is NOT a treatment option for a radial ganglion?
    A. Observation
    B. Closed rupture
    C. Aspiration and injection of tetracycline
    D. Excision

**Answer: C**

Treatment options for a radial ganglion include no directed care, closed rupture by impact, hypodermic needle aspiration plus steroid injection, and operative excision. Rupture by digital pressure or with a swift blow is unnecessarily traumatic and has little chance of long-term success. Aspiration and steroid instillation may be of considerable value, particularly when the expanding lesion has not been diagnosed or is associated with discomfort. At the dorsal wrist, the most common site of origin is from the scapholunate interosseous ligament, and the smaller, occult ganglion may account for a significant amount of dorsal wrist pain, particularly in the female teenage population. Volar ganglions are most commonly situated between the flexor carpi radialis tendon and the radial artery, at or just proximal to the wrist, near the radioscaphoid joint. Most arise from the radiocarpal or intercarpal capsule. Aspiration with injection may be entirely curative for the flexor sheath ganglion that appears as a 3- to 10-mm hard mass at or just distal to the metacarpophalangeal joint flexion crease. Aspiration and injection of the mucous cyst distal interphalangeal joint ganglion is less likely to be curative. Repeated drainage at this site increases the risk of joint contamination and secondary sepsis. Surgical excision must include the capsular base origin, sometimes referred to as the stalk or root. (See Schwartz 8th ed., p 1782.)

11. Which of the following statements about fractures of the carpal scaphoid is correct?
    A. Displacement of 1–2 mm may result in nonunion at the fracture site.
    B. Fractures through the proximal third of the bone are complicated by aseptic necrosis of the distal fragment.
    C. The fracture is caused by a fall on the back of the hand (wrist in flexion).
    D. Tenderness over the 2nd metacarpal is a characteristic physical finding.
    E. When a fracture is suspected, bony injury can be accurately assessed with initial X-ray examination.

**Answer: A**

Carpal scaphoid (navicular) fracture results from a fall on an outstretched hand. Tenderness in the anatomic snuffbox is a characteristic finding. With a suggestive history and snuffbox tenderness, the injury should be treated initially as a fracture regardless of initial X-ray findings. The fracture line may not be evident until some bony resorption has developed in 2 or 3 weeks. The proximal part of the bone receives its arterial supply from the distal part of the bone, and it is the proximal fragment that may develop avascular necrosis after a fracture through the proximal part of the bone. Even a very small amount of displacement, if uncorrected, may lead to nonunion at the fracture site. (See Schwartz 7th ed.)

12. Which of the following statements concerning wound closure after amputation through the finger is correct?
    A. Bone shortening and primary wound closure should no longer be considered.
    B. Composite replacement of the amputated skin and pulp usually functions as a temporary biologic dressing.
    C. Full-thickness skin grafts afford adequate protection over exposed bone.
    D. If local flaps are required, the finger will be insensate.
    E. Microvascular reimplantation is the appropriate management of adults with a clean amputation through the distal phalanx.

**Answer: B**

Bone shortening and primary wound closure is appropriate as a method that provides rapid recovery at the price of some finger shortening. Composite replacement of amputated skin and pulp may be considered in young children, but the replaced part usually undergoes superficial necrosis. It should be considered a biologic dressing. Either partial-thickness or full-thickness skin grafts are successfully done under local anesthesia, but skin grafting does not satisfactorily protect bone. When feasible, local flaps from the proximal part of the injured finger supply padding, vascularity, and sensation. Microvascular techniques allow digit reimplantation, which would otherwise be impossible. (See Schwartz 7th ed.)

# CHAPTER 44

# Plastic and Reconstructive Surgery

1. The most common area of the mandible to be fractured is the
   A. Condyle
   B. Ramus
   C. Angle
   D. Body

**Answer: A**

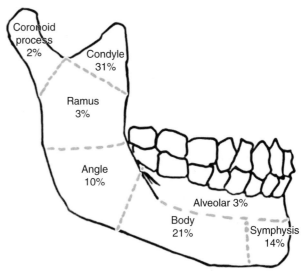

**FIG. 44-1.** *Mandibular fractures: location and distribution.* (See Schwartz 8th ed., p 1806.)

2. Treatment of a 3-mm displaced fracture of the anterior wall of the frontal sinus is
   A. Observation
   B. Antibiotics alone
   C. Open reduction
   D. Open reduction, demucosalization, and packing of fat into the sinus

**Answer: C**

The most common surgical approach to the frontal sinus is through a coronal incision. Treatment of frontal sinus fractures is predicated on the number of walls involved and the status of the nasofrontal duct (Fig. 44-34). In nondisplaced anterior wall fractures, no treatment is indicated. If the anterior wall is displaced, then elevation and recontouring of the anterior table is executed. The patient should be observed for any sinus opacification or obstruction. If the nasofrontal duct is involved in the fracture, one can assume that this is a dysfunctional sinus. Therefore, the sinus must be demucosalized, the nasofrontal duct must be plugged with bone graft, and sinus cavity obliterated with cancellous bone or fat. The technique of frontal sinus exenteration or removal of the anterior table, with demucosalization plugging of the ducts, is an antediluvian procedure not routinely performed because of the significant contour deformity. (See Schwartz 8th ed., p 1807.)

3. Which of the following is the best treatment of a septal hematoma in a patient with a nasal fracture?
   A. Observation
   B. Aspiration of the hematoma
   C. Closed reduction of the fracture and aspiration of the hematoma
   D. Operative repair of the fracture

**Answer: B**
The nose is the most commonly fractured facial region. The nose is either laterally or posteriorly displaced, and the fracture may involve the cartilaginous septum, or both the nasal bones and septum. Patients commonly present with swelling, nasal deformity, epistaxis, septal deviation, and/or crepitus on palpation. Intranasal inspection should be performed, and if a septal hematoma is noted, it should be percutaneously drained. Diagnosis by computed tomography (CT) scan is not obligatory but is implemented to rule out other injuries. Immediate treatment consists of reduction of both the pyramid and septum, followed by nasal splinting. In spite of early reduction, there is usually a residual deformity or deviations, which will require formal rhinoplasty in an elective setting after swelling and bruising have resided. (See Schwartz 8th ed., p 1807.)

4. A 40-year-old woman develops severe lymphedema involving the right calf and foot after receiving radiation therapy to metastatic lymph nodes in the inguinal region and the femoral triangle. The most appropriate management of this problem is
   A. Microsurgical lymphaticovenous anastomoses in the affected area
   B. Staged excision of subcutaneous tissue and excess skin
   C. Subcutaneous placement of an omental flap into the upper calf
   D. Use of an individually fitted compressive garment on the calf and foot

**Answer: D**
Lymphedema is a frustrating problem. There have been many surgical procedures suggested, including all of those listed, but none of them have a high success rate. Palliation is in order. This is best supplied by elevating the limb to minimize the swelling, followed by rigorous use of an individually fitted compressive garment. (See Schwartz 7th ed.)

5. Three days after an accident in which a 25-year-old woman suffers a maxillary and mandibular fracture, she develops facial nerve palsy with oral incompetence and slurred speech. The facial nerve problem should be managed by
   A. Facial nerve graft
   B. Facial nerve suture
   C. Nonoperative management
   D. Transfer of part of the masseter muscle to the oral commissure

**Answer: C**
When facial nerve palsy is incomplete or late in appearance, the nerve injury is partial. With observation, the palsy will regress over time, and intervention is not required. The operative techniques listed may be necessary with a complete nerve injury. (See Schwartz 7th ed.)

6. Which of the following statements concerning cleft lip and cleft palate is true?
   A. Cleft lip is a midline failure of lip closure.
   B. Development of cleft lip is related to environmental factors and not to familial tendencies.
   C. Deformities of the nose occur in approximately 50% of patients who have a cleft lip.
   D. Middle ear infections are common among patients with cleft palate.

**Answer: D**
The incidence of cleft palate, cleft lip, or both is variously reported as 1 in 1000 to 1 in 2500 live births in the United States. If a parent or sibling has a cleft lip, the chance of a subsequent child's being born with the same defect is higher. Cleft lip may be unilateral or bilateral when the nasomedial and nasolateral processes fail to unite during embryologic development. Cleft palate is due to isolated failure of palatal process fusion. Almost all cleft lips, even minor ones, are associated with nasal distortions, and many plastic surgeons advocate rhinoplasty at the time of repair of the cleft lip. Malocclusion is a uniform problem, and all patients with cleft palates have drainage problems

of the middle ear, which may lead to recurrent ear infections. Normal speech is achieved in more than 75% of cases of corrective surgery in which the cleft palate is closed entirely by the age of 12 to 14 months. (See Schwartz 7th ed.)

7. Each of the following statements about meshed skin grafts is correct EXCEPT
   A. They allow egress of fluid collections under the graft.
   B. They contour well over irregular surfaces.
   C. They contract to the same degree as a grafted sheet of skin.
   D. They permit coverage of large areas.

**Answer: C**
Meshed grafts are useful because they permit coverage of large injured areas like burn wounds. They contour better than sheets of skin over irregular surfaces, and they are well adapted to granulatory wounds because they permit the escape of fluid or purulent drainage without major graft loss. They contract more than a sheet of skin, however, and may produce more prominent scarring. (See Schwartz 7th ed.)

8. When a subcutaneous tissue expander is placed, each of the following effects occur EXCEPT
   A. Collagen fibers are reoriented
   B. Collagen synthesis occurs
   C. Dermal thickness increases
   D. Melanocyte activity increases

**Answer: C**
When a tissue expander is placed, collagen fibers are reoriented to parallel the expansion force, and collagen synthesis increases. Melanocyte activity is increased, and this may account for the hyperpigmentation seen in expanded tissue. Skin vascularity is increased in much the same way as when a skin flap is delayed. The tissue covering the expander initially appears thick, probably from tissue edema, but over time the dermis becomes thinner than normal. (See Schwartz 7th ed.)

# CHAPTER 45

# Surgical Considerations in the Elderly

1. Which of the following is a criterion used for risk assessment in elderly patients in the Revised Goldman Classification?
   A. Age >70 years
   B. Electrocardiogram other than normal sinus rhythm
   C. Poor general health status
   D. Preoperative insulin therapy

**Answer: D**

Revised Goldman Classification (1 point each)

- History of heart failure
- History of ischemic heart disease
- History of cerebrovascular disease
- Preoperative insulin therapy
- Preoperative creatinine >2
- High-risk surgery

0 points: 0.5% cardiac morbidity risk
1 point: 1.3%
2 points: 3.6%
3 points: 9.1%

**Table 45-1.**
**Original and Modified Goldman's Criteria for Preoperative Assessment of the Elderly Surgical Patient to Determine Perioperative Risk of Cardiac Event**

| Original Goldman Classification | Points |
| --- | --- |
| Age >70 years | 5 |
| Myocardial infarction in previous 6 months | 10 |
| Presence of $S_3$ gallop or jugular venous distention | 11 |
| Valvular aortic stenosis | 3 |
| Electrocardiogram rhythm other than normal sinus | 7 |
| Presence of >5 PVCs/min any time prior to surgery | 7 |
| Poor general health status | 3 |
| Intra-abdominal, intrathoracic, or aortic procedure | 3 |
| Emergency surgery | 4 |
| Total possible points: | 53 |

| Revised Goldman Classification | Points |
| --- | --- |
| History of heart failure | 1 |
| History of ischemic heart disease | 1 |
| History of cerebrovascular disease | 1 |
| Preoperative insulin therapy | 1 |
| Preoperative serum creatinine ≥2 mg/dL | 1 |
| High-risk surgery | 1 |
| Total possible points: | 6 |

PVC = premature ventricular contraction.
Source: Adapted from Goldman L, et al: Multifactorial index of cardiac risk in noncardiac surgical procedures. *N Engl J Med* 297:845, 1977; and Lee TH, et al: Derivation and prospective validation of a simple index of cardiac risk of major noncardiac surgery. *Circulation* 100:1043, 1999.
See Schwartz 8th ed., p 1838.

2. Glomerular filtration rate in a healthy 80-year-old patient
   A. Is the same as age 40 years
   B. Is 80–90% of age 40 years
   C. Is 50–75% of age 40 years
   D. Is 30–45% of age 40 years

**Answer: C**
Elderly surgical patients also are at increased risk of renal compromise in the perioperative period. The physiologic changes in renal function in these patients increase the susceptibility to renal ischemia perioperatively as well as to nephrotoxic agents. This functional decline with age is caused by glomerular damage and sclerosis leading to a decreased glomerular filtration rate (GFR). The GFR decreases by approximately 1 mL/min for every year over the age of 40. The GFR for a healthy 80-year-old patient is one half to two thirds of the value at age 30 years. (See Schwartz 8th ed., p 1836.)

3. A 92-year-old woman undergoing a breast biopsy who has 2/6 positive risk factors on the Revised Goldman Classification has what risk of a postoperative cardiac event?
   A. ~0.5%
   B. ~1.5%
   C. ~3.5%
   D. ~5.0%

**Answer: C**
Cardiac complications are the leading cause of perioperative complications and death in surgical patients of all age groups, but particularly among the elderly who may have underlying cardiac disease in addition to normal physiologic decline (Table 45-2). Myocardial infarction or congestive heart failure comprises one quarter of all cardiac complications and perioperative deaths in elderly patients. Therefore, identifying correctable and uncorrectable cardiovascular disease is critical prior to elective surgical intervention. The cardiac risk in elderly surgical patients has been best demonstrated by Goldman's criteria, which assigned a total of 53 risk points for various cardiac risk factors known in noncardiac surgery (Table 45-1). This criteria was later simplified to six variables that determine preoperative cardiac risk (see Table 45-1). Using this new model, an elderly patient with no risk factors has a cardiac morbidity rate of 0.5%, one factor will raise it to 1.3%, two factors to 3.6%, and three factors to 9.1%. This is a much simpler system to use than the original "criteria." (See Schwartz 8th ed., p 1836.)

4. The optimal treatment for a 3-cm breast cancer with a single palpable axillary node in an 85-year-old woman is
   A. Observation
   B. Lumpectomy alone
   C. Lumpectomy with axillary dissection
   D. Mastectomy

**Answer: C**
The estimated mortality for a patient 70 years of age or older undergoing a mastectomy is less than 1%. Elderly women should be offered, and typically prefer, breast-conserving surgery. It has been suggested that elderly women have a low rate of recurrence after lumpectomy, axillary dissection, and radiotherapy, making this a viable option. Radiation therapy is well tolerated by elderly women, with a minimal increase in morbidity and mortality, when added to breast-conserving procedures. Despite the success of this combination therapy, elderly women often do not receive radiation therapy; this is likely a result of reluctance by providers to refer them.

Routine axillary lymph node dissection with breast-conserving surgery remains controversial in elderly patients. There has been a trend toward providing adjuvant therapy with tamoxifen to patients with node-positive and node-negative disease, making axillary lymph node dissection (ALND) unnecessary. Furthermore, because ALND is associated with some morbidity, elderly women are considered at greater risk of chronic lymph edema and decreased shoulder mobility. The latter can be worsened by comorbidities, including neurologic dysfunction and degenerative arthritis. In patients with clinically node-negative status, the axillary field also can be added to the radiation port to provide local control rates equivalent to those achieved with axillary dissection. However, ALND remains necessary in patients with clinically palpable axillary lymph nodes for adequate local control. (See Schwartz 8th ed., p 1839.)

5. The prognosis for elderly patients with thyroid cancer is
   A. Worse than younger patients
   B. The same as younger patients
   C. Better than younger patients
   D. There are no data

**Answer: A**

Papillary carcinoma in elderly patients tends to be sporadic with a bell-shape distribution of age at presentation, occurring primarily in patients age 30 to 59 years. The incidence of papillary carcinoma decreases in patients older than 60 years of age. However, patients older than 60 years of age have increased risk of local recurrence and for the development of distant metastases. Metastatic disease may be more common in this population secondary to delayed referral for surgical intervention because of the misconception that the surgeon will be unwilling to operate on an elderly patient with thyroid disease. Age is also a prognostic indicator for patients with follicular carcinoma. There is a 2.2 times increased risk of mortality from follicular carcinoma per 20 years of increasing age. Therefore, prognosis for elderly patients with differentiated thyroid carcinomas is worse when compared to younger counterparts. The higher prevalence of vascular invasion and extracapsular extension among older patients is in part responsible for the poorer prognosis in geriatric patients. Advancing age leads to increased mortality risk for patients with thyroid cancer and is demonstrated by the AMES (age, metastases, extent of primary tumor, and size of tumor) classification system developed by the Lahey Clinic (Table 45-4). (See Schwartz 8th ed., p 1839.)

6. A common presenting symptom in elderly patients with hyperparathyroidism is
   A. Fracture
   B. Dementia
   C. Renal stones
   D. Skin changes

**Answer: B**

Approximately 2% of the geriatric population, including 3% of women 75 years of age or older, will develop primary hyperparathyroidism. Geriatric patients are usually referred to surgery only when advanced disease is present because of concerns regarding the risks of surgery, but low rates of morbidity and negligible mortality combined with high cure rates of approximately 95 to 98% make parathyroidectomy safe and effective.

Elderly patients are especially prone to developing mental manifestations of hyperparathyroidism that may be severe enough to produce a dementia-like state. There often is a significant improvement in mental status after parathyroidectomy. Another specific symptom of hyperparathyroidism that may easily be mistaken for osteoporosis and can be present in postmenopausal, elderly women is orthopedic disease, specifically back pain and possibly the occurrence of vertebral fractures. This pain can be of moderate intensity, leading to impaired mobility and severely affecting the quality of life of elderly patients. The decreased bone density observed in elderly patients with hyperparathyroidism tends to improve during the first 2 years after successful parathyroid surgery. (See Schwartz 8th ed., p 1840.)

7. The most common etiology for trauma in elderly people is
   A. Abuse
   B. Motor vehicle accidents
   C. Auto-pedestrian accidents
   D. Falls

**Answer: D**

Geriatric patients older than 65 years of age currently account for approximately 23% of total hospital trauma admissions—many of which are multisystem and life-threatening. This percentage is expected to rise to as high as 40%, making this a growing concern for potential long-term morbidity, mortality, rehabilitation, and cost.

The most common mechanism for injuries in the elderly is from falls, which account for approximately 20% of severe injuries. Many underlying chronic and acute diseases common to elderly patients place them at increased risk for falls. These diseases include postural hypotension leading to syncopal "drop attacks," dysrhythmia from sick sinus syndrome, autonomic dysfunction from polypharmacy with improper dosage of antihypertensive or oral hypoglycemic agents resulting in hypotension, and hypoglycemia. (See Schwartz 8th ed., pp 1841–42.)

# CHAPTER 46

# Anesthesia of the Surgical Patient

1. Amide local anesthetics are metabolized
   A. In the liver
   B. In the kidney
   C. By hydrolysis
   D. By urinary excretion only

**Answer: A**
Local anesthetics are divided into two groups based on their chemical structure: the amides and the esters. In general, the amides are metabolized in the liver and the esters are metabolized by plasma cholinesterases, which yield metabolites with slightly higher allergic potential than the amides (Table 46-2). (See Schwartz 8th ed., p 1854.)

2. The toxic dose of bupivacaine is
   A. 2 mg/kg
   B. 3 mg/kg
   C. 4 mg/kg
   D. 5 mg/kg

**Answer: B**
With increasingly elevated plasma levels of local anesthetics, progression to hypotension, increased P-R intervals, bradycardia, and cardiac arrest may occur. Bupivacaine is more cardiotoxic than other local anesthetics. It has a direct effect on ventricular muscle, and because it is more lipid soluble than lidocaine, it binds tightly to sodium channels (it is called the fast-in, slow-out local anesthetic). Patients who have received an inadvertent intravascular injection of bupivacaine have experienced profound hypotension, ventricular tachycardia and fibrillation, and complete atrioventricular heart block that is extremely refractory to treatment. The toxic dose of lidocaine is approximately 5 mg/kg; that of bupivacaine is approximately 3 mg/kg. (See Schwartz 8th ed., p 1856.)

3. Epidural anesthesia
   A. Has a more rapid onset than spinal anesthesia
   B. Requires a smaller volume of anesthetic agent than spinal anesthesia
   C. Has a higher risk of post-procedure headache than spinal anesthesia if there is an inadvertent puncture of the dura
   D. Eliminates the risk of high block with unconsciousness and respiratory depression seen with spinal anesthesia

**Answer: C**
Complications are similar to those of spinal anesthesia. Inadvertent injection of local anesthetic into a dural tear will result in a high block, manifesting as unconsciousness, severe hypotension, and respiratory paralysis requiring immediate aggressive hemodynamic management and control of the airway. Indwelling catheters are often placed through introducers into the epidural space, allowing an intermittent or continuous technique, as opposed to the single-shot method of spinal anesthesia. By necessity, the epidural-introducing needles are of a much larger diameter (17- or 18-gauge) than spinal needles, and accidental dural puncture more often results in a severe headache that may last up to 10 days if left untreated. (See Schwartz 8th ed., p 1857.)

4. Malignant hyperthermia
   A. Is more common in children than adults
   B. Is most commonly triggered by neuromuscular-blocking agents
   C. Is invariably associated with an increase in body temperature
   D. Results in an increased serum calcium level

**Answer: A**

Malignant hyperthermia (MH) is a life-threatening, acute disorder, developing during or after general anesthesia. The clinical incidence of malignant hyperthermia is about 1:12,000 in children and 1:40,000 in adults. A genetic predisposition and one or more triggering agents are necessary to evoke MH. Triggering agents include all volatile anesthetics (e.g., halothane, enflurane, isoflurane, sevoflurane, and desflurane), and the depolarizing muscle relaxant succinylcholine. Volatile anesthetics and/or succinylcholine cause a rise in the myoplasmic calcium concentration in susceptible patients, resulting in persistent muscle contraction. The classic MH crisis entails a hypermetabolic state, tachycardia, and the elevation of end-tidal $CO_2$ in the face of constant minute ventilation. Respiratory and metabolic acidosis and muscle rigidity follow, as well as rhabdomyolysis, arrhythmias, hyperkalemia, and sudden cardiac arrest. A rise in temperature is often a late sign of MH. (See Schwartz 8th ed., p 1871.)

5. Which of the following is an early symptom of lidocaine toxicity?
   A. Ventricular tachycardia
   B. Bradycardia
   C. Tinnitus
   D. Stridor

**Answer: C**

As plasma concentration of local anesthetic rises, symptoms progress from restlessness to complaints of tinnitus. Slurred speech, seizures, and unconsciousness follow. Cessation of the seizure via administration of a benzodiazepine or thiopental and maintenance of the airway is the immediate treatment. If the seizure persists, the trachea must be intubated with a cuffed endotracheal tube to guard against pulmonary aspiration of stomach contents. (See Schwartz 8th ed., p 1856.)

6. Which of the following intravenous agents has analgesic properties?
   A. Propofol
   B. Diazepam
   C. Etomidate
   D. Ketamine

**Answer: D**

The intravenous agents that produce unconsciousness and amnesia are frequently used for the induction of general anesthesia. They include barbiturates, benzodiazepines, propofol, etomidate, and ketamine. Except for ketamine, the following agents have no analgesic properties, nor do they cause paralysis or muscle relaxation. (See Schwartz 8th ed., p 1857.)

7. Propofol
   A. Has a medium to long duration of action
   B. Has a high incidence of nausea and vomiting
   C. Is a bronchodilator
   D. Does not cause hypotension

**Answer: C**

Propofol is an alkylated phenol that inhibits synaptic transmission through its effects at the gamma-aminobutyric acid (GABA) receptor. With a short duration, rapid recovery, and low incidence of nausea and vomiting, it has emerged as the agent of choice for ambulatory and minor general surgery. Additionally, propofol has bronchodilatory properties which make its use attractive in asthmatic patients and smokers. Propofol may cause hypotension, and should be used cautiously in patients with suspected hypovolemia and/or coronary artery disease (CAD), the latter of which may not tolerate a sudden drop in blood pressure. It can be used as a continuous infusion for sedation in the intensive care unit setting. Propofol is an irritant and frequently causes pain on injection. (See Schwartz 8th ed., p 1857.)

8. Ketamine should not be used in patients with
   A. Myocardial ischemia
   B. Reactive airway disease
   C. Acute hypovolemia
   D. Benzodiazepine overdose

**Answer: A**

Ketamine differs from other intravenous agents in that it produces analgesia as well as amnesia. Its principal action is on the N-methyl-D-aspartate (NMDA) receptor; it has no action on the gamma-aminobutyric acid (GABA) receptor. It is a dissociative anesthetic, producing a cataleptic gaze with nystagmus. Patients may associate this with delirium and hallucinations while regaining consciousness. The addition of benzodiazepines has been shown to prevent these side effects. Ketamine can increase heart rate and blood pressure which may cause myocardial ischemia in patients with coronary artery disease (CAD). Ketamine is useful in acutely hypovolemic patients to maintain blood pressure via sympathetic stimulation, but is a direct myocardial depressant in patients who are catecholamine depleted. Ketamine is a bronchodilator, making it useful for asthmatic patients, and rarely is associated with allergic reactions. (See Schwartz 8th ed., p 1857.)

9. Which of the following is the least likely to produce respiratory depression when given in an equianalgesic dose?
   A. Morphine
   B. Hydromorphone
   C. Fentanyl
   D. None of the above

**Answer: D**

The commonly used opioids—morphine, codeine, oxymorphone, meperidine, and the fentanyl-based compounds—act centrally on μ-receptors in the brain and spinal cord. The main side effects of opioids are euphoria, sedation, constipation, and respiratory depression, which also are mediated by the same μ-receptors in a dose-dependent fashion. Although opioids have differing potencies required for effective analgesia, equianalgesic doses of opioids result in equal degrees of respiratory depression. Thus there is no completely safe opioid analgesic. The synthetic opioids fentanyl, and its analogs sufentanil, alfentanil, and remifentanil, are commonly used in the operating room. They differ pharmacokinetically in their lipid solubility, tissue binding, and elimination profiles, and therefore have differing potencies and durations of action. Remifentanil is remarkable in that it undergoes rapid hydrolysis that is unaffected by sex, age, weight, or renal or hepatic function, even after prolonged infusion. Recovery is within minutes, but there is little residual postoperative analgesia. (See Schwartz 8th ed., p. 1857.)

10. Succinylcholine
    A. Is metabolized by the liver
    B. Is the neuromuscular blocker of choice for ophthalmologic surgery
    C. Can lead to hyperkalemia
    D. Has a duration of action of approximately 30 min

**Answer: C**

Although the rapid onset (<60 seconds) and rapid offset (5 to 8 minutes) make succinylcholine ideal for management of the airway in certain situations, total body muscle fasciculations can cause postoperative aches and pains, an elevation in serum potassium levels, and an increase in intraocular and intragastric pressure. Its use in patients with burns or traumatic tissue injuries may result in a high enough rise in serum potassium levels to produce arrhythmias and cardiac arrest. Unlike other neuromuscular blocking agents, the effects of succinylcholine cannot be reversed. Succinylcholine is rapidly hydrolyzed by plasma cholinesterase, also referred to as pseudocholinesterase. There are many reasons for a patient to have low pseudocholinesterase levels, such as liver disease, concomitant use of other drugs, pregnancy, and cancer. These factors are usually not clinically problematic, delaying return of motor function only by several minutes. Some patients have a genetic disorder manifesting as atypical plasma cholinesterase; the atypical enzyme has less-than-normal activity, and/or the patient has extremely low levels of the enzyme. The incidence of the homozygous form is approximately one in 3000; the effects of a single dose of succinylcholine may last several hours instead of several minutes. Treatment is to keep the patient sedated and unaware he or she is paralyzed, continue mechanical ventilation, test the return of motor function with a peripheral nerve stimulator, and extubate the patient only after he or she has fully regained motor strength. Two separate blood tests must be drawn: pseudocholinesterase level to determine the amount of enzyme present, and dibucaine number, which indicates the quality of the enzyme. Patients with laboratory-confirmed abnormal pseudocholinesterase levels and/or dibucaine numbers should be counseled to avoid succinylcholine as well as mivacurium, which is also hydrolyzed by pseudocholinesterase. First-degree family members should also be tested. Succinylcholine is the only intravenous triggering agent of malignant hyperthermia discussed [in Schwartz 8th ed., Malignant Hyperthermia, p 1871]. (See Schwartz 8th ed., p 1858.)

11. The shortest-acting nondepolarizing agent is
    A. Pancuronium
    B. Vecuronium
    C. Atracurium
    D. Mivacurium

**Answer: D**

There are several competitive nondepolarizing agents available for clinical use. The longest-acting is pancuronium, which is excreted almost completely unchanged by the kidney. Intermediate-duration neuromuscular blockers include vecuronium and rocuronium, which are metabolized by both the kidneys and liver, and atracurium and cis-atracurium, which undergo breakdown in plasma known as Hofmann elimination. The agent with shortest duration is mivacurium, the only nondepolarizer that is metabolized by plasma cholinesterase, and like succinylcholine, is subject to the same prolonged blockade in patients with plasma cholinesterase deficiency. All non-depolarizers reversibly bind to the postsynaptic terminal in the neuromuscular junction and prevent acetylcholine from depolarizing the muscle. Muscle blockade occurs without fasciculation and without the subsequent side effects seen with succinylcholine. The most commonly used agents of this type and their advantages and disadvantages are listed in Table 46-3. (See Schwartz 8th ed., p 1858.)

12. Which of the following inhalational agents is most likely to induce liver injury?
    A. Halothane
    B. Enflurane
    C. Desflurane
    D. Isoflurane

**Answer: A**

The coexisting presence of liver disease may influence the selection of volatile anesthetics. Halothane is the anesthetic most studied regarding possible hepatotoxicity. Halothane hepatitis occurs rarely (approximately 1:25,000 patients) and may have an immune-mediated mechanism stimulated by repeated exposures to halothane. Halothane, enflurane, isoflurane, and desflurane all yield a reactive oxidative trifluoroacetyl halide and may be cross-reactive, but the magnitude of metabolism of the volatile anesthetics is a probable factor in the ability to cause hepatitis. Halothane is metabolized 20%, enflurane 2%, isoflurane 0.2%, and desflurane 0.02%; desflurane probably has the least potential for liver injury. Sevoflurane does not yield any trifluoroacetylated metabolites and is unlikely to cause hepatitis. (See Schwartz 8th ed., p 1862.)

13. Nitroglycerin must be given sublingually because
    A. Nitroglycerin is hydrolyzed in the wall of the intestine.
    B. Nitroglycerin is metabolized in the liver through the portal circulation.
    C. Nitroglycerin is more effective with the rapid absorption seen in sublingual administration.
    D. Nitroglycerin is activated by salivary enzymes.

**Answer: A**
Drug elimination varies widely; some drugs are excreted unchanged by the body, some decompose via plasma enzymes, and some are degraded by organ-based enzymes in the liver. Many drugs rely on multiple pathways for elimination (i.e., metabolized by liver enzymes then excreted by the kidney). When a drug is given orally, it reaches the liver via the portal circulation and is partially metabolized before reaching the systemic circulation. This is why an oral dose of a drug often must be much higher than an equally effective intravenous dose. Some drugs (e.g., nitroglycerin) are hydrolyzed presystemically in the gut wall and must be administered sublingually to achieve an effective concentration. (See Schwartz 8th ed., p 1854.)

14. Which of the following is a local anesthetic of the amide group?
    A. Benzocaine
    B. Procaine
    C. Tetracaine
    D. Bupivacaine

**Answer: D**
Lidocaine, bupivacaine, mepivacaine, prilocaine, and ropivacaine have in common an amide linkage between a benzene ring and a hydrocarbon chain, which in turn is attached to a tertiary amine. The benzene ring confers lipid solubility for penetration of nerve membranes, and the tertiary amine attached to the hydrocarbon chain makes these local anesthetics water soluble. Lidocaine has a more rapid onset and is shorter acting than bupivacaine; however, both are widely used for tissue infiltration, regional nerve blocks, and spinal and epidural anesthesia. Ropivacaine is the most recently introduced local anesthetic. It is clinically similar to bupivacaine in that it has a slow onset and a long duration, but is less cardiotoxic. All amides are 95% metabolized in the liver, with 5% excreted unchanged by the kidneys. (See Schwartz 8th ed., p 1854.)

15. Which of the following is a depolarizing agent?
    A. Pancuronium
    B. Atracurium
    C. Vecuronium
    D. Succinylcholine

**Answer: D**
There is one commonly used depolarizing neuromuscular blocker—succinylcholine. This agent binds to acetylcholine receptors on the postjunctional membrane in the neuromuscular junction and causes depolarization of muscle fibers. (See Schwartz 8th ed., p 1858.)

16. The therapeutic index of a drug is defined by
    A. Median effective dose ($ED_{50}$)/lethal dose ($LD_{50}$)
    B. $LD_{50}/ED_{50}$
    C. $ED_{50} < 0.5$
    D. $ED_{50} > 0.5$

**Answer: B**
The lethal dose ($LD_{50}$) of a drug produces death in 50% of animals to which it is given. The ratio of the lethal dose and effective dose, $LD_{50}/ED_{50}$, is the therapeutic index. A drug with a high therapeutic index is safer than a drug with a low or narrow therapeutic index. (See Schwartz 8th ed., p 1854.)

17. The initial toxicity of most local anesthetics is
    A. Cardiac
    B. Neural
    C. Hepatic
    D. Renal

**Answer: B**

Toxicity of local anesthetics results from absorption into the bloodstream or from inadvertent direct intravascular injection. Toxicity manifests first in the more sensitive central nervous system, and then the cardiovascular system. (See Schwartz 8th ed., p 1856.)

18. Lidocaine with epinephrine
    A. Is the preferred anesthetic for pediatric circumcisions because of its longer duration
    B. Has the same onset of nerve block as plain epinephrine
    C. Causes local vasoconstriction
    D. Requires the same dose as plain lidocaine for an equivalent effect

**Answer: C**

Epinephrine has one physiologic and several clinical effects when added to local anesthetics. Epinephrine is a vasoconstrictor, and by reducing local bleeding, molecules of the local anesthetic remain in proximity to the nerve for a longer time period. Onset of the nerve block is faster, the quality of the block is improved, the duration is longer, and less local anesthetic will be absorbed into the bloodstream, thereby reducing toxicity. Although epinephrine 1:200,000 (5 μg/mL) added to a local anesthetic for infiltration will greatly lengthen the time of analgesia, epinephrine-containing solutions should not be injected into body parts with end-arteries such as toes or fingers, as vasoconstriction may lead to ischemia or loss of a digit. When added to the local anesthetic, sodium bicarbonate will raise the pH, favoring the non-ionized uncharged form of the molecule. This speeds the onset of the block, especially in local anesthetics that are mixed with epinephrine. The pH of such solutions is around 4.5, therefore the addition of sodium bicarbonate results in a relatively large increase in pH. (See Schwartz 8th ed., p 1856.)

19. Headache after spinal anesthesia occurs in what percentage of patients?
    A. <0.5%
    B. 1%
    C. 5%
    D. 10%

**Answer: B**

Possible complications include hypotension, especially if the patient is not adequately prehydrated; high spinal block requires immediate airway management; and postdural puncture headache sometimes occurs. Spinal headache is related to the diameter and configuration of the spinal needle, and can be reduced to approximately 1% with the use of a small 25- or 27-gauge needle. (See Schwartz 8th ed., p 1856.)

# CHAPTER 47

# ACGME Core Competencies

*Note to Reader:* This chapter is found only in *Schwartz's Manual of Surgery*, 8th ed., and not in *Schwartz's Principles of Surgery*, 8th ed.

1. What are the six core competencies?
   A. Patient care, medical knowledge, practice based learning, interpersonal and communication skills, professionalism, systems based practice
   B. Education, patient care, professionalism, practice based learning, medical knowledge, systems based practice
   C. Patient care, ethics, interpersonal and communication skills, professionalism, education, medical knowledge
   D. Research, medical knowledge, patient care, systems based practice, professionalism, time management

**Answer: A**

The six core competencies include six specific areas that have been designated as critical for resident training. Each surgical training program must provide an environment that is conducive for training of these six core competencies as well as proper assessment of that training. The areas of training include:

- **Patient Care.** Residents must be able to provide patient care that is compassionate, appropriate, and effective for the treatment of health problems and the promotion of health.
- **Medical Knowledge.** Residents must demonstrate knowledge about established and evolving biomedical, clinical, and cognate (e.g., epidemiological and social-behavioral) sciences and the application of this knowledge to patient care.
- **Practice Based Learning and Improvement.** Residents must be able to investigate and evaluate their patient care practices, appraise and assimilate scientific evidence, and improve their patient care practices.
- **Interprofessional and Communication Skills.** Residents must be able to demonstrate interpersonal and communication skills that result in effective information exchange and teaming with patients, their patients' families, and professional associates.
- **Professionalism.** Residents must demonstrate a commitment to carrying out professional responsibilities, adherence to ethical principles, and sensitivity to a diverse patient population.
- **Systems Based Practice.** Residents must demonstrate an awareness of and responsiveness to the larger context and system of health care and the ability to effectively call on system resources to provide care that is of optimal value. (See Schwartz Manual 8th ed., pp 1223–25.)

2. Which governing body is responsible for the mandates for the core competencies?
   A. American Board of Surgery
   B. ACGME (Accreditation Council of Graduate Medical Education)
   C. Congress
   D. Resident review committee

**Answer: B**

ACGME, Accreditation Council for Graduate Medical Education. (See Schwartz Manual 8th ed., p 1223.)

3. Which statement about patient care as a core competency is true?
   A. Patient care as a core competency in surgical training is currently observed through mentorship, especially during the late stages of training
   B. Patient care can most efficiently be learned by spending as much time in the hospital, on rounds, and in the operating room as possible to maximize learning
   C. The employment of physician extenders (e.g., physician assistants) would greatly hinder the learning of patient care as a core competency in the training of a surgical resident
   D. None of the above

**Answer: D**
Patient care is the foundation for the practice of clinical medicine and must be addressed early on in the stages of a trainee's professional development. In the past, patient care has been observed through mentorship by time spent with attending physicians, on the wards, or in the operating room. However, this model of training requires numerous hours in the hospital that cannot be accomplished due to work hour restrictions. So how does the resident learn compassionate and respectful patient care in this new era of surgical training? The application of resident time motion studies may aid in properly allocating time to high-yield patient care. For example, residents would participate in high-yield operations with attending physicians who have a dedication to teaching. This scenario would allow the resident to maximize his or her time in the hospital by participating in an environment that teaches excellent patient care. Furthermore, the employment of increased numbers of physician extenders (e.g., physician assistants) would improve the educational and patient care experiences of trainees by allowing surgical residents to focus on high-yield tasks instead of performing tasks that do not add to the learning experience. (See Schwartz Manual 8th ed., pp 1225–26.)

4. Which of the following statements is true?
   A. The 2nd core competency, medical knowledge, was created to require that "residents must demonstrate knowledge about established and evolving biomedical, clinical, and cognate (e.g., epidemiological and social-behavioral) sciences [as well as] the application of this knowledge to patient care."
   B. Because of the rapidly advancing medical research environment in the 80-hour week, surgical trainees are no longer required to learn basic physiology and biology of different diseases.
   C. Medical knowledge as a core competency does not apply to surgical training.
   D. As of this date, there are no novel techniques that can be taught to residents to help them assimilate the growing medical knowledge and research.

**Answer: A**
Residents must demonstrate knowledge about established and evolving biomedical, clinical, and cognate (e.g., epidemiological and social-behavioral) sciences as well as the application of this knowledge to patient care. Answers B, C, and D are contrary to what the 2nd core competency is about. (See Schwartz Manual 8th ed., p 1226.)

5. Which of the following statements accurately describes "professionalism" as a core competency?
   A. Residents must communicate effectively and demonstrate caring and respectful behaviors when interacting with patients.
   B. Residents must gather essential and accurate information about patients.
   C. Residents must develop and carry out patient management plans.
   D. Residents must demonstrate sensitivity and responsiveness to a patient's culture, age, gender, and disabilities.

**Answer: D**
The core competency of professionalism states that "residents must demonstrate a commitment to carrying out professional responsibilities, adherence to ethical principles, and sensitivity to a diverse patient population." The trainee should demonstrate respect, compassion, and integrity while involved in patient care. (See Schwartz Manual 8th ed., pp 1227–28.)

6. Which of the following statements does NOT describe "systems based practice"?
   A. Residents must know how types of medical practice and delivery systems differ from one another.
   B. Residents must practice cost-effective health care and resource allocation that does not compromise quality of care.
   C. Residents must advocate for quality patient care and assist patients in dealing with system complexities.
   D. Residents must use information technology to manage information and access on-line medical information to support their own education.

**Answer: D**
Residents must demonstrate an awareness of and responsiveness to the larger context and system of health care and the ability to effectively call on system resources to provide care that is of optimal value. (See Schwartz Manual 8th ed., pp 1228–29.)

7. To be an effective team leader, the surgeon must be able to effectively communicate with
   A. Consultants
   B. Nurses
   C. Patients
   D. All of the above

**Answer: D**
To be an effective team leader, the surgeon must be able to effectively communicate with all team members, such as consultants and ancillary health care personnel. (See Schwartz Manual 8th ed., p 1227.)

8. Understanding of the interaction between the individual medical practice and health care system refers to what core competency?
   A. Professionalism
   B. Patient care
   C. Systems based practice
   D. Medical knowledge

**Answer: C**
One of the goals of this core competency is to teach residents how to acknowledge the importance of understanding that each individual medical practice is a component of the entire health care system and that each individual practice impacts the overall delivery and access of health care. (See Schwartz Manual 8th ed., pp 1228–29.)

9. Application of systems based practice can be facilitated mainly by
   A. Demonstrating principles of ethical behavior
   B. Applying up-to-date medical knowledge
   C. Improving communication skills
   D. Incorporating in training systems individuals who have specialized in health care management and are able to analyze the important components of the health care delivery system to surgical trainees

**Answer: D**
Recent reports have demonstrated that surgeons feel deficient in the understanding of the public health and business aspect of surgery. These principles can be taught through mentoring by individuals who have an expertise in health care delivery systems and overall health care management. (See Schwartz Manual 8th ed., pp 1228–29.)

# Index

Note: Page numbers followed by *t* indicate tables; those followed by *f* indicate figures.